T0275916

William Hunter and the eighteenth-century medical world

William Hunter

and the
eighteenth-century medical world

EDITED BY

W. F. BYNUM and ROY PORTER
Wellcome Institute for the History of Medicine, London

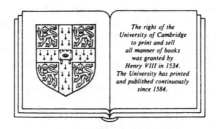

The right of the
University of Cambridge
to print and sell
all manner of books
was granted by
Henry VIII in 1534.
The University has printed
and published continuously
since 1584.

CAMBRIDGE UNIVERSITY PRESS
Cambridge
London   New York   New Rochelle
Melbourne   Sydney

PUBLISHED BY THE PRESS SYNDICATE OF THE UNIVERSITY OF CAMBRIDGE
The Pitt Building, Trumpington Street, Cambridge, United Kingdom

CAMBRIDGE UNIVERSITY PRESS
The Edinburgh Building, Cambridge CB2 2RU, UK
40 West 20th Street, New York NY 10011–4211, USA
477 Williamstown Road, Port Melbourne, VIC 3207, Australia
Ruiz de Alarcón 13, 28014 Madrid, Spain
Dock House, The Waterfront, Cape Town 8001, South Africa

http://www.cambridge.org

© Cambridge University Press 1985

First published 1985
First paperback edition 2002

A catalogue record for this book is available from the British Library

Library of Congress Cataloguing in Publication data
Main entry under title:
William Hunter and the eighteenth-century medical
world.
"The essays in this volume are revised versions
of papers given at an international symposium to
mark the two hundredth anniversary of the death of
William Hunter, held at the Wellcome Institute for
the History of Medicine in London from 29 June to
1 July 1983" – Acknowledgements.
Includes index.
1. Medicine – Europe – History – 18th century –
Congresses.   2. Hunter, William, 1718–1783 – Congresses.
I. Bynum, W. F. (William F.), 1943–   . II. Porter,
Roy, 1946–   . [DNLM: 1. History of Medicine,
18th Century – congresses.   2. Hunter, William, 1718–
1783.   3. Physicians – biography.   4. Physicians –
congresses. WZ 100 W717 1983]
R484.W55   1985   610′.94   84-21378

ISBN 0 521 26806 0 hardback
ISBN 0 521 52517 9 paperback

CONTENTS

v

CONTRIBUTORS

C. HELEN BROCK read natural sciences at Cambridge University. During World War II she worked in the Audio Frequency Laboratory, the Royal Aircraft Establishment, Farnborough, the RAF Physiological Laboratory, the Royal Navy Physiological Laboratory and the Insect Infestation Department of the Ministry of Food. After the war she conducted research on structural materials in animals, cancer, animal reproduction and applied psychology. Until her recent retirement, she was Honorary Research Fellow, Department of History of Science, Glasgow University. Her current research interests include James Douglas, MD, FRS, and William Hunter, MD, FRS, as well as medicine in North America in the eighteenth century.

W. F. BYNUM is Head of the Academic Unit at the Wellcome Institute for the History of Medicine and the Unit of the History of Medicine, Department of Anatomy and Embryology, University College, London. He holds an MD from Yale University and a PhD from Cambridge University. He has published on many aspects of medicine and the life sciences since the seventeenth century and has edited several books, including (with E. J. Browne and R. S. Porter) *A Dictionary of the History of Science* (1981). He is co-editor of *Medical History*.

FRANÇOIS DUCHESNEAU is Professor of Philosophy and History of Science and Head of the Philosophy Department at the Université de Montréal. He holds an Agrégation de Philosophie and a Doctorat d'Etat ès-lettres et sciences humaines from the Université de Paris-I. He is the author of *L'empirisme de Locke* (1973) and *La Physiologie des Lumières: empirisme, modèles et théories* (1982). His current research interests relate to physiological theories of the eighteenth and nineteenth centuries, as well as to topics in the philosophy of science.

TOBY GELFAND is Associate Professor in the Faculty of Health Sciences, University of Ottawa (Hannah Chair) and the Department of History. Born in Philadelphia in 1942, he took his PhD in the history of medicine at the Johns

vii

Hopkins University. He is the author of *Professionalizing Modern Medicine: Paris Surgeons and Medical Science and Institutions in the Eighteenth Century* (1980) and articles in *Bulletin of the History of Medicine, Medical History, Revue d'Histoire Moderne et Contemporaine, Histoire Sociale – Social History,* and he has taught at the University of Minnesota and Princeton University. He is currently working on late nineteenth-century medical discourse in France and the Jews.

JOHANNA GEYER-KORDESCH, MA, PhD, is Medical Historian at the Institut für Theorie und Geschichte der Medizin at the University of Münster, Federal Republic of Germany. She studied at Oberlin College, the University of Massachusetts, Amherst, and the Universities of Freiburg im Breisgau and Vienna. She was a Wellcome Trust Research Fellow at the Wellcome Unit for the History of Medicine at Oxford University. She has published mainly on Pietism and medicine in eighteenth-century Germany and is currently writing a monograph on Georg Ernst Stahl. In 1982, together with Wolfgang Eckart, she edited *Heilberufe und Kranke im 17. und 18. Jahrhundert: Die Quellen- und Forschungsituation.*

L. J. JORDANOVA, who has been Lecturer in History at the University of Essex since 1980, teaches courses on the history of science and medicine and on the history of the family. She is particularly interested in the use of visual materials in cultural history. She is writing a book entitled *Family and Ideology in Eighteenth-Century France and Britain.* Other research areas include French science and medicine from 1770 to 1830 and eighteenth-century art. Among her publications are *Lamarck* (1984), *Images of the Earth* (1979, co-editor and contributor) and articles on French biomedical sciences and on the scientific construction of gender.

OTHMAR KEEL worked at the Institut d'Histoire des Sciences et des Techniques of the Université de Paris with Georges Canguilhem. For the past six years he has been part of the staff of the Institut d'Histoire et de Sociopolitique des Sciences of the Université de Montréal. He is the author of *La généalogie de l'histopathologie: Une révision déchirante* (1979). His research in recent years has been financed by the Canada Council, the Social Science Research Council of Canada, the Fonds FCAC of the Ministère de l'Education of Quebec, the Fonds CAFIR of the Université de Montréal and the Fonds National Suisse de la Recherche Scientifique. He is currently researching the history of the biomedical sciences in Europe in the eighteenth and nineteenth centuries, as well as the history and socio-politics of health in Quebec and the rest of Canada.

JOAN LANE, a former Wellcome Fellow, is a research fellow at the Centre for the Study of Social History at the University of Warwick. She has published on English apprenticeship, on eighteenth-century parish medical services and on the administration of the Old Poor Law. She established and teaches a course on the social history of medicine in England. A graduate of the University of Wales and with a University of Birmingham doctorate, she is currently investigating the relationship between eighteenth-century medical practitioners and their patients from the evidence of contemporary diaries and correspondence.

CHRISTOPHER LAWRENCE, formerly a general medical practitioner in the Shetland Islands, is currently a lecturer in the history of medicine at the Wellcome Institute. He has completed a PhD thesis on medicine in the Scottish Enlightenment and has published on various aspects of Scottish medicine. He also works on late nineteenth- and early twentieth-century physiology, pathology and clinical medicine with particular reference to the use of technology in medicine.

ANGUS McLAREN is Professor of History at the University of Victoria, British Columbia, where he has taught since 1975. Earlier he held teaching positions at the University of Calgary and Grinnell College and was a senior associate fellow at St Antony's College, Oxford. His published work includes *Birth Control in Nineteenth Century England* (1978), *Sexuality and Social Order: The Debate over the Fertility of Women and Workers in France, 1770–1920* (1983) and *Reproductive Rituals: The Perception of Fertility in Britain, 1500–1800* (1984).

ROY PORTER is Senior Lecturer at the Wellcome Institute for the History of Medicine, London. After working early on the history of the earth sciences and writing *The Making of Geology*, he has subsequently researched in parallel into social history (*English Society in the Eighteenth Century* [1982]) and the social dimensions of the history of medicine. He is currently working on the early history of psychiatry in Britain, on quackery and on the lay experience of illness and doctors.

W. D. IAN ROLFE is Deputy Director and Senior Keeper in Geology at the Hunterian Museum of Glasgow University. Born in Essex and a graduate of Birmingham University, he was subsequently demonstrator at Keele University. A Fulbright Scholarship took him thereafter to Harvard University's Museum of Comparative Zoology for two years, and he was Visiting Scientist at the Field Museum, Chicago, in 1981. As a palaeontologist, his main interest is in Palaeozoic arthropods, but he has published on more general topics and edited several geological journals, as well as a popular volume of *Geological Howlers*.

EDWARD SHORTER, Professor of History at the University of Toronto, is the author of *Strikes in France* (1974, with Charles Tilly), *The Making of the Modern Family* (1975) and *A History of Women's Bodies* (1982).

ADRIAN WILSON teaches history of medicine in the Cambridge Wellcome Unit. His book *A Safe Deliverance: Changing Rites of Childbirth in Early-Modern England* is to be published by Cambridge University Press.

ACKNOWLEDGEMENTS

The essays in this volume are revised versions of papers given at an international symposium to mark the two hundredth anniversary of the death of William Hunter, held at the Wellcome Institute for the History of Medicine in London from 29 June to 1 July 1983. That symposium would have been impossible without the aid of a generous grant from the Wellcome Trustees, to whom we are most grateful. The occasion was made more memorable by a splendid exhibition on William Hunter and his world mounted by William Schupbach, Curator of the Iconographic Collections at the Wellcome Institute. In our planning we benefited enormously from the knowledge and enthusiasm of Helen Brock. Steven Emberton and Frieda Houser handled the administrative arrangements with admirable efficiency. At Cambridge University Press, Richard Ziemacki has always been encouraging and helpful. Jean Runciman prepared the index with her customary professionalism.

INTRODUCTION

For too long William Hunter has been eclipsed in the historical record by his brother John. John Hunter of course deserves fame in his own right, and historians have studied him extensively for his pioneering work on such diverse topics as gunshot wounds, venereal disease, physiological surgery and the nature of the blood.[1] But to some extent John's reputation may less be a reflection of his superior historical importance than of the symbolic meaning his image has come to have. As Jacyna stressed recently, whenever nineteenth-century surgeons felt the need to vindicate their craft, demonstrating its scientific nature, its character as progressive knowledge, its supreme human importance, they invoked John Hunter as founding father and patron saint.[2] And they did so knowing they had a trump card in John's personality: honest, fresh, direct, bluff, full of enthusiasm for knowledge, a tireless seeker after truth.

It is not our intent here to debunk John. Far from it. In fact, Chapter 9, by François Duchesneau, examines John Hunter's significance in the physiological thought of his time. We seek rather to spotlight his elder brother William. A more enigmatic man, indeed; one who, despite his enormous success and rise to fame and riches; despite his notable anatomy school and his thousands of grateful pupils, clearly cut an ambiguous figure in his own times (almost none of his medical colleagues attended his funeral) and failed to capture the imagination of succeeding generations of surgeons and obstetricians, or provide them with a serviceable icon to worship and ideal to emulate. Significantly the Hunterian Society commemorates John, not William. Nor

1 For a recent assessment of John Hunter, with extensive bibliographical apparatus, see Stephen J. Cross, 'John Hunter, the Animal Economy, and Late Eighteenth Century Physiological Discourse', *Studies in the History of Biology* V (1981), 1–110.
2 L. S. Jacyna, 'Images of John Hunter in the Nineteenth Century', *History of Science* XXI (1983), 85–108.

have scholars treated William generously.[3] No full-length, scholarly biography of William has ever appeared, though Peachey's volume is extremely valuable, Sir Charles Illingworth's study is illuminating, and we can now welcome and greatly profit from Helen Brock's edition of Samuel Foart Simmons's eighteenth-century biography.[4] Nor has any edition of his letters ever been printed (though it is a project on which Helen Brock has been working, which, it is hoped, will shortly see light of day). Moreover, William Hunter's medical and scientific publications have never been reprinted, and his unpublished lecture notes have in general been neglected.[5]

All this is peculiar in view of the fact that William Hunter not only made rather impressive positive contributions to medical knowledge (his work on the lymphatic system was, in his own words, 'the greatest discovery, both in physiology and in pathology, that Anatomy has suggested, since the discovery of the circulation'), but perhaps more significantly played innovatory and influential roles in many of the most critical new trends in medicine during the Enlightenment. His pioneering of the private anatomy school was a key development in the reshaping of British medical education in the era before its domination by the teaching hospital and the university medical school. His insistence on teaching anatomy through direct student dissection of cadavers helped to transform the medico-scientific standing of the surgical profession. His involvement with the plastic and figurative arts performed a similar function, elevating the figure of physician as guardian of culture and presaging the complex dialectic of the arts and sciences so integral to romanticism.[6] Finally, William Hunter's enormous eminence and prestige as obstetrician and instructor in the art were crucial in the emergence of midwifery as a preserve of male physicians – a shift significant far beyond medicine itself, since it is a key index of occupational power struggle between the sexes, and male–female rivalry in general in the field of professional services.

In all these fields – medical education, the advancement of surgery, the cultural standing of the medical profession, the particular significance for women's history of the male doctor–female patient rela-

3   For instance, Lester King's pioneering exploration of the eighteenth-century medical world has left William Hunter largely untouched. His *The Medical World of the Eighteenth Century* (Chicago, 1958) contains only three brief references to Hunter.
4   George Peachey, *A Memoir of William and John Hunter* (Plymouth, 1924); Sir Charles Illingworth, *The Story of William Hunter* (Edinburgh, 1967); S. F. Simmons and John Hunter, *William Hunter, 1718–1783*, ed. C. H. Brock (Glasgow, 1983).
5   But see the facsimile printing of Charles White's notes on *William Hunter's Lectures of Anatomy* (Amsterdam, 1972).
6   See Martin Kemp, *Dr. William Hunter at the Royal Academy of Arts* (Glasgow, 1975).

tionship in obstetrics and gynaecology – William Hunter's importance has been recognised, but only in a rather shadowy way. There are perhaps three important reasons for this. First, there has been a simple lack of information about his life and works. Several of the essays in this collection aim in their distinct ways to remedy this defect. Thus Roy Porter puts Hunter into his entrepreneurial niche; Helen Brock offers the first analysis of that *sine qua non* of Hunter's standing, his wealth; Adrian Wilson gives us a scrutiny of Hunter's unpublished obstetrical lectures; and Ian Rolfe examines Hunter's outlooks on scientific knowledge and his views on the place of life in the cosmos.

Second, Hunter does not really fit into the stereotypes of the medical man or medical scientist with which medical historians commonly work. He was not a university medical professor, a shrewd clinician, the benevolent autocrat of a hospital, or – unlike his contemporary and correspondent Albrecht von Haller – a tireless producer of research papers and textbooks. Neither a Boerhaave, a Cullen, a Haller, a Mead, a Sloane nor an Ashley Cooper – then what sort of a medical man *was* William Hunter? Several contributors argue that historians often hamper themselves with anachronistic or inappropriate models of medicine, implicitly borrowed from the nineteenth century. Joan Lane shows how important apprenticeship was to the medical world of the eighteenth century; W. F. Bynum and Toby Gelfand show that the London hospital scene of Hunter's day was very different from the picture of High Victorian hospital medicine evoked recently by Jeanne Peterson.[7] Edward Shorter demonstrates how we misconstrue the responses of women in labour to the new man-midwife, if we apply the slogans of the present-day feminist rejection of intrusive, hospital-based, 'high-tech' obstetrics. And, for his part, Angus McLaren demonstrates what erroneous views of Enlightenment sexuality we carry away, if we look through the blinkers of our Victorian forebears (though L. J. Jordanova's essay reaffirms the central power of basic traditional sexual stereotyping).

The third reason why it is difficult to put William Hunter in his context is that so much of the background fine texture of eighteenth-century medicine remains to be explored. Compared with medicine in the age of Harvey and the founding of the Royal Society, or with Victorian 'scientific' medicine – medicine after the 'birth of the clinic'[8] – the eighteenth century has suffered real neglect. This volume can-

7 Jeanne Peterson, *The Medical Profession in Mid-Victorian London* (Berkeley, 1978).
8 The phrase of course is Michel Foucault's, *The Birth of the Clinic*, trans. A. M. S. Smith (London, 1973).

not in itself rectify this situation – though drawing attention to the neglect of major areas of the history of Enlightenment medicine will, it is hoped, stimulate future research efforts. But certain of the contributions, which do not touch directly on the career of William Hunter, do explore major new developments in the broader medical world of the eighteenth century (for example Othmar Keel's wide-ranging examination of eighteenth-century clinical teaching, Christopher Lawrence's chapter on medical education in Edinburgh, and Johanna Geyer-Kordesch's parallel study of German medical education), and so help to illuminate some aspects of this era just before the recognisably 'modern' nineteenth-century medical world.

PART I. LIFE

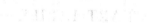

1

William Hunter: a surgeon and a gentleman

ROY PORTER

In 1794 the Reverend Thomas Gisborne published his ponderous 900-page *Enquiry into the Duties of Men in the Higher and Middle Classes of Society in Great Britain*.[1] Though devoting sixty-six pages to the physician's vocation, Gisborne made no mention of the surgeon. Not surprisingly, perhaps; in disdaining to stoop to surgery, he was merely perpetuating time-hallowed snobberies. Being not a mental but a manual craft, utilising hand not head, might not mind, the cutter's art neither was for gentlemen born, nor did it confer gentility. In medicine's scale of honour, only physic was fit for gentlemen.

Mainstream histories of medicine confirm that such honorific ideals were mirrors of occupational reality. They expound how healing was traditionally compartmentalised by statute, station and status into a three-tiered hierarchy, in which the vocation of physic lorded it over the art of surgery, which in turn was a cut above the apothecary's shopkeeper trade.[2] Well into the nineteenth century, as Holloway

---

1 T. Gisborne, *An Enquiry into the Duties of Men in the Higher and Middle Classes of Society in Great Britain Resulting from their Respective Stations, Professions and Employments*, 4th ed., 2 vols. (London, 1797), II, pp. 132–98 (1st ed., 1794).
2 Cf. I. Waddington, 'General Practitioners and Consultants in Early Nineteenth Century England: The Sociology of an Intra-Professional Conflict', in J. Woodward and D. Richards (eds.), *Health Care and Popular Medicine in Nineteenth-Century England* (London, 1977), 164–88, p. 165: 'As noted above, the three legally recognised types of practitioner in England were physicians, surgeons and apothecaries. These three groups were organised in a hierarchical structure, with physicians forming the "first class of medical practitioner in rank and legal pre-eminence". By the early nineteenth century, the practice of the physician was held to be 'properly confined to the prescribing of medicines to be compounded by the apothecary, and in superintending operations performed by surgeons in order to prescribe what was necessary to the general health of the patient, or to counteract any internal disease.' See also L. S. King, *The Medical World of the Eighteenth Century* (Chicago, 1958); A. Chaplin, *Medicine in England during the Reign of George III* (London, 1919), and at a more popular level, G. Williams, *The Age of Agony* (London, 1975), and Williams, *The Age of Miracles* (London, 1981).

and Peterson have reiterated,[3] establishment spokesmen such as Sir Henry Halford still snootily upheld against would-be medical 'levellers' the exclusive alliance of physic with gentility; and – scholars argue – it was not till the long-drawn-out restructuring around consultants and GPs in early Victorian times, a shift signalled by the 1858 Medical Registration Act, that the old caste system of rank finally gave away to the career open to talent.

For the aspiring Georgian practitioner craving respect and glory, Gisborne's message was thus clear: Become a physician. Ideally, one should start with good blood; one's parents should preferably be English, Anglican and affluent. A liberal university education would then breed a scholar and a gentleman,[4] but the Oxbridge MD would further prove the 'open sesame' enabling a man, once set up in the metropolis where the choice patients and fat fees were, to leap-frog the licentiate, the mere outworks of that citadel of physic, the Royal College of Physicians, and jump straight into its inner sanctum, the fellowship, an ascent perhaps culminating in collegiate office and power. Such dignities would inevitably go hand-in-glove with acquiring titled and even royal patients. Such was the *cursus honorum* followed by Baker, Battie, Heberden, Baillie, Halford and others – all men achieving cachet in high society and the rewards of perhaps £10,000 a year, the bankroll of a pinched peer. For the élite of gentlemen physicians were indeed big fish, though this has implicitly been denied by scholars such as the Parrys, informed, or misinformed, by the sociology of professionalisation, who suggest that glittering prizes materialised thanks only to the processes of professional consolidation and 'collective upward social mobility' that the nineteenth century brought.[5] Before then, writes Ian Inkster, 'even in the London setting the medical man was occupationally marginal . . . the situation would have provided at best a marginal occupational identity for those who came within its influences'[6] – a view

---

3 S. Holloway, 'Medical Education in England, 1830–1858: A Sociological Analysis', *History*, LXIX (1964), 299–344; M. J. Peterson, *The Medical Profession in Mid-Victorian London* (Berkeley, 1978).
4 Presumably this is the reason why William Hunter sent his younger brother, John, to St. Mary's Hall, Oxford, in 1755, and so minutely supervised Matthew Baillie's passage through Balliol. See Hunter-Baillie papers, Royal College of Surgeons.
5 N. Parry and J. Parry, *The Rise of the Medical Profession: A Study of Collective Social Mobility* (London, 1976).
6 I. Inkster, 'Marginal Men: Aspects of the Social Role of the Medical Community in Sheffield, 1790–1850', in Woodward and Richards, *Health Care and Popular Medicine in Nineteenth-Century England*, 128–63, p. 129. The notion of marginality is questioned in Paul Weindling, 'The British Mineralogical Society: A Case Study in Science and Social Improvement', in I. Inkster and J. Morrell (eds.), *Metropolis and Province: Science in British Culture 1780–1850* (London, 1983), pp. 120–50.

echoed by Michael Durey,[7] who has averred that even 'in the early nineteenth century medicine was not a prestigious occupation'. Such readings smack, however, of teleological preconceptions about the rise of the professions, and do not seem to fit the facts. After all, as early as the reign of Anne, as Geoffrey Holmes reminds us, top-notch physicians such as Sloane, Radcliffe and Mead were pocketing more than many lords, making friends in high places and amongst the classiest literati coteries, and building up breath-taking art, book and natural history collections, Sloane bequeathing his to the nation as the British Museum.[8] For the cream at least, physic was a royal road to riches, rank and respect.[9]

But what of William Hunter? A hasty glimpse at his assault on the social climber's mountain suggests he at least was bound to get bogged down in the morasses of marginality.[10] Born in 1718, seventh of ten children – and not even the eldest son – with a father who, as a retired grain merchant, was, though not penurious, not exactly polished, William Hunter had his start in life in the wrong country – Scotland – in the wrong religion – Presbyterianism. In 1731 he matriculated at the wrong university – Glasgow – destined for the wrong profession – his father meant him as an oblation for the ministry.[11] Backing out, he left without a degree and edged crablike into

---

7 M. Durey, 'Medical Elites, the General Practitioner and Patient Power in Britain during the Cholera Epidemic of 1831–2', in Inkster and Morrell, *Metropolis and Province*, 257–78, p. 258.
8 See G. Holmes, *Augustan England: Professions, State, and Society 1680–1730* (London, 1982), and J. F. Kett, 'Provincial Medical Practice in England, 1730–1815', *Journal of the History of Medicine*, XIX (1964), 17–29.
9 For anecdotes of the wealth of doctors see [W. MacMichael], *Lives of British Physicians* (London, 1857), and *The Gold-Headed Cane* (London, 1884); C. D. O'Malley, 'The English Physician in the Eighteenth Century', in H. T. Swedenberg, Jr. (ed.), *England in the Restoration and Early Eighteenth Century* (Berkeley, 1972), pp. 145–60; D'Arcy Power, 'The Fees of our Ancestors', in *Selected Writings 1877–1930* (Oxford, 1931), pp. 95–102.
10 For biography see Samuel Foart Simmons, *The Life and Writings of the Late Dr. William Hunter* (London, 1783). This has been reissued, together with John Hunter's marginal notes and an important reassessment by C. H. Brock, in *William Hunter 1718–1783* (Glasgow, 1983); R. Hingston Fox, *William Hunter, Anatomist, Physician, Obstetrician with Notices of his Friends* (London, 1901); Sir Charles Illingworth, *The Story of William Hunter* (Edinburgh, 1967); Jane M. Oppenheimer, *New Aspects of John and William Hunter* (New York, 1946); G. C. Peachey, *Memoir of William and John Hunter* (Plymouth, 1924); John Young, 'William Hunter', in *Record of the Ninth Jubilee of the University of Glasgow* (Glasgow, 1901), pp. 97–119; P. Huard, 'William Hunter (1718–83)', *History of Medicine*, VIII (1958), 3–13; J. M. Munro Kerr, 'William Hunter, his Life, Personality and Achievements', *Scottish Medical Journal*, II (1957), 372–8.
11 Fenwick Beekman, 'Long Calderwood, the Birthplace of the Hunters', *Bulletin of the New York Academy of Medicine*, 2nd ser., XIX (1943), 849–64; also 'William Hunter's Education at Glasgow, 1731–1736', *Bulletin of the History of Medicine*, XV (1944), 284–97; 'William Hunter's Early Medical Education', *Journal of the History of Medicine*, V (1950), 72–84; 'Teacher and Pupil: the Brothers William and John Hunter from 1748–1760', *Bulletin of the History of Medicine*, XXVIII (1954), 501–14.

medicine, joining the humble surgical branch in 1736 by becoming assistant to William Cullen in wee provincial Hamilton. Even when his career horizons widened on migrating to London in 1740 to complete his surgical training, the obstacle race surely continued. 'No Scots' agitation, always a-bubble, soon boiled over during the second Jacobite rising of 1745, and once more in the 1760s due to John Bull's loathing of George III's toady, the earl of Bute, a courtier Hunter eyed up as a patron. But animosity also ran high against 'those rascals the surgeons', sporadic antisurgeon riots being directed against their infamous and often illegal traffic in bodies for dissection.[12] Anatomising was, after all, Hogarth's ultimate stage of cruelty.

Hunter, moreover, gravitated towards the unsavoury trade of man-midwifery, probably as a result of lodging with what Mrs Nihell called the 'great horse-god-mother of a he-midwife', the 'nightman', William Smellie.[13] Feminists have stressed what disreputable work it was – the ploy of marginal men to annex what had traditionally been women's work. Man-midwifery was a branch of 'quackery' particularly unscrupulous because (as Margaret Connor Versluysen assures us) with their intrusive and infected forceps, their labours were 'usually fatal' – and no wonder, given pompous, bumbling, 'instrumentarian' operators such as Laurence Sterne's Dr Slop.[14] So ignominious was this cowboy trade that when Hunter disfranchised himself from the Company of Surgeons, he found that, on joining the College of Physicians, he was ineligible, as an *accoucheur*, for the fellowship.[15] His attempts to take the College by storm in the 1760s through the agitations of a ginger group, the Society of Collegiate Physicians, formed to bully the Royal College into opening up the fellowship, failed dismally; the rebuff was never reversed.[16]

12 The phrase is in John Gay's *Beggar's Opera* (London, 1728). See P. Linebaugh, 'The Tyburn Riot against the Surgeons', in D. Hay, P. Linebaugh, E. P. Thompson (eds.), *Albion's Fatal Tree* (London, 1975), pp. 65–118.
13 See R. W. Johnston, *William Smellie* (Edinburgh, 1952).
14 See J. Donnison, *Midwives and Medical Men* (London, 1977); J. E. Donegan, *Women and Men Midwives* (Westport, Conn., 1978); S. Romalis, *Childbirth* (Austin, Texas, 1981); Margaret Connor Versluysen, 'Midwives, Medical Men and "Poor Women Labouring of Child"; Lying-In Hospitals in Eighteenth Century London', in H. Roberts (ed.), *Women, Health and Reproduction* (London, 1981), 18–49, p. 31. For a counterblast see E. Shorter, *A History of Women's Bodies* (New York, 1982).
15 See Donnison, *Midwives and Medical Men*, p. 42.
16 L. G. Stevenson, 'The Siege of Warwick Lane, Together with a Brief History of the Society of Collegiate Physicians, 1767–98, *Journal of the History of Medicine*, VII (1952), 105–21; B. C. Corner, 'Dr. Melchisedech Broadbrim and the Playwright', *Journal of the History of Medicine*, VII (1952), 122–35; I. Waddington, 'The Struggle to Reform the Royal College of Physicians, 1767–1771: A Sociological Analysis', *Medical History*, XVII (1973), 107–26; B. Hamilton, 'The Medical Professions in the Eighteenth Century', *Economic History Review*, 2nd ser., IV (1951), 141–69.

Told thus, Hunter's story does, indeed, read like a cruel sport, a sombre Johnsonian parable of the vanity of human wishes, or the innocent abroad whose naïve ambition was crossed by spite, prejudice and the insolence of office, confirmation – were such necessary – of how the complacent nepotistic *ancien régime* house of oligarchy barred the outsider. Yet the tale as I have edited it is, of course, a travesty of what really counted in William Hunter's triumphal surgeon's progress. For, though not born with the silver key in his mouth which would automatically have opened all the doors leading up to a top hospital appointment, the council of the Royal College and perhaps even a knighthood, Hunter enjoyed a real success story, becoming the doyen of his profession. His claims to fame are familiar enough. Unrivalled excellence in anatomical lecturing, begun in 1746, won him a secure annual income of several hundred guineas and cohorts of protégés attracted by his renown as an anatomist-breeder, and gave him a forum for his physiological discoveries. Largely through obstetrics, he built up an ultra-fashionable practice, including amongst his patients the Pitts, Hertfords, Lady Ossory, the Fitzroys, the earl of Sandwich, Lord North, the Coutts, and the Hollands. On the recommendation of Sir Caesar Hawkins, he was appointed Physician-in-Extraordinary to Queen Charlotte in 1762, supervising all her many subsequent lyings-in[17] and winning intimacy in high places (Samuel Johnson credited him with 'good intelligence' at Court).[18] And he complemented his sway amongst the Quality by moving easily within the artistic and intellectual élites of the metropolis. His familiarity with cultural lions such as Samuel Johnson, Henry Fielding,[19] Joshua Reynolds,[20] Hester Thrale, Charles Burney, David Hume[21] and Horace Walpole was officially recognised in fellowships at the Royal Society and the Society of Antiquaries, and by his appointment in 1769 as anatomy professor at the newly established Royal Academy.

All this of course registered in his bank balance, Hunter making, as his first biographer, Simmons, put it, 'immense gains' and accruing

17   J. Peel, 'William Hunter – Royal Accoucheur', *Transactions of the Hunterian Society*, XXVIII (1969–70), 53–65; Brock, *William Hunter*, p. 17; a marginal note of John Hunter's reads, 'In the year 17 [*sic*] he was imployed to lay the Princess of Brunswick, and his manner pleased the Dowager Princess of Wales and Lady Bute that they both recommended him to the Queen.'
18   Oppenheimer, *New Aspects of John and William Hunter*, p. 157.
19   H. Fielding, *A Voyage to Lisbon* (Everyman Library ed., London, 1964), p. 209: Fielding is tapped for dropsy by 'my friend Mr. Hunter'.
20   M. Kemp, *Dr William Hunter at the Royal Academy* (Glasgow, 1975), p. 22. Kemp notes Hunter received a personal copy of Reynolds's *Discourses*.
21   For Hunter's contacts with Hume see Hunter Papers H 117, Glasgow University Library.

'vast riches'.[22] The precise sources and grand total of his takings are not known, but as early as the 1760s he was, it seems, pulling in more than £10,000 a year. And as the times demanded, he astutely manicured his upstart riches into respectability. After toying with the idea of sinking some £20,000 into an estate –a rare move for a medical man – he chose perhaps a more prudent and enduring seal to his fame: He laid out his fortune on an astonishing collection of specimens, paintings, books, medals and above all coins (did coin-collecting have its psychological appeal? certainly his brother judged that 'whatever he was really attached to, he was in the strictest sense a miser')[23] – a collection bequeathed to his alma mater as a memorial to his success, taste and public spirit. Though (as his sister Dorothea admitted) through lacking frankness and generosity William did not freely win love ('glib' was Smellie's word),[24] his accomplishments, address and Chesterfieldian decorum certainly commanded respect and opened doors. In contrast to his bluff brother John, no one could doubt that William bore the port of gentleman, the ultimate accolade being a two-page *Gentleman's Magazine* obituary.[25]

How then did the one-time provincial Scottish surgeon's apprentice, who never had the title of FRCP or a prestige hospital appointment, so successfully deliver himself into the charmed circles? The sombre Dr Johnson opined that the destiny of practitioners lay in the palm of fate:

A physician in a great city [he wrote in his *Life of Akenside*] seems to be the mere plaything of fortune; his degree of reputation is for the most part totally casual; they that employ him know his excellence; they that reject him know not his deficience. By any acute observer, who had looked at the transactions of the medical world for the last half century, a very curious book might be written on the Fortune of Physicians.[26]

Hunter disagreed point-blank; eminence in medicine was causal not casual, won by merit not blind chance. In a spirit that reminds us that he was a compatriot and acquaintance of Adam Smith, Hunter enjoined *virtù*, offering himself as living proof to his students that in life's market-place, Smilesian self-help was the key to success:

22 Anonymous obituary (in fact by Simmons) in *Gentleman's Magazine*, LIII, no. I (1783), 365–6. See C. Helen Brock, Chap. 2, this volume.
23 Brock, *William Hunter*, p. 8.
24 Ibid., p. 49.
25 *Gentleman's Magazine*, LIII, no. I (1783), 365–6.
26 Samuel Johnson, *The Works of the English Poets*, 21 vols. (London, 1810), XIV, p. 54.

I firmly believe, that it is in your power [he addressed his pupils] not only to *chuse*, but to *have*, which rank you please in the world. An opinion the child of spleen and idleness, has been propagated, which has done infinite prejudice to science, as well as to virtue. They would have us believe that merit is neglected, and that ignorance and knavery triumph in this world. Now, in our profession it seems incontestable, that the man of abilities and diligence always succeeds. Ability, indeed, is not the only requisite; and a man may fail, who has nothing besides to recommend him; or has some great disqualifications either of head or heart. But sick people are so desirous of life and health, that they always look out for ability; and surely the man who is really able in his profession, will have the best chance of being thought so. In my opinion, a young man cannot cultivate a more important truth than this, that merit is sure of its reward in this world.[27]

Hunter's claim that there was room at the top and the rat race was to the swift should not be simply dismissed out of hand as the smug congratulation of the self-made man who worshipped his maker, nor merely as student pep-talk humbug, challenging them to fly at the eagle. Every practitioner could be his own midwife, giving birth to fame and fortune – that was his own experience. Having formed from youth (as Simmons phrased it) a 'consciousness of the superiority of his talents',[28] he played the Hogarthian industrious apprentice, and performed word-perfect. Spurred (in brother John's words) by ambition 'to be at the head of his profession',[29] he drove himself unstintingly, sustaining a lecture course at his anatomy school that ran from October to May, six days a week, for two or more hours a day, quite aside from the backroom labours of 'putting my own hand to the knife' in performing dissections and making preparations, his wide-ranging scientific researches, and his extensive and taxing obstetrical practice, to say nothing of his passion for collecting.[30] It is characteristic of his tenacity that he died in March 1783 on the job, rising off

---

27 [William Hunter], *Two Introductory Lectures, Delivered by Dr William Hunter* (London, 1784), pp. 102–3. Compare the notes to Hunter's student lectures at the Royal Academy, in which he urges students, 'take pains and you will become ornaments' and cannot 'fail of success'; 'genius', he says, must be 'shooting up to its fullest magnitudes' for 'the prize is most certainly within reach – and it is not less than immortality!' Hunter papers H 46, Glasgow University Library.
28 Brock, *William Hunter*, p. 4.
29 Ibid., p. 8.
30 Of course much of the routine labour was done by assistants; yet the vast organisational work involved in running the anatomy school should not be underestimated.

his sick-bed to begin a new lecture course on the operative part of
surgery, collapsing, and expiring ten days afterwards.

Hunter applauded 'regulated ambition':[31] His own was unblush-
ing. As his brother put it:

   When he began to practice midwifery, he was like most other
   young beginners desirous of getting on in his profession, as
   also he was desirous of acquiring a fortune sufficient to place
   him in easy and independent circumstances. His industry was
   attended with the desired success and he soon became the
   most distinguished of his profession.[32]

Nor did he have any compunction about gauging achievement by
gain (he wrote of his Scottish friends, 'they ought to pray for my
prosperity in the world').[33] He knew the power of money – it bought
respect and independence – and never squandered it. Though generous to a few (he lent money, for example, to Tobias Smollett and
waived repayment),[34] Hunter was generally ruled by prudence, apparently declining to attend patients who could not afford his full fee.
He was also sparing in his philanthropy, according to John, pitying
none 'who had been the cause of their own misery'.[35] He thus saw it
as his duty not to extend loans to the ne'er-do-well son of his master,
James Douglas, because one should not encourage a fool in his fol-
ly.[36] Yet neither, as Simmons phrased it, did he allow 'his economy to
interfere when the dignity . . . of his character' was at stake.[37]

   In other words, Hunter studied advancement; he aimed at peer-
group and public honour, and was sidetracked by nothing – neither
by la dolce vita (he ate frugally, dining in public on just an egg – surely
a pregnant symbolic gesture! – rarely entertaining and even then
offering but two dishes),[38] nor, unlike many of his patients, by sexual

31 Two Introductory Lectures, p. 102.
32 Brock, William Hunter, p. 24.
33 Brock, William Hunter, pp. 43–45, has sensible words about his attitudes
towards wealth and fame. John Hunter similarly knew the importance of money in
securing independence. Cf. letter of May 1788 quoted in S. Paget, John Hunter
(London, 1897), p. 181: 'Dear Jenner, – I have been going to write to you some time
past, but business and a very severe indisposition for three weeks past has
prevented me; but when two guineas rouse me, I cannot resist'. For the William
Hunter quotation see Royal College of Surgeons, Hunter-Baillie papers, 2.5.
34 See G. S. Rousseau, Tobias Smollett: Essays of Two Decades (Edinburgh, 1982).
35 An instance of his tightness with his bawbees is that on election to the Scottish
Society of Antiquaries he wrote excusing the fact that he was not offering a money
donation: 'If I had not myself more children than I can provide for, I would send it a
present in money.' Hunter was of course childless. Hunter Papers H 496, Glasgow
University Library.
36 J. Oppenheimer, 'A Note on William Hunter and Tobias Smollett', Journal of the
History of Medicine, II (1947), 481–6, p. 484.
37 Brock, William Hunter, p. 28.
38 Brock, William Hunter, p. 41.

intrigue and marriage ties (the only occasion he perhaps contemplated matrimony was, in the nursery-tale way, to his master's daughter, Martha Jane Douglas). He did have a loved one, however; that was 'my darling London',[39] an Eldorado of which, like Dr Johnson, he never tired. Nothing could drag him away from town, neither the prospect of the high road north to serve with Cullen – his initial undertaking – nor the arguments of his ageing father,[40] nor even the entreaties of his mother dying of cancer (her wish for him to journey to see her was, he wrote to Cullen, 'a very bad scheme . . . I hope she will consider better of it . . . it is really a whim begot by sickness and low spirits').[41] When Boswell reached London, he was 'all life and joy';[42] I doubt that William ever lost control like that, but the prospect certainly excited him: 'I want to tell you', he wrote to Cullen in 1748, 'many things about colleges, hospitals, professorships, chariots, wives, etc. I'm busy forming a plan for being an author. In short, my head is full of a thousand things.'[43] And, once settled, he seized every chance to shin up the greasy pole to success. Thus within a year of arriving, he quit the homespun Smellie household – it lacked refinement and reeked of Scotticisms – exchanging it for the hospitality of the urbane and Anglicized Dr James Douglas, who was by then drawing some £4,000 a year, partly from midwifery, and had assembled a library including some 557 editions of Horace.[44]

Thus one can track the young surgeon's progress. But is there not something implausibly 'chapbook' in this tale of the triumph of Will, the heroic young outsider, excluded from the Citadel, battling to the top, against the odds, a chapbook perhaps called *Anatomy his Destiny?* Yes, indeed; but our sense of incongruity arises from half-sleep expectations about the anatomy of medicine in that period, its structure, power centres and career patterns, assumptions too often parroting historiographical myths or anachronistically back-projected from modern sociological theory. To begin with, our hoary belief that surgery was infra dig. needs radical modification. Certainly, as Jacyna has shown,[45] it was not till later that surgery was accorded scientific status. Yet throughout the eighteenth century it was rising in rewards

39 In a letter to his elder brother James, quoted in Paget, *John Hunter*, p. 41.
40 Brock, *William Hunter*, p. 2.
41 Brock, *William Hunter*, p. 44.
42 F. A. Pottle (ed.), *Boswell's London Journal* (London, 1950), p. 43.
43 Letter to Cullen, 1748, quoted in Paget, *John Hunter*, p. 45.
44 K. B. Thomas, *James Douglas of the Pouch and his Pupil William Hunter* (London, 1964).
45 L. S. Jacyna, 'Images of John Hunter in the Nineteenth Century', *History of Science*, XXI (1983), 85–108.

and esteem, both in the provinces, where, Holmes suggests, the surgeon-apothecary was already the fledgling general practitioner, and
in the metropolis where new voluntary hospitals opened a flood of
valuable appointments.[46] The surgeon's role as smallpox inoculator
and manager of venereal infections; the vast improvements in lithoto-
my; the prominence and precious experience that war gave to army
and navy surgeons; the thorough anatomy training and university
qualifications of many Scottish-educated surgeons – all enhanced the
surgeon's craft in the public eye.[47] From early in the century with
men such as Cowper and Cheselden,[48] through Bromfield, Caesar
Hawkins, *père et fils*, Adair, Tomkins, Gunning, up to the Hunters
and the debonair Percivall Pott,[49] an élite of surgeons commanded
respect as authors in scientific anatomy, as men of fortune[50] (Cheselden could allegedly charge up to £500 for cutting for the stone), and
as friends of culture (Cheselden was an intimate of Pope and had a
hand in designing Putney Bridge). The likes of William Hunter in the
London of 1740s would not need to feel trapped; with his dreams of
'colleges, hospitals, professorships, chariots, wives etc', well might
he feel his prospects were sunnier than many a physician's.[51]

   A similar, revisionist, story also needs telling for the man-midwife.
We tend to identify this grotesque beast of prey through his foes –
haranguing midwives such as Elizabeth Nihell,[52] disdainful satirists
like Laurence Sterne, and prurient moralists like Philip Thicknesse,[53]
with his nightmare vision of obstetricians as hypocrite lechers, 'men
of feeling', forever 'touching'. But was this trashing not mere envy, as
William Hunter himself believed, writing to Cullen on the publication
of Frank Nicholls's anonymous tirade against man-midwife butch-
ers:[54] 'Physic is in a strange ferment here. The practitioners in mid-

46 Holmes, *Augustan England*, pp. 234ff. For hospitals see Bynum, chap. 4, this
volume.
47 J. Dobson, 'Barber into Surgeon', *Annals of the Royal College of Surgeons of
England*, LIV (1974), 84–91.
48 Sir Z. Cope, *William Cheselden* (Edinburgh, 1953).
49 J. Dobson, 'Percivall Pott', *Annals of the Royal College of Surgeons of England*, L
(1972), 54–65.
50 Sir Z. Cope, 'William Cheselden and the Separation of the Barbers from the
Surgeons', *Annals of the Royal College of Surgeons of England*, XII (1953), 1–13; A. M.
Carr-Saunders and P. A. Wilson, *The Professions* (Oxford, 1933), pp. 74ff.
51 Sir C. N. Morgan, 'Surgery and Surgeons in 18th century London', *Annals of the
Royal College of Surgeons of England*, XLII (1968), 1–36.
52 E. Nihill, *A Treatise on the Art of Midwifery* (London, 1760); cf. B. This, *La Requête
des Enfants à Naître* (Paris, 1982).
53 P. Thicknesse, *Man Midwifery Analysed* (London, 1764); cf. P. Gosse, *Dr Viper*
(London, 1952).
54 [F. Nicholls], *The Petition of the Unborn Babes to the Censors of the Royal College of
Physicians of London* (London, 1751).

wifery have been virulently attacked, but by a madman; and in that scuffle I have had a blow too, obliquely; the reason is, we get money, our antagonists none. May the dispute, therefore, long continue.'[55] Feminist historians have seen *accoucheurs* as a motley, marginal crew, forceps wedged in the door. But the reality seems far different. For man-midwifery was already deeply entrenched in England, Frank Nicholls reckoning, with paranoid exaggeration, that hundreds of operators were already swarming in London by mid-century. And because having a male operator in attendance first became popular amongst society ladies, obstetrics was inevitably (as Simmons put it) 'lucrative',[56] its upper end becoming a fashionable branch of medicine, as the careers of Sir David Hamilton,[57] John Birch, Francis Sandys, James Douglas and Sir Richard Manningham testify. (Manningham, a bishop's son, netted about £4,000 a year.)[58] The trusted velvety obstetrician won gratitude and an entrée into intimacy, becoming an accomplice to sexual secrets and scandals, attending on the mistresses of peers (as Hunter did, for example, with Lord Sandwich's Miss Ray) and managing the clandestine confinements of the *jeunesse dorée* (he once secretly delivered a peer's unmarried daughter of twins and organised their admission into the Foundling Hospital).[59] When William Hunter opted for obstetrics, it was not a desperate remedy in an overcrowded profession, but testimony to his nose for rich pickings and for access to the boudoirs of the great. No wonder, supping at his favourite London Scottish coffee house, he

55 J. Thomson, *An Account of the Life, Lectures and Writings of William Cullen*, 2 vols. (Edinburgh, 1832–59), I, p. 544.
56 Brock, *William Hunter*, p. 8.
57 P. Roberts (ed.), *The Diary of Sir David Hamilton 1709–1714* (Oxford, 1975).
58 One recalls that Mrs Shandy wanted Dr Manningham but he was too busy. L. Sterne, *Tristram Shandy* (Harmondsworth, 1979), pp. 71, 75.
59 See W. Wadd, *Mems Maxims and Memoirs* (London, 1827), p. 283: 'Dr. William Hunter used to relate the following anecdote. During the American war, he was consulted by the daughter of a Peer, who confessed herself pregnant, and requested his assistance; he advised her to retire for a time to the house of some confidential friend; she said that it was impossible, as her father would not suffer her to be absent from him a single day. Some of the servants were, therefore, let into the secret, and the Doctor made his arrangement with the Treasurer of the Foundling Hospital for the reception of the child, for which he was to pay £100. – The lady was desired to weigh well if she could bear pain, without alarming the family by her cries; she said "Yes," – and she kept her word. At the usual period, she was delivered, not of one child only, but of twins. The Doctor bearing the two children, was conducted by a French servant through the kitchen and left to ascend the area steps into the street. Luckily the lady's-maid recollected that the door of the area might perhaps be locked; and she followed the doctor just in time to prevent his being detained at the gate. He deposited the children at the Foundling Hospital, and paid for each £100. The father of the children was a Colonel of the army, who went with his regiment to America, and died there. The mother afterwards married a person of her own rank.'

made its habitual toast, 'May no English nobleman venture out of the
world without a Scottish physician, as I am sure there are none who
venture in.'[60] In a society where lyings-in were occasions for brilliant
display, obstetrics proved William Hunter's short cut to fashionable
practice, as Horace Walpole's witty observation of 1759 on society
gambling bears witness:

> Loo is mounted to its zenith; the parties last till one and two
> in the morning. We played at Lady Hertford's last week, the
> last night of her lying-in, till deep into Sunday morning, after
> she and her lord were retired. It is now adjourned to Mrs.
> Fitzroy's, whose child the town called Pamela. I proposed,
> that instead of receiving cards for assemblies, one should
> send in a morning to Dr. Hunter's, the man-midwife, to know
> where there is loo that evening.[61]

Yet one might object that this sunshine cameo of the beau monde
opening its arms to the *accoucheur* is falsified by the diehard hostility
of both medical colleges to that newfangled traffic. Quite the contrary. What this shows is just the reverse – the ineffectual, sclerotic,
one is tempted to say, marginal, posture of the College of Physicians
and above all, the Company of Surgeons, limping along lamely from
its formation in 1745 to its winding up in 1799. For these institutions
had become unrepresentative of the social realities of London medicine (after all, the Royal College had a mere fifty-four fellows and
twenty-four licentiates in mid-century, barely half the tally of those
who were actually practising physic in the metropolis). They lacked
the collective will and authority to dominate practice. They offered
scant medical instruction; yet neither were they energetic in policing
practice, summonsing few unlicensed practitioners or even brazen
quacks. For they had become essentially inward-looking, cliques that,
in the age of the club, provided honours and sociability for their own
members, while encroaching less upon the affairs of the medical
market-place (beyond provoking by their mere presence). Although
William Hunter tried briefly to storm the Physicians, in actual fact the
colleges were remarkably irrelevant to the patterning and progress of
his career. If we are fixated on the picture of hermetically sealed caste
divides between the ranks of medicine, we would do well to remember with what ease William Hunter quit the Surgeons in 1756
and became a licentiate of the Physicians, all at the cost of a footling
fine.

Entrenched historiographical traditions, I wish to suggest, focus

60 Quoted in Oppenheimer, *New Aspects of John and William Hunter*, p. 125.
61 Ibid., p. 123.

our attention too much on the more institutional, formal and public dimensions of medicine. Old-style scholarship gave us worthy histories of the colleges[62] and hospitals.[63] We now also have accounts of the growth of medical education, medical police and the clinic, and of the development of public health legislation, locally and nationally,[64] leading finally to the welfare state and the National Health Service. And paralleling these, historical sociology has been preoccupied with 'medicalisation' and the constitution of medicine as a profession, with its organised and corporate power seen as engines of collective upward social mobility.[65] This has involved, at the macro level, analyses of professional dominance; and in case-studies it has yielded fine accounts of intraprofessional rivalry and the 'struggle for reform', for example, the analyses by Waddington and Holloway of conflicts between the Company of Apothecaries and the College of Physicians.[66] The unspoken assumption behind this focus is that medicine's crucial dimension is the public and corporate. Exploring the politics of health is thus the worthiest labour for the historian. Lord spare us from being thought mere biographers or, still worse, hagiographers![67]

I have no quarrel with these priorities, even if they have left us without a history of general practitioners, to say nothing of studies of sufferers and patients. Yet our fondness for institutional affiliation,

---

62 For example, Sir G. Clark, *A History of the Royal College of Physicians of London*, 2 vols. (Oxford, 1964–72); Z. Cope, *The History of the Royal College of Surgeons of England* (London, 1959); W. Munk, *The Roll of the Royal College of Physicians of London*, 2d ed., 3 vols. (London, 1878); S. Young, *The Annals of the Barber Surgeons* (London, 1890).
63 For example, H. C. Cameron, *Mr Guy's Hospital 1726–1948* (London, 1954); A. E. Clark-Kennedy, *London Pride: The Story of a Voluntary Hospital* (London, 1979); J. Blomfield, *St George's 1733–1933* (London, 1933).
64 For introductions to this literature see J. Woodward and D. Richards, 'Towards a Social History of Medicine', in their *Health Care and Popular Medicine*, 15–55; M. Pelling, 'Medicine since 1500', in P. Corsi and P. Weindling (eds.), *Information Sources in the History of Science and Medicine* (London, 1983), 379–410; C. Webster, 'The Historiography of Medicine', in ibid., 29–43; M. MacDonald, 'Anthropological Perspectives on the History of Science and Medicine', in ibid., 81–98; and L. J. Jordanova, 'The Social Sciences and History of Science and Medicine', in ibid., 81–98.
65 See, e.g., E. Freidson, *Profession of Medicine* (New York, 1972); T. J. Johnson, *Professions and Power* (London, 1972); M. S. Larson, *The Rise of Professionalism* (London, 1977); N. L. Parry and J. Parry, *Rise of the Medical Profession;* D. Mechanic, *Medical Sociology: A Selective View* (New York, 1968); and the recent reassessment of this literature in R. Dingwall and P. Lewis (eds.), *The Sociology of the Professions* (London, 1983).
66 See, e.g., Waddington, 'General Practitioners and Consultants'; 'The Struggle to Reform the Royal College of Physicians'; S. W. F. Holloway, 'The Apothecaries' Act, 1815: A Reinterpretation', *Medical History*, X (1966), 107–29, 221–36.
67 For a defence see T. Hankins, 'In Defence of Biography: The Use of Biography in the History of Science', *History of Science*, XVII (1979), 1–16.

the occupational caste system and the gross anatomy of the profession risks putting the cart before the horse, reducing individual doctors to pawns in deeper strategies, forgetting that even pawns have power to advance into queens; foreclosing even on the possibility that career-making can be a very personal business, opportunistically manipulating qualifications and institutions as they serve their turn. The solution to the paradoxes of William Hunter's career, I believe, will come from distancing ourselves from institutional and professional history, and scrutinising individual career-building. In this we can profit from Jewson's extremely suggestive, if rather abstract, paper on 'Medical Knowledge and the Patronage System',[68] and from the socio-economic history and Namierite political analysis upon which he drew.

Jewson argued that English medicine before the birth of the clinic was client dominated. Practitioners shaped their careers and won their identity more through interaction with the laity than through colleague control within the vocational hierarchy. Unless we accept the persuasiveness of this interpretation, it is hard to make sense of a century in which – to the scandal of physicians – certain apothecaries and midwives could make thousands of pounds a year, swaggering around in carriages;[69] a provincial surgeon such as Daniel Sutton[70] could pocket £6,000 a year from his inoculating business, and quacks and medical showmen such as Chevalier Taylor,[71] 'Spot' Ward, Mrs Mapp and James Graham[72] could command fashionable clienteles, public acclaim and ample fortunes.

In this patient-orientated milieu, of course, the price of favour was often deference, and hence later struggles to professionalise and shelter under institutional carapaces were the practitioner's escape from lay tutelege. But patronage and face-to-face contact also lay the career market extremely open, effervescent with opportunities. George Saintsbury wrote of 'the peace of the Augustans',[73] and we tend to think of Old England as a closed, exclusive, oligarchic landscape of decaying institutions and corrupt practice. There is some truth in

68   N. Jewson, 'Medical Knowledge and the Patronage System in Eighteenth Century England', Sociology, XIII (1974), 369–85.
69   See Hamilton, 'Medical Profession in the Eighteenth Century', 159, 161.
70   D. van Zwanenberg, 'The Suttons and the Business of Inoculation', Medical History, XXII (1978), 71–82.
71   A. D. Wright, 'The Quacks of John Hunter's Time', Transactions of the Hunterian Society, XI (1952–3), 68–84.
72   Roy Porter, 'The Sexual Politics of James Graham', British Journal for Eighteenth Century Studies, V (1982), 199–206.
73   See Roy Porter, English Society in the Eighteenth Century (Harmondsworth, 1982), chap. 3.

that. But the economy was buoyant, culture and leisure were becoming commercialised, and improvements in markets and media were spreading taste and fashion; and all these made for a fluid, consumer- and service-orientated, acquisitive society of plenty and panache, full of golden opportunities for the enterprising to thrust themselves up in the interstices like luxuriant weeds through the cracks.[74] Maybe it was in fact the professional order of the Victorian era, with its vaunted career 'open to talent', which ironically became 'closed', clogged by the restrictive professional practices arising from over-production of highly qualified men.[75] Seen in the light of lay patronage and entrepreneurial responses to an opportunity economy, the enigmas of William Hunter's meteoric career dissolve, and fresh perspectives open on the medical market-place of the mid-eighteenth century.

William Hunter saw medicine as an enterprise in a competitive environment. This idea, implicit in his practice, is quite overt in his lectures.[76] Hunter needs to be viewed not in terms of professional elevators, collective mobility and so forth, but rather in the light of entrepreneurship.[77] From 1747 the base of his business was his anatomy school, an enterprise essentially self-created, self-owned and self-managed right up to his death. Who can say he would have wanted it any differently? Never did he hold, seek or express regrets at not having a prestigious hospital appointment (his attachments were minor: surgeon-midwife to the Middlesex Hosptial in 1748 and surgeon-*accoucheur* at the British Lying-in Hosptial in Brownlow Street, Long Acre, in 1749). Such a post would presumably have cramped his autonomy, his *Lehrfreiheit* – perhaps leading to recriminations similar to those embroiling his brother John at St George's.[78] Nor did he ever cast eyes at academe like his former mentor Cullen, for whom a chair at Glasgow was a welcome escape from provincial practice. Only once did he propose abandoning his private anatomy school, when, in 1763, he petitioned Lord Bute to donate a prestige site for a National School of Anatomy, which he would build and equip. But Hunter's astute plan amounted in essence to crowning his private school with a royal crest, for he would

---

74 See H. Perkin, *The Origins of Modern English Society* (London, 1969); A. Mac-Farlane, *The Origins of English Individualism* (Oxford, 1978); Roy Porter, *English Society in the Eighteenth Century*; J. B. Morrell, 'Individualism and the Structure of British Science in 1830', *Historical Studies in the Physical Sciences*, III (1971), 183–204.
75 A point nicely made in W. Reader, *Professional Men* (London, 1966).
76 [William Hunter], *Two Introductory Lectures*.
77 Perkin, *Origins of Modern English Society*, has a good discussion of the 'professional' and 'enterpreneurial' ideals. My suggestion is that many 'professionals' were themselves 'entrepreneurial'.
78 See Paget, *John Hunter*, pp. 194ff.

retain control of its management and profits. When this proposal met
with silence, Hunter briefly contemplated going into partnership
with Cullen,[79] to run another private medical school ('to make our
neighbours stare'),[80] this time in Glasgow, and presumably in rivalry
with the university – hardly a serious proposal, as private anatomy
schools needed bodies galore, for which London was the only large
mart. Overall, public institutions had nothing to offer Hunter.[81]

Rather, from 1746 to his death, Hunter used his private anatomy
school as his base, physical and symbolic.[82] He was by no means the
first London private anatomy lecturer, for as Peachey showed,[83] at
least twenty-six other lecturers had preceded him, seizing from the
somnolent Barber-Surgeons' Company the office of anatomy demonstration. But Hunter did it consummately well, lecturing with command, in a voice free of empty rhetoric and Scotticisms, to an audience often exceeding a hundred,[84] which occasionally included
such luminaries as Gibbon, Adam Smith, Edmund Burke and 'Jupi-
ter' Carlyle. Theatrically uniting self-display yet self-concealment, lecturing was perhaps his forte, as his *Gentleman's Magazine* obituarist
judged:

> To consider him as a teacher, is to view him in his most amia-
> ble character; perspicuity, unaffected modesty, and a desire
> of being useful, were his peculiar characteristics; and, of all
> others, he was most happy in blending the utile with the
> dulce, by introducing apposite and pleasing stories, to illus-
> trate and enliven the more abstruse and jejune parts of
> anatomy; thus fixing the attention of the volatile and the
> giddy, and enriching the minds of all with useful
> knowledge.[85]

Hunter offered a more comprehensive course than his rivals. Where-

---

79 J. H. Teacher, *Catalogue of the Anatomical and Pathological Preparations in the Hunterian Museum, University of Glasgow*, 2 vols. (Glasgow, 1900), p. LXXI; cf. Peachey, *Memoir of William and John Hunter*, pp. 120–1.
80 Thomson, *William Cullen*, I, p. 151.
81 It is possible though that the titles helped to promote his lectures. A student manuscript of his lectures bears the title 'Lectures Anatomical and Chirurgical by William Hunter Physician Extraordinary to her Majesty Professor of Anatomy to the Royal Academy and fellow of the Royal and Antiquarian Societies 1775'. Hunter Papers H 506, Glasgow University Library.
82 Stuart Craig Thomson, 'The Great Windmill Street School', *Bulletin of the History of Medicine*, XII (1942), 377–91. The career of Smellie, who never held a hospital appointment but lectured extensively, makes a good parallel.
83 Peachey, *Memoir of William and John Hunter*, pp. 8ff; Inkster, in Inkster and Morrell, *Marginal Men*, p. 133.
84 Paget, *John Hunter*, p. 61.
85 *Gentleman's Magazine*, LIII, no. I (1793), 365–6. Simmons wrote that Hunter was 'never happier than employed in delivering a lecture'. Brock, *William Hunter*, p. 6.

as for example, Frank Nicholls, whose lectures Hunter had attended, scuttled through the bare bones of anatomy in about thirty sessions,[86] Hunter delivered over a hundred (astonishingly good value at seven guineas). He possessed London's best array of dry and wet preparations and models, and as a bonus taught his pupils the art of making preparations.[87] And he had two final trump cards. Securing – by business talent – a plentiful supply of corpses, he alone was able to advertise teaching anatomy 'in the French manner',[88] giving individual students cadavers to dissect. Whereas Nicholls had been demonstrating his entire course from just a couple of bodies,[89] George Fordyce was able to testify that as one of Hunter's men he personally had dissected three.[90] Living in an age when it was agreed that 'the young Surgeon must be an accurate anatomist',[91] Hunter was of course lucky to hit the scene at just the right moment. Earlier in the century the Barber-Surgeons' Company had rapped Cheselden over the knuckles for privately teaching anatomy from corpses contrary to

86   Teacher, *Catalogue of Preparations* p. LXIII: 'To describe Hunter's courses as anatomy lectures conveys a very inadequate idea of what they were. They embraced anatomy, physiology, and pathology, and also courses of operative surgery and midwifery. The autumn course of 1775 (MS. no. 42 c. 25) consisted of 112 meetings, which is probably about the average, and extended over about three and a half months. The lectures were given daily, Saturdays as well as week days, and extra evening lectures had to be added to make up this number in that brief time. William Hunter delivered most of the day lectures himself; it was a regular engagement with him; but the evening lectures, and certain of the day ones were left to his partner, who also had to lecture if "The Doctor" happened to be called away on urgent business, or were indisposed. Of the 112 lectures, 2 were the introductory ones; 80 were devoted to what was included under the term anatomy; 15 were on operative surgery; 3 on the making of preparations and embalming (a subject to which William Hunter had devoted a good deal of attention); and the remaining 12 on midwifery, about half of them being anatomical. The importance of these courses can hardly be overestimated; with the exception of chemistry and materia medica, they were the whole of what may be described as the science part of a medical curriculum in those days.'
87   Brock, *William Hunter*.
88   For the French manner see T. Gelfand, ' "The Paris Manner" of Dissection: Student Anatomical Dissection in Early Eighteenth Century Paris', *Bulletin of the History of Medicine*, XLVI (1972), 99–130, and chap. 5, this volume; for Hunter's studies in Paris with Ferrein in 1743–4, see Peachey, *Memoir of William and John Hunter*, pp. 44–5.
89   Brock, *William Hunter*, p. 3.
90   Teacher, *Catalogue of Preparations* p. LXVII.
91   R. Campbell, *The London Tradesman* (London, 1747), p. 50: 'The young Surgeon must be an accurate Anatomist, not only a speculative but practical Anatomist; without which he must turn out a mere Bungler. It is not sufficient for him to attend Anatomical Lectures, and see two or three Subjects cursorily dissected; but he must put his Hand to it himself, and be able to dissect every Part, with the same Accuracy that the Professor performs.' A letter of William Shippen's to William Hewson (24 May 1771) states 'the study of anatomy is thought more necessary every day'. Hunter Papers H 504, Glasgow University Library.

their privilege; but the parting of the Barbers and Surgeons in 1745 left the Surgeons' Company without a dissecting theatre or the collective will to promote lecturing (top surgeons feared it would 'interfere with private courses').[92] Moreover an act of 1752, legalising dissection of the corpses of all executed felons, effectively put Hunter's lectures above-board.[93]

Second, Hunter's lectures pulled in the crowds because he had major advances in anatomy and obstetrics to impart – for example his understanding of the lymphatics as the body's absorbent system – reserved for the privileged ears of his auditors. The fact that he communicated his anatomical teaching not in textbooks but as lectures, delivered orally but never printed, shows how far his self-image as captain of an anatomy school shaped Hunter's identity, even in his approach to the standing of knowledge.[94] Hunter did not see himself primarily as a sage, as a solitary genius, a public servant or savant, as a collaborator within a fraternal egalitarian, gift-giving community of truth-seekers governed by proto-Mertonian imperatives of universalism, communism, disinterestedness and organised scepticism.[95] Rather he epitomised a proprietorial attitude towards knowledge. He was an owner, producer and packager of medico-scientific truth; it was his capital and stock. He distributed this commodity freely within the anatomy school – where it was literally embodied in the skeletons and preparations – to those paying to hear; it was not broadcast at all to those beyond the walls. It was not for any 'hermetic', Rosicrucian, reason that Hunter kept his teachings 'secret', fearing pollution by the profane (though, knowing how controversial dissection was, he warned students to keep mum in front of the vulgar).[96] Rather,

92 Leading surgeons themselves were averse to the Company's setting up lectures in competition. See P. Roberts, The Diary of Sir David Hamilton, 1709–1714 (Oxford, 1975), p. 125. The famous reformer of the Surgeons' Company, Gunning, opposed a school of anatomy at the Hall because it would 'interfere with private courses'.
93 Peachey, Memoir of William and John Hunter, p. 5; Cope, 'William Cheselden'.
94 Most of Hunter's published papers were on technical aspects of medicine, such as the following published in Medical Observations and Inquiries: 'The History of an Aneurysm of the Aorta with Some Remarks on Aneurysms in General', I (1757), p. 323; 'The History of an Emphysema, Followed by a Remark on the Cellular Membrane and Some of its Diseases', II (1761), p. 17; 'An Account of a Diseased Tibia as a Supplement to [Dr Mackenzie's Account of Separation of Part of the Thigh Bone]', II (1761), p. 303.
95 For some of these images of the scientist, see R. K. Merton, 'The Institutional Imperatives of Science', in Barry Barnes (ed.), Sociology of Science (Harmondsworth, 1972), pp. 65–79, and Barry Barnes and David Edge, Science in Context (Milton Keynes, 1982), Introduction, pp. 1–12.
96 Two Introductory Lectures, p. 113: 'In a country where liberty disposes the people to licentiousness and outrage, and where Anatomists are not legally supplied with dead bodies, particular care should be taken, to avoid given offence to the populace, or to the prejudices of our neighbours. Therefore it is to be hoped, that you will be upon your guard; and, out of doors, speak with caution of what may be passing here.'

with Hunter, as with other contemporary lecturers such as Joseph Black, reserving his teachings for the lecture-hall was for the hard-headed business reason of preserving the trade mystery.[97] Publication in books, subject to rampant pirating, would have cheapened the goods, reduced pupil demand and the face-to-face homage of students, and thereby risked economic suicide.[98] In any case, viewing his school, rather like the lyceums of classical philosophers, as a self-defining community of the *cognoscenti*, Hunter regarded unfolding his discoveries within the walls of his 'private college' a bona fide form of 'publication'.[99]

Hunter fiercely defended his rights to his findings as private property like everything else in his anatomy theatre. When fellow anatomists such as Alexander Monro *secundus*[100] and Percivall Pott[101] published discoveries to which he claimed priority, his response was remorseless. At last he launched into print, asserting his own intellectual property in his savagely sarcastic *Medical Commentaries* (1762).[102] He backed his claims by elaborate documentation of prior 'publication' (i.e. before his own private lecture audience), supported by copious affidavits from his epigoni, and by innuendos about Monro's

97 Hunter had apparently promised his pupils he would publish his lectures, but never did. See Hunter Papers H 45, Glasgow University Library.
98 The sour Jesse Foot considered it sharp practice on the part of John Hunter to lecture privately for profit, instead of gratis at hospitals. See Paget, *John Hunter*, p, 105: 'Instead of lecturing at the hospital, free of expense to its pupils, as was done by Pott, and of openly imparting his system to those who were desirous of increasing the stock of surgical knowledge, Mr. Hunter could by lecturing at home shut out every one capable of comparing his dogmas with established doctrines, infuse without contradiction his principles into the minds of his pupils, and take their money into the bargain.'
99 In his *Life of John Hunter* (London, 1794), Jesse Foot disputed Hunter's claim to 'publication': 'What they were desirous of being considered as a publication, was only a demonstration' (p. 20). For the war of words surrounding the ethics of proprietorship in knowledge see 'Facts Relating to the Dispute between Dr. Hunter and Dr. Munro', *Critical Review*, IV (1757), 437–9; IV (1757), 523–8; IV (1757), 529–39; V (1758), 312–15.
100 N. B. Eales, 'The History of Lymphatic System, with Special Reference to the Hunter-Monro Controversy', *Journal of the History of Medicine*, XXIX (1974), 280–94; M. M. Ravitch, 'Invective in Surgery: William Hunter versus Monro Primus, Monro Secundus and Percivall Pott', *Bulletin of the New York Academy of Medicine*, L (1974), 797–816; Lilian Lindsay, 'Medical Polemics from Hunter to Owen', *Proceedings of the Royal Society of Medicine*, XXXVI (1942), 113–8.
101 Ravitch, 'Invective in Surgery'; Dobson, 'Percivall Pott'.
102 William Hunter, *Medical Commentaries. Part 1. Containing a Plain and Direct Answer to Professor Monro, jun., Interspersed with Remarks on the Structure, Functions and Diseases of Several Parts of the Human Body* (London, 1762). Paget, *John Hunter*, p. 56, wrote that it was 'one of the strangest books that a physician or a surgeon ever wrote. From beginning to end, it is an incessant attack on those who discovered what the brothers also discovered; every device of italic types, notes of exclamation, and long quotations, interrogation and interjection, heavy sarcasm, charges of stupidity, falsehood, and flagrant theft [was employed].'

industrial espionage (Monro's friends allegedly had attended Hunter's lectures and reported back). Yet Hunter simultaneously expounded an explicit psycho-sociology of how such priority feuds, literary larceny and rancorous jealousy over 'just rights' inevitably formed the imperative order of the commerce in knowledge; dog eats dog was inscribed in the melancholy of anatomy:[103]

> It is remarkable that there is scarce a considerable character in anatomy, that is not connected with some warm controversy. Anatomists have ever been engaged in contention. And indeed, if a man has not such a degree of enthusiasm, and love of the art, as will make him impatient of unreasonable opposition, and of encroachments upon his discoveries and his reputation, he will hardly become considerable in anatomy, or in any other branch of natural knowledge.[104]

Hobbesian self-assertion, 'emulation and contention',[105] Hunter suggested, were especially marked amongst anatomists, because 'the passive submission of dead bodies, their common objects, may render them less able to bear contradiction'.[106] In any case why *should* one submit, in a business in which 'most philosophers, most great men, most anatomists, and most other men of eminence lie like the devil'?[107]

But Hunter's proprietorial claims extended further, beyond his personal researches, to embrace all investigations undertaken within his patrimony. Though he could be scrupulous in acknowledging the

103 Hunter's psycho-sociological analysis of the inbuilt nature of controversy is evident in his Scottish Enlightenment vision of social progress. See *Two Introductory Lectures*, p. 52: 'Here it may be useful, as well as entertaining to observe that novelties, and improvement of course, have always become subjects of emulation and contention, between young men, and the old. In the exercise of the mind, as well as of the body, young men are quick, eager, ambitious of being distinguished, and often rash. In adopting new opinion, they have not to struggle with the habitual influence of a contrary opinion, to which they have long adapted all their other reasonings. Young men have likewise, very commonly, no dislike to pull down the magisterial dictates of age; and old men can seldom bear, what they think an inversion of the natural order of things, that youth should instruct age. Of all men, teachers of every kind, bear this with the least patience. For that reason, we see in fact, that the seniors of schools, colleges and universities, have generally been the most obstinate in shutting out light, and claiming a birth-right for opinion, as for property.'
104 William Hunter, *Medical Commentaries* (London, 1767), supplement, p. iii.
105 Ibid., p. 52.
106 Brock, *William Hunter*, p. 13. Hunter was a notably touchy man, who in his brother John's words 'did not make sufficient allowance for the natural frailty of human nature' (Brock, p. 28). He quarrelled with Smellie, Smollett, and not least the illustrator of his *Human Gravid Uterus*, van Rymsdyk; see B. Corner, 'Dr. Ibis and the Artist: a Side Line on Hunter's Atlas, *The Gravid Uterus*', *Journal of the History of Medicine*, VI (1951), 1–21.
107 Teacher, *Catalogue of Preparations*, p. LVII.

contributions of assistants,[108] his relations with his underlings generally plunged into cantankerous wrangling, with their claims to property in preparations or research done under his employ being dismissed by him as embezzlement. Such long shadows were cast by Hunter's lordly proprietorialness over the fruits of their minds and hands that, as late as 1780, John was still moved to stake claims to discoveries concerning the placental circulation made under William's roof in 1754, more than twenty-five years earlier, claims in this case warped by time but which led to a total breach between the brothers and a surgeon's unkindest cut of all, William's cutting John utterly out of his will, the ultimate symbolic exercise of property rights.[109] The force of William's patriarchal claims to absolute property rights as master in his own house is conveyed by the tone of his assertion, before his doubtless suitably awed students, of priority in the discovery of the lymphatic system, 'the greatest discovery both in physiology and in pathology, that Anatomy had suggested, since the discovery of the circulation' (and 'in merit Harvey's rank must be comparatively low indeed').[110] Having discovered the system, he explained, he set about proving its universality:

> Accordingly, my brother, Mr John Hunter, whom I bred to practical Anatomy, and who worked for me, and attended my dissecting-room, and read some lectures for me many years, found some lymphatics, first in birds, and then in a crocodile.
>
> Next, Mr Hewson, whom I first bred to Anatomy, and then took into my house to work for me, and under my direction, in practical Anatomy, to attend my dissecting-room, and read

---

108   R. H. Major, 'William Hewson, the Hunters and Benjamin Franklin', *Journal of the History of Medicine*, VIII (1953), 324–8. Brock, *William Hunter*, pp. 49–50: 'Hewson found Hunter's behaviour inexplicable varying from condemnation to praise of the same work. He also found Hunter's strict and narrow interpretation of the terms of the contract of partnership between them unreasonable, for Hunter assumed ownership of all the anatomical preparations made by Hewson and all his experimental results, and claimed that all Hewson's time should be at his disposal. Furthermore, Hewson, who paid Hunter for his board and lodging, had to pay him for the use of the museum and was not allowed access to Hunter's library.' For contemporary redefinitions of the law on fringe benefits and embezzling see Porter, *English Society in the Eighteenth Century*, chap. 3.
109   W. I. C. Morris, 'Brotherly Love: An Essay on the Personal Relations between William Hunter and his Brother John', *Medical History*, III (1959), 20–32; E. A. Schuman, 'William Hunter's Teaching on Obstetrics and Infant Care', *Transactions and Studies of the College of Physicians of Philadelphia*, IX (1941), 155–83.
110   *Two Introductory Lectures*, p. 53. Note that Hunter had no high opinion of Harvey (p. 44): 'In merit, Harvey's rank must be comparatively low indeed. So much had been discovered by others, that little more was left for him to do, than to dress it up into a system; and that, every judge in such matters will allow, required no extraordinary talents.' See K. B. Thomas, 'William Hunter on Harvey', *Medical History*, IX (1965), 279–86.

some lectures as my partner, which he did for a number of
years; Mr Hewson, I say, by a continued course of observations demonstrated the lymphatics and lacteals both in birds
and fishes, which confirmed the use of importance of the
absorbent system in the human body; and in comparative
Anatomy was one of the greatest improvements that could
have been made, to establish the universality of nature's laws
in animal bodies.

And, last of all, Mr Cruikshank, whom I likewise bred to
Anatomy, and took into my house upon the same plan, with
the opportunities which he has had in this place, and by
being particularly attentive to the lymphatic system, my desire, has traced the ramifications of that system in almost
every part of the body; and from his dissections, figures have
been made, which, with what I had before, will enable us to
publish (we hope, in a little time) a full account of the whole
system illustrated by accurate engravings.[111]

I have been arguing that in the open and pluralistic medical world of
the eighteenth century, when corporate controls were weak, when
the English universities slumbered and the London medical colleges
had effectively given up instruction, yet before the teaching hospital
materialised, ownership of his pre-eminent anatomy school gave
Hunter an immense fiefdom: freedom and leverage against colleague
or institutional control, a fortress from which to do battle against
rivals, and posses of acolytes, retainers loyal at least out of respect
and advantage if not exactly love.[112] It created a private medical business,[113] but it also endowed him with public visibility, difficult to be
matched by the mere clinical physician, gold-headed cane and all.
The Great Windmill Street anatomy school and museum was an impressive edifice abutting onto the fashionable West End, yet in the
thick of those many other dazzling shows of London that Richard
Altick has so graphically evoked,[114] two minutes away from that

111 Two Introductory Lectures, pp. 60–1.
112 There is plenty of evidence of deep student respect for Hunter, and gratitude
for his lectures. See Brock, William Hunter, p. 37, and the letters in Hunter H 45,
Glasgow University Library. Yet his eminent medical colleagues were evidently less
warm. There was no public funeral or memorial, no large biography; no society was
named after him.
113 A parallel instance of the medical right to private property was that making
and vending proprietary medicines did not at all seem unethical. John Hunter
recommended Edward Jenner to go into the business. Paget, John Hunter, p. 165:
'Dear Jenner, – I am puffing off your tartar as the tartar of all tartars, and have
given it to several physicians to make trial, but have had no account yet of the
success. Had you not better let a bookseller have it to sell, as Glass of Oxford did
his magnesia? Let it be called Jenner's Tartar Emetic, or anybody's else that you
please. If that mode will do, I will speak to some, viz, Newberry, & c.'
114 R. Altick, The Shows of London (Cambridge, Mass., 1978).

other pupil of Cullen's, the 'master-quack', James Graham, demonstrating his own anatomy, mud-bathing naked in Panton Street, and five minutes' walk from the Royal Academy in Pall Mall, where Hunter displayed anatomy to a different, expert yet stylish audience. Cultural historians have long been characterising Georgian society as one dominated by ostentation, symbolic performance, street theatre and ritual display;[115] and historians of science, seeking the key to eighteenth-century natural philosophy, have recently argued that its preoccupations with ocular demonstration, experiment and spectacle were not just the crowd-pulling bag of tricks of the itinerant populariser, but the very heart of the enterprise, laying nature open to the people. William Hunter belongs to that moment.[116]

Amongst the medical world, Hunter skirted public institutions and subordination to his peers, building a private apanage round his students. Turning to the laity, however, he sought visibility amongst a much wider audience of patients and the polite. Throughout the century doctors were noted for their show,[117] combining self-advertisement with the conspicuous consumption[118] that marked success. 'A physician', wrote Henry Fielding, 'can no more prescribe without a full wig, than without a fee';[119] and, as Hunter had been well aware when he mused about chariots, every carriage told a story. Mead and Radcliffe had swaggered in their coaches-and-six, accompanied by running footmen, for as the contemporary verse put it, 'The carriage marks the peer's degree / And almost tells the doctor's fee.'[120] William Hunter made himself a master of those arts both of camouflage and of conspicuousness, which, rightly compounded, assured public entrée and applause.[121] On the one hand, he masked and ingratiated himself by obliterating his Scottish accent; by mouthing

115   See D. Jarrett, *England in the Age of Hogarth* (London, 1974); J. H. Plumb, *The Commercialization of Leisure in Eighteenth Century England* (Reading, 1973); J. Brewer, 'Commercialization and Politics', in N. McKendrick, John Brewer, and J. H. Plumb, *The Birth of a Consumer Society* (London, 1982); R. Paulson, *Popular and Polite Culture in the Age of Hogarth and Fielding* (Notre Dame, Ind., 1979).
116   S. Schaffer, 'Natural Philosophy and Public Spectacle in the Eighteenth Century', *History of Science*, XXI (1983), 1–43; and 'Natural Philosophy', in G. S. Rousseau and Roy Porter (eds.), *The Ferment of Knowledge* (Cambridge, 1980), pp. 53–92.
117   MacMichael, *Gold-Headed Cane*; Wadd, *Mems Maxims and Memoirs*; Jewson, 'Medical Knowledge and the Patronage System', p. 376.
118   See N. McKendrick, 'Commercialization and the Economy', in McKendrick et al., *Birth of a Consumer Society*, pp. 9–196.
119   O'Malley, in Swedenberg, *England in the Restoration*, p. 154.
120   Ibid.
121   On the idea of building an identity see P. M. Spacks, *Imagining a Self* (Cambridge, Mass., 1976); R. Sennett, *The Fall of Public Man* (Cambridge, 1976), and more generally, E. Goffman, *The Presentation of Self in Everyday Life* (Harmondsworth, 1969).

religious pieties in his lectures (though perhaps not a believer him-
self); and by trimming his politics to suit his betters.[122] An erstwhile
Whig, mingling in court circles and with politicians such as Lord
North led him to more ministerialist sentiments, to the scorn of his
Whig friend, Horace Walpole, who accused him of peddling 'political
anatomy' from the dais.[123]

Yet he also excelled in display. The cultural gloss preferred by
physicians early in the century was that of the man of letters or coffee-
house wit, an image cultivated by Drs Garth, Arbuthnot, Blackmore,
Mandeville, Akenside and Cheyne.[124] It is perhaps significant that
Hunter did not try that veneer. By his day authorship had lost its
cachet, as the pastime of the amateur had sunk into the trade of the
hacks: Dr Goldsmith and Hunter's debtor, Dr Smollett, were dire
warnings on his doorstep of the calamities of authors. Perhaps authorship was also too controversial. Though ever ready to put the
knife in faculty rivals, as a *social* animal Hunter glided through the
fashionable world with never a cross word. Hence, perhaps, his
choice to be celebrated by collecting, building up vast hoards of
coins,[125] medals, paintings, manuscripts,[126] as well as medical and
natural history specimens, and winning a nonpareil reputation for
connoisseurship, discrimination and scholarship. Collecting was his
symbolic act of assimilation into the values of high society, literally
acquiring culture, while, as with the anatomy school, annexing tangible objects of control.[127] As he revealingly wrote to Cullen in 1768,
'My affairs go well. I am, I believe, the happiest of all men. At present
I am sinking money so fast that I am rather embarrassed. I am now
collecting in the largest sense of the word.'[128] A dissector amongst the
medics, he was a collector with the laity, heaping up dependants,
objects, patients, glory. And above all, what he collected were the
trappings of civilisation: coins, or cash elevated into culture; medals,
or fame immortalised; and paintings, or anatomy dignified in art.
Hunter was deeply involved in painting, sitting frequently himself,

122 Oppenheimer, *New Aspects of John and William Hunter*, pp. 150ff.
123 Brock, *William Hunter*, p. 55.
124 W. R. LeFanu, 'The Lost Half Century in English Medicine, 1700–1750',
Bulletin of the History of Medicine, XLVI (1972), 319–48.
125 Anne S. Robertson, 'Some Treasures of the Hunter Coin Cabinet', *Scottish
Society for the History of Medicine Report of Proceedings* (1953–4), 7.
126 Sir George Macdonald, *Greek Coins in the Hunterian Collection* (Glasgow, 1899);
R. O. MacKenna, 'The Library of William Hunter', *Scottish Society for the History of
Medicine Proceedings* (1966–7), 11–12, 15; R. O. MacKenna, 'William Hunter as a
Book Collector', ibid. (1953–4), 5–7, 9–10.
127 Sir Charles Illingworth, 'The Erudition of William Hunter. His Notes on Early
Greek Printed Books', *Scottish Medical Journal*, XVI (1971), 290–2.
128 Thomson, *William Cullen*, I, pp. 554–5.

courting artists such as Ramsay, Strange and Reynolds ('I am pretty much acquainted with all of our best artists and live in friendship with them', he wrote to Cullen in 1768),[129] and taking his responsibilities seriously as professor at the Royal Academy,[130] expounding in his lectures how anatomy was indeed the foundation stone of art. It is perhaps no accidentt that Hunter's *magnum opus*, his *Treatise on the Human Gravid Uterus*, is essentially a work of medical illustration in the Vesalian tradition. For the man who professionally used artistry in wax and acid, plaster and turpentine to preserve his corpses, also knew how to deploy art to immortalise his rank as a gentleman. His raw brother John, with a more scientific bent, turned his back on culture and walked with nature, presenting an uncouth face but conducting exhaustive research into the natural world.[131] William, however, chose culture, not nature and, as he expounded in his *Introductory Lectures*, saw anatomy and art co-flourishing amongst geniuses such as his heroes Leonardo and Vesalius,[132] under enlightened patronage ('scarce any science or art requires the protection of a prince more than anatomy'), as touchstones of the progress of civilisation.[133]

I have argued that to grasp Hunter's success we must shift our gaze from the profession and its chartered institutions, and cast him onto a different stage, as an entrepreneur, carving out his own domain. Much as his upstart contemporaries Garrick and Reynolds created spaces for themselves – theatre owner-managership in one case, the Royal Academy in the other – to give themselves leverage against professional rivals, platforms for public visibility, yet also freedom from the more servile forms of patron control, so Hunter deployed his anatomy school and his obstetrics as platforms for winning wealth and fame yet also independence.[134] Neither is comparison with an-

---

129 Kemp, *Dr William Hunter;* Kemp notes that Hunter performed dissections at the Academy; Sir R. Smith, 'The Hunters and the Arts', *Annals of the Royal College of Surgeons of England*, LVII (1975), 117–32; S. C. Hutchinson, *The History of the Royal Academy* (London, 1968); Jane Oppenheimer, 'John and William Hunter and Some Contemporaries in Literature and Art', *Bulletin of the History of Medicine*, XXIII (1949), 21–47.
130 Brock, *William Hunter*, p. 58.
131 Jacyna, 'Images of John Hunter'.
132 Martin Kemp, 'Dr William Hunter on the Windsor Leonardos and his Volume of Drawings Attributed to Pietro da Cortona', *Burlington Magazine*, CXVIII (1976), 144–8.
133 *Two Introductory Lectures*, p. 117.
134 See D. Jarrett, *The Ingenious Mr Hogarth* (London, 1976); M. Foss, *The Age of Patronage* (London, 1972); J. Saunders, *The Profession of English Letters* (Toronto, 1964). Contemporaries obviously saw Hunter's theatre and Garrick's theatre as rivals. Hunter found his audience going off to hear Garrick in preference to him, and so moved his lecture time from five to two o'clock. Brock, *William Hunter*, p. 65.

other contemporary – Josiah Wedgwood – fanciful, a man who built his own factory and battled with competitors yet who never forgot that his livelihood hinged upon exquisite sensitivity to taste and fashion.[135]

Yet to cast Hunter as the rugged individualist is to risk manufacturing fresh myths. We now understand better how even the entrepreneurs of the early Industrial Revolution were less self-made than they made out. Men like Wedgwood arose not *ex nihilo* but climbed on the backs of traditions of craft skill, networks of protection, relations and credit, tapping funds of expertise and finance. Hunter must be seen likewise; he won independence, but did so by climbing up the ladder of mutuality and dependence.[136]

It may have been a stroke of luck that the surgeon Hunter's family knew was William Cullen. But thereafter little in his career was not carefully managed by himself and shepherded by contacts. He came to London in 1740 not a wide-eyed provincial lad, but clutching a reference from Cullen to Smellie, the leading obstetrician, and with other letters of introduction to James Douglas.[137] Between them, Smellie and Douglas familiarised the young Hunter with the Scottish medical community in London: William Pitcairn, Tobias Smollett,[138] John Armstrong, William Wilkie, John Pringle, Thomas Dickson, John Clephane and others. Moving cuckoo-like into Douglas's household in 1741, Hunter eventually became his heir apparent. A famed midwife-physician, rich, cultivated and respected, Douglas was fortunately also aged sixty-eight.[139] Hunter eventually supplanted his wastrel son, for whom he acted as tutor for several years, became engaged to Douglas's daughter, and nearly took over the practice of his brother John on his death. When old Douglas died in 1742, Hunter literally cast himself as being designated successor by the laying on of hands, through apostolic succession:[140]

> Early next morning I was call'd at his desire, when he thought himself pretty easy. I went in, he snatch'd my hand and spoke a few words, with too great affection for his giddy disorder. Immediately his fancy wandered, and tho' he could not talk

135 Cf. McKendrick, in McKendrick et al., *Birth of a Consumer Society*.
136 J. Brewer, in McKendrick et al., *Birth of a Consumer Society*.
137 T. H. Sellors, 'John Hunter – the Scotsman in London', *Transactions of the Hunterian Society*, XLI (1972–3), 197–209.
138 Oppenheimer, *New Aspects of John and William Hunter*; L. M. Knapp, *The Letters of Tobias Smollett* (Oxford, 1970).
139 Thomas, *James Douglas*, p. XIV.
140 Peachey, *Memoir of William and John Hunter*, p. 74. Peachey somewhat misquotes the letter, which is in the Hunter-Baillie papers, Royal College of Surgeons, 2.3.

sensibly, yet he still knew me and would not let me go out of the room. I sat on his bed till after noon when he expired with his hand locked in mine . . . On his death bed he acquainted the family that he had promised I should go to Paris and that I must go. At present I sleep and eat with the young Dr his son, and in harvest I go to France with him if a war does not prevent our intension for one season. I have the happiness of being agreeable to the whole family so far as I can guess by their behaviour. . . . After I come from Paris I have a scheme laid out of settling here, and certainly nobody can say that it will not succeed.

Indeed, greatness being thrust upon him, the continuing patronage of the Douglas family – his widow let William share their household for eight years – allowed him to assume Douglas's mantle. In his early lecture courses Hunter made use of Douglas's preparations and notes, which he inherited along with Douglas's medical books.[141] And most of Hunter's early research interests, such as his investigations into aneurysms, placental circulation and the gravid uterus, followed up problems Douglas had been working on. In a way faintly prefiguring Everard Home's succession to John, William Hunter undertook to publish Douglas's *magnum opus* on osteology – he was still guiltily promising to do so to his lecture audience twenty years later – but never quite got round to it.[142] A surrogate son, Hunter thus inherited Douglas's business and his goodwill, soon enhancing it by scooping up the collections and preparations of Sandys and Bromfield for £200.[143] Skilful at manipulating situations to his advantage, no wonder he wrote, 'I have the pleasure of thinking that every soul of my acquaintance wishes me well and would be ready to serve me.'[144]

As well as receiving patronage, Hunter was also grand enough to dispense it. 'I shall always think it the happiness of riches to support relations', he proclaimed to his elder brother in 1742 with breathtaking gravity and bravura for a twenty-four year old.[145] He was as good as his word. He brought on both his elder and younger brothers as his assistants, and his sister Dorothea as housekeeper, as well as encouraging other Scots such as William Cruikshank to come south to

141 Thomas, *James Douglas*, p. XIV; Brock, *William Hunter*, pp. 60–1.
142 *Two Introductory Lectures*, p. 57.
143 Brock, *William Hunter* p. 25.
144 Paget, *John Hunter*, p. 40. Amongst the various importuning letters in Hunter's correspondence is one from Sylvester Douglas (2 Feb. 1766) craving 'countenance and protection'. Hunter-Baillie papers, Royal College of Surgeons, 1.28.
145 For Hewson's characterisation of his work under Hunter as 'drudging' see Hunter Papers H 494, Glasgow University Library.

'drudge' in the business as protégés. In the household-centred micro-economy of the world we have lost, Hunter ran a family business upon a domestic basis, living on the premises; and like a good patriarch he enforced the dependency of his surrogate 'sons' – symbolically punishing William Hewson by dismissal soon after he married, and rewarding the pliant Matthew Baillie by bequeathing him his anatomy school by a right in entail, as it were: Baillie and Cruikshank were to have thirty years' use of Hunter's legacy before it passed to Glasgow University. It is significant that in his negotiations with Glasgow to clarify the handover, Baillie declined to surrender the preparations and injections.[146] A chip off the Hunterian block, he knew these were indeed his livelihood: 'I cannot live without lectures.' Indeed, the anatomy school of Great Windmill Street later changed hands several times, passing to Wilson and Bell down to the 1830s, when the challenge of the efficient teaching hospital put paid to the private teaching patrimony. Hunter's career shows how medical men could forge independence, but only through effectively milking informal support systems and ties of connection.

Thus we have the rise to success and gentility of 'Goody Hunter',[147] as Horace Walpole dubbed him, a man who lived, in Simmons's words, 'in the midst of a crowd, master of himself and of his own pursuits'.[148] Medical historians should pay due attention to the elements of his judgement: the importance of the crowd – both the faculty and the public; mastery, or the techniques of control of self and others; and pursuits of surgeons and gentlemen.

146 Teacher, *Catalogue of Preparations*, p. LXXIII.
147 Oppenheimer, *New Aspects of John and William Hunter*, p. 155.
148 Brock, *William Hunter*.

2

The happiness of riches

C. HELEN BROCK

William Hunter's father, John, was a laird and farmer at Long Calder-wood, East Kilbride, in Lanarkshire. But farming in East Kilbride was far from profitable, for the soil and the climate were unsuitable.[1] John Hunter was of an anxious temper and lay awake at night worrying over the expenses of his family.[2] So William, born in 1718 and the fifth surviving child, was brought up in an atmosphere of financial anxiety and I suspect early learnt respect for money and extreme care in its expenditure: a lesson well learnt and remembered through life.

Primary education, though not free, was cheap. Even in 1791 a grounding in reading, writing, arithmetic and Latin could be obtained locally for 5s. 8d. a quarter.[3] But higher education was another matter, and after William and his older brother James had attended the local Latin School, John Hunter was forced to sell off land[4] to provide the premium for James's legal apprenticeship in Edinburgh and William's education at Glasgow in preparation for entering the church.[5] There was nothing at the university to incite William to either extravagance or envy at the wealth of others, for as yet, in 1731, neither Glasgow nor Scotland generally had profited by the Act of Union with England, and living standards in the country were very low. Though plain living was in order at the university so too was high thinking, and students, at the hands of a remarkable and outstanding body of professors and in particular Francis Hutcheson, professor of moral philosophy, not only learnt to think for themselves but had 'awakened in

---

1   Sir John Sinclair, *Statistical Account of Scotland 1791–1799*, new ed. (Wakefield, 1973), vol. VII. East Kilbride, Lanarkshire.
2   Notes in Matthew Baillie's handwriting. Hunter-Baillie Papers, Royal College of Surgeons of England, vol. 6, fol. 21.
3   Sinclair, *Statistical Account of Scotland*.
4   Notes by Matthew Baillie, Hunter-Baillie Papers, vol. 6, fol. 21.
5   Account of the Hunter family by Joanna Baillie. Hunter-Baillie Papers vol. 6, fol. 19.

them a taste for literature, fine art and all that was ornamental and useful in human life'.[6] So well did William respond to the teaching that, his mind set free, he embraced the heresies of Arius,[7] and thus the church was not for him. After five years he left the university without a degree and without a profession. Encouraged, I suspect by his father, who was anxious not to have an unemployed son on his hands, he applied, unsuccessfully, to become the local schoolmaster.[8] William may not have regretted that church and school were not for him, both poorly paid professions, the schoolmaster often not paid at all. But if William, at this time, had secret ambitions, nothing is known of them. William Cullen, a friend of the family, in medical practice at nearby Hamilton, offered to take him as an assistant. Though previously William had shown no interest in medicine, under Cullen's influence he found, in medicine, a profession to which he was prepared to devote his life, but as yet he did not realise its full potentialities. So well did the two of them agree that they decided to go into partnership, with William taking over surgery and midwifery, for which he required further education. In 1738 he went to Edinburgh mainly to attend the anatomy lectures of Alexander Monro *primus*. Edinburgh, the capital city, was certainly more sophisticated than Glasgow, but William apparently saw there nothing that weaned him from the commitment to become a provincial doctor.

Edinburgh could offer little practical experience in surgery or midwifery, so in 1740, William went to London as assistant to Cullen's friend, William Smellie, recently established there in midwifery practice and planning to lecture on the subject. Here William entered a new world. Smellie's business took him mainly to the poorer parts of London but he saw all round him what wealth could achieve. He had come south with letters of introduction to various Scottish doctors who had established themselves successfully in the city and he realised how possible it was for even a Scots doctor to earn a good living in London.

Amongst his letters of introduction was one from his friend, Robert Foulis, printer in Glasgow, to Dr James Douglas[9] an outstanding Scots physician, man-midwife and anatomist and equally dis-

6   Francis Hutcheson, *A System of Moral Philosophy* to which is added some account of the life of the author by W. Leechman (Glasgow, 1755).
7   Account of the Hunter family by Joanna Baillie. Hunter-Baillie Papers, vol. 6 fol. 19.
8   George R. Mather, *Two great Scotsmen: the brothers William and John Hunter* (Glasgow, 1893).
9   Samuel Foart Simmons and John Hunter, *William Hunter 1718–1783*, ed. C. H. Brock (Glasgow, 1983).

tinguished as a comparative anatomist, botanist, grammarian, phoneticist and authority on Horace. He was a Fellow of the Royal Society and of the Royal College of Physicians. William called on him, Douglas took a liking to him, and as he had recently lost his anatomy assistant, James Parsons, offered William the job with the added duty of tutoring his son. William weighed the plain, unpretentious Smellie against the influential Douglas and found Smellie wanting. The temptation to accept Douglas's offer was overwhelming but it would mean breaking the arrangement with Cullen. Letters to Scotland were hastily dispatched. Cullen, seeing possible advantages to William, absolved him from the proposed partnership. William's father, true to form, saw possible financial disaster ahead and bade him

> Consider well what you do, with Cullen you may be very comfortably settled and make money and if you miss this opportunity now, you cannot be sure of it another time. Dr. Douglas's kind offer is only for a time. He may die before you come home or are settled, and leave you without friends at a great enough uncertainty. I suppose now you know very well the difference between the expense of living at home and abroad, and that perhaps cloaths and pocket money may cost you more than your whole expenses at home would do. You know my willingness to assist you, but you know too that already I have gone fully as far as my numerous family will allow of. You must now do something for yourself.[10]

Fully self-confident, what he did for himself was accept Douglas's offer and join the Douglas household in the autumn of 1741. What the financial arrangements with Douglas were is not known. His father died in October 1741, and his mother had from time to time to supplement what Douglas paid him,[11] in particular, so that he could become a surgical pupil at St George's Hospital.

William quickly established himself on a very friendly basis in the Douglas household, but he had not been there a year before what William's father had feared happened. James Douglas died, but he died with his hand in William's and not before he had made the family promise that William would be sent, with the son William George, to study in Paris.[12]

The war between France and Britain prevented the visit taking place at once, so William stayed on with the Douglas family, and,

10 John Hunter senior to William Hunter. 28 July 1741. Hunter-Baillie Papers, vol. 1 fol. 51.
11 Samuel Foart Simmons and John Hunter, *William Hunter*.
12 William Hunter to his mother, 3 June 1742, Hunter-Baillie Papers, vol. 2, fol. 3.

now only committed to tutoring the son, was able to take a few patients, some possibly former patients of James Douglas.

The battle of Dettingen in June 1743, and the resulting peace, enabled William and William George to leave for Paris in time for the start of the autumn lectures. Before the journey he settled all his affairs except payment of his tailor to whom he had to give a note of hand. But it was essential to be properly dressed for the part he hoped to play in life. Already he was beginning to speculate on the dividend he might receive from his excellent medical education and his own determination. Writing home the night before he left he asked his family to pray, not for his safety, but for his prosperity, excusing such a request by saying, 'I shall always think it the happiness of riches to support relations, not only to assist them but to make them the sharer in the greatest prosperity.'[13] But he was by now well aware that this was not the only happiness to be gained from riches.

His time in Paris was spent profitably, extending his knowledge of anatomy and surgery and making good use of the opportunities there for dissecting, so essential for understanding anatomy. Renewed hostilities between France and Britain drove the two back to London in 1744, and William again took up his residence with the Douglases.

His education now complete, it was necessary to plan his future. No idea of returning to Scotland entered his mind. All was directed to remaining in his 'darling London'. Besides practice as surgeon and man-midwife for which he had been trained, he saw an opening in teaching anatomy and set about preparing lectures and the necessary demonstration material. He announced his first course to start in October 1746 at which students 'would have the opportunity of learning the art of dissecting during the whole winter session in the same manner as in Paris'.

It is unlikely that at this first course he had more than ten or fifteen students, who paid three guineas for the course. His takings cannot have been more than £40 out of which he had to pay for the rent of premises, cadavers and possibly for assistance. For the course, repeated twice a year, the profits were small. Even in 1770, when his reputation was at its height, he cleared only £540 of which half was paid over to his partner in the lectures, William Hewson.[14] Obviously anatomy lecturing was not going to make his fortune. It was only his sense of duty to the public that kept him lecturing to the end of his life.

13 William Hunter to James Hunter, 17 September 1743. Hunter-Baillie Papers, vol. 2, fol. 5.
14 William Hewson's account of his dispute with William Hunter. Transcription American Philosophical Society. Philadelphia.

In 1747 he became a member of the Company of Surgeons; in 1748 surgeon, man-midwife to the Middlesex Hospital and in 1749 to the newly founded Lying-in Hospital. Hospital appointments carried no salary but they confirmed his position as a man-midwife and for the next ten years his reputation was built on his skill in surgery and midwifery. By the summer of 1748 he was able to afford a visit to Holland and Paris,[15] returning in time for his autumn course of lectures and to welcome to London his brother John, aged twenty and as yet without a profession, for now he was in a financial position to take John off his mother's hands.

Things continued to go well with him and in 1749 he was able to leave the Douglas household where he had continued to live and had been joined there by John. He took premises in Covent Garden. Ever cautious, aware that there was strong opposition in some quarters to the dissection of human bodies, he had written into his lease that if his next-door neighbour, Lord Archer, disturbed his lectures, making his premises useless to him, he would give up his tenancy at six months' notice.[16]

James Hunter had died in 1745, and now William was head of the family, but it was not till 1750 that he went north to attend to family business. While he was there Glasgow University conferred on him a doctorate of medicine.[17] Now he was qualified as a physician, but because he was prospering as a surgeon, it was another six years before he disenfranchised himself from the Company of Surgeons and became a licentiate of the Royal College of Physicians,[18] at which his surgeon colleagues heaved a sigh of relief for he was becoming too successful for their comfort.[19] With the retirement of Dr Francis Sandys and the death of Sir Richard Manningham, he now rose to the head of midwifery practice.

With his ever-growing reputation and strict economy he was beginning to accumulate savings. In 1753 he started speculating in a modest way in government stock.[20] In 1754 and in 1755 he was able to make considerable purchases at the sale of Dr Richard Mead's library and museum and in 1754 purchased land round Long Calderwood to

15 William Hunter to William Cullen, 20 September 1748. John Thomson, *An Account of the Life, Lectures and Letters of William Cullen M.D.* (Edinburgh, 1832–59), 2 vols., vol. 1.
16 *Survey of London*, vol. XXXVI. The Parish of St Paul, Covent Garden (London, 1970).
17 W. Innes Anderson, *A Roll of the Graduates of the University of Glasgow* (Glasgow, 1898).
18 G. C. Peachey, *Memoir of William and John Hunter* (Plymouth, 1924).
19 Samuel Foart Simmons and John Hunter, *William Hunter*.
20 Bank of England, records of William Hunter's holdings of government stock.

replace what his father had to sell to pay for his and James's education. In 1756 he felt the need of a bank and opened an account with
Drummond's Bank, now Drummond's Branch of the Royal Bank of
Scotland, Charing Cross, which still holds the record of his account.
From then on there is a great deal of information about William's
finances, but by no means all is revealed for some of his deals are
known not to have gone through the bank.

William's mother died in 1752 and his surviving sister came south
to live with him in London. Presumably the farm was let, but is
unlikely to have augmented his income, any profits being used for
farm improvements.[21]

There is no record of fees charged by William. John said that as his
reputation increased he put his charge up to ten guineas a delivery.[22]
His bank account often records receipts of £100 or 100 guineas, suggesting that for some attendances he charged considerably more.

By now he was making a comfortable living but could not be described as rich. There were, of course, short cuts to wealth, if one was
lucky. Between 1759 and 1762 he bought over £14,000 of government
stock, which he held only briefly but which entitled him to state
lottery tickets. Unfortunately no prize lists for these years survive.
Between these years the credit side of his bank account leapt from
£2,222 in 1759 to £31,000 in 1762, in modern equivalent nearly
£1,000,000. After this he lost interest in the lotteries, though he continued to speculate in government stock.

The year 1762 was all together a fortunate one for him. After being
on call at the birth of the queen's first child, he was later that year
appointed Physician-in-Extraordinary to Queen Charlotte, which
brought him £200 a year.

Now he was a wealthy man, but his first idea was not the promotion of his relatives to prosperity. His sister in 1758 had married James
Baillie, Minister of Shotts and later of Bothwell. William made her an
allowance of £100 a year.[23] This was a useful addition to the salary of
a parish minister and latterly of a Glasgow professor but was hardly
likely to promote a feeling of the greatest prosperity. When James
Baillie died in 1778 William allowed Dorothea and her three children
to live at Long Calderwood but did not increase her allowance. He
assumed responsibility for the higher education of his nephew, Mat-

21 James Baillie to William Hunter, 27 October 1770. Hunter Papers H 248,
Hunterian Manuscripts, Hunterian Library, Glasgow University (refers to repairs to
the house at Long Calderwood and on 15 November 1778), Hunter-Baillie Papers,
vol. 1 fol. 5 (refers to plantings at Long Calderwood).
22 Samuel Foart Simmons and John Hunter, *William Hunter.*
23 William Hunter's bank account. Drummond's Branch, Royal Bank of Scotland,
Charing Cross, London.

thew Baillie, after he had helped him to a Snell exhibition from Glasgow to Balliol, Oxford,[24] and obtained a Warner Scholarship for him from the archbishop of Canterbury.[25] Nor in his will did he leave much to his nephew for he told him that he had derived too much pleasure from making his own fortune to deprive him of doing the same.[26]

After John returned from the army in 1763 and set up in practice on his own, he is known to have been, on occasion, short of money. William's bank account records various payments to John up to the time of his marriage, but what for is not known.[27]

William was much more concerned with a scheme that he hoped would not only be useful to the public but also immortalise his name, that is, the gift to the nation of a public school of anatomy. At his own expense he would build and equip the school if the government would provide the land on which to build it. In 1763 he presented the plan to the government through Lord Bute, but Bute fell from power soon after and handed the matter to his successor, Mr Grenville. Grenville did nothing about it and William, becoming impatient, got Caesar Hawkins in 1764 to present on his behalf a petition to the king. Another year passed and still there was no response to his offer and William withdrew it.[28] Greatly hurt, for a time he thought of leaving London. Still wishing 'to do something that shall be mentioned when the few years I have to live are gone', he wrote to William Cullen, who had just been disappointed in his hope to become professor of the practice of physic at Edinburgh, suggesting that they should join to establish a school of medicine in Glasgow.[29] Nothing came of this suggestion. Next William thought to retire to an estate in Scotland. One was found for him at Alloa, for which the asking price was £22,000. When the deeds were sent to him he found them to be defective.[30] Probably he realised that, after all, he could not leave his 'darling London'. He decided, instead, to establish a private anatomy school in the City. He commissioned his friend Robert Mylne, the architect of Blackfriars Bridge and the Lying-in Hospital, to convert

24 Matthew Baillie to William Hunter, 9 February 1779. Hunter-Baillie Papers, vol. 7, fol. 18, which may suggest that William Hunter canvassed his friends at Glasgow University on behalf of Matthew Baillie.
25 Archbishop of Canterbury to William Hunter, 24 March 1780. Hunter-Baillie Papers, vol. 1, fol. 21.
26 Matthew Baillie, *Works*, with an account of his life by Jas. Wardrop. 2 vols. (London, 1825).
27 William Hunter's bank account, Drummond's Branch.
28 William Hunter, *Two Introductory Lectures Delivered by Dr. Hunter to his Last Class of Anatomy Lectures* (London, 1784).
29 William Hunter to William Cullen, April 1765. J. Thomson, *William Cullen.*
30 Samuel Foart Simmons and John Hunter, *William Hunter.*

premises in Great Windmill Street to provide a lecture theatre, dissecting and preparation rooms, living accommodation and a large museum room for he had also decided to indulge his cultural interests and become a serious collector.

In 1766 Clive sent back from India a communication suggesting greatly improved profits from a reorganisation of the administration of the East India Company.[31] This led to heavy speculation in East India Company stock, in which William joined, buying and selling again as the price rose only to buy again as the price rose still higher. His accumulating profits[32] and his general financial well-being gave him great satisfaction and in 1768 he wrote to William Cullen: 'My affairs go well . . . I am, I believe, the happiest of all men. At present I am sinking money so fast I am rather embarrassed. I am now collecting in the largest sense of the word.'[33]

This again was a fortunate year for him, for on the king's recommendation, he was appointed Professor of Anatomy at the newly created Royal Academy of Arts, though this was worth only £30 per annum.[34]

The East India Company stock crash came in 1770. The price fell from £275 to £192 and William lost some £2,000.[35] After that neither East India nor government stock attracted him. Instead he put his money on long-term investment in mortgages on land in Scotland, which at the time of his death amounted to £16,000.[36] But he did not cease to speculate, for his bank account shows large payments to stockbrokers, chief amongst whom was John Maddison of Charing Cross, to whom he paid £19,000 over ten years.[37]

Though he lived surrounded by a magnificent library and a fine collection of pictures, well, if soberly, dressed (for appearances were important), maintaining a carriage (for this was a necessity for his business), his general style of living was very modest. When he dined with a club of Scottish physicians that met at the British Coffee-House, his meal consisted of a couple of eggs and a glass of claret.[38] Dining at home he never had more than one dish, and even when he

31   Dame Lucy Stuart Sutherland, *The East India Company in Eighteenth-Century Politics* (Oxford, 1952).
32   East India Company Record of Stockholders. India Office Library.
33   William Hunter to William Cullen. 1768. J. Thomson, *William Cullen.*
34   S. C. Hutchison, *The History of the Royal Academy* (London, 1968).
35   East India Company Record of Stockholders.
36   Account of the charge and discharge of Dr William Hunter's estate. Hunter-Baillie Papers, vol. 6, fol. 37.
37   William Hunter's bank account, Drummond's Branch.
38   Alexander Carlyle, *Autobiography* (Edinburgh, 1860).

had guests he never regaled them with more than two.[39] He wrote to Dr Cuming at Dorchester to thank and scold him for sending him a hare, 'for one that never eats him self or has ever any body to eat with him except they prefer cheese or cowheel to game'.[40]

Doubtless his household was run with the strictest economy. William Hewson, his partner in the lectures, who lived with him till his marriage, complained that he had to pay for his board and lodging and for the use of the museum and as an employee was not allowed to use the library.[41]

There is only one record of a donation to charity in William's bank account, but this may be deceptive for John said that William's charitable acts were made in 'the quietest way possible'.[42] But Hewson reported that William was not prepared to treat any that were not able to pay his full fees.[43]

All that could be accumulated from his parsimony and speculations was put into his museum. His agents attended auctions in England and on the Continent. Friends and acquaintances sought for him at home and abroad collectors willing to part with their collections. Several must have regretted entering into negotiations with him for he always believed he was being cheated and dealings often became acrimonious. Having grounds for thinking he had been tricked into agreeing to buy the Peralta coin collection, he found that his agent, but not he, could be prosecuted for the agreed sum, so he refused to pay for the collection. Finally this was arranged satisfactorily.[44] Poor Sir William Hamilton did not get off so lightly. He had the offer of what he thought was a very fine collection of coins. He sent William a catalogue of it and suggested he buy it for £330. William neglected to reply by return of post as requested and Hamilton, being pressed by the vendor, bought it for William, trusting he would take it, but since it was bought without William's consent, Hamilton offered to make good any loss on the deal. William paid £330 into Hamilton's bank account. When the collection arrived in London it was found not to be worth £100 and was finally auctioned for £83, and William called on Hamilton, not only to pay back the difference between what he had

39   W. MacMichael, *Lives of the British Physicians* (London, 1830).
40   William Hunter to Dr Cuming, 7 December 1781. Copy in the Pulteney Correspondence, Linnean Society, London.
41   William Hewson, account of dispute with William Hunter.
42   Samuel Foart Simmons and John Hunter, *William Hunter.*
43   William Hewson, account of dispute with William Hunter.
44   Correspondence between William Hunter and Louis Dutens. Hunter Papers H 269–96.

paid him and what the coins fetched at auction, but also to pay freight charges, customs fees and auctioneer's commission. Hamilton who was already overdrawn at his bank could only 'try to think as little as possible about his loss'.[45]

William agreed to purchase for £230 from Arthur Dawes coins from his brother's collection that filled gaps in his cabinet. All coins that were duplicated in William's collection were to be returned to Dawes. When the duplicates were returned, Dawes was 'deeply chagrined' to find that William had taken all the valuable coins, sometimes nine or ten of the same coin, and returned only worthless items. In the ensuing dispute William justified his action in an extremely brusque manner, explaining his conception of duplicates, which did not allow the slightest variation between two coins, and pointing out that the whole collection was worth only £200 though Dawes maintained he had been offered £270 for it.[46]

There were happier results from his dealings with l'Abbé Barthelemy, curator of the collection of the king of France, with whom William exchanged duplicates. When a vacancy occurred amongst foreign members of the Royal Academy of Science in Paris, the king recommended William to fill the vacancy.[47]

On books, coins, pictures, minerals, fossils, natural history specimens and his anatomical preparations, Dr Brocklesby reported William had spent £100,000,[48] by present-day reckoning about £3,000,000. In those days William could buy a Rembrandt for £12 and an Aldine Plato of 1513 for only £15.15.0. He built up the finest coin collection after that of the king of France, a library of 10,000 volumes with some 500 incunabula and five Caxtons, over 600 manuscripts, many of them great treasures: fifty pictures of importance, and the finest collection of shells after that of the duchess of Portland.

At his introductory lecture at the opening, in 1767, of his anatomy school in Great Windmill Street, he told his students, who sat there surrounded by all the signs of wealth, that money was of no use to him except for acquiring and communicating science.[49]

He more than once said that he collected for pleasure. What he derived from his collections was not the happiness of a miser gloating over his hidden treasure. Not only was his library a source of material

45   Correspondence between William Hunter and Sir William Hamilton. Hunter Papers H 326–9.
46   Correspondence between William Hunter and Arthur Dawes. Hunter Papers H 249–52.
47   Ainelot to M. de Condorcet, 3 February 1782. Académie des Sciences. Paris.
48   *Letters of Samuel Johnson*, ed. George Birkbeck Hill, 2 vols. (Oxford, 1892), II, p. 437.
49   William Hunter, *Two Introductory Lectures*.

to feed his own interests in such subjects as classical bibliography and medical history, but his library and museum were available to any friends or scholars who could make use of them. Edward Harwood who worked in the library preparing his *View of the various editions of the Greek and Roman Classics* (1775) records important contributions by William to the subject. Others borrowed books from the library, including Benjamin West the artist, Thomas Astle the palaeographer, and William's medical colleagues; the St Aubyn family used it as a general lending library.[50] James Barry, engaged on a great mural for the Society of Arts, hoped William could lend him coins with the heads of Pericles and Lycurgus.[51] William, unfortunately, could not oblige and so Barry had to base the head of Pericles in the *Crowning of the Victors at Olympia* on Lord Chatham. But he gave public expression to his gratitude to 'Dr. Hunter for the great assistance my pictures had received from the use of his most extensive and valuable Collections'.[52]

George Fordyce was allowed to take samples for analysis from the mineral collection.[53] He worked out a classification of minerals based on chemical composition that he applied in arranging William's collection for him,[54] a rational arrangement that was destroyed when the minerals were taken to Glasgow and Professor Jameson was brought over from Edinburgh to rearrange them according to the much less rational Wernerian system.[55] John Bedford devised his classification of iron ores from William's museum and this led Lord Townshend, Master-General of the Ordnance, to appoint Bedford to advise on ores suitable for casting cannon.[56]

Charles Combe advised William on the purchase of coins and catalogued the collection for him and in so doing revolutionised the recording of coins.[57] J. C. Fabricius arranged the insects and found amongst them a number of nondescript species that he added to his *Species Insectorum* (1781). And the whole museum was a spectacle that

50 William Hunter. Record of books borrowed from the library. Hunterian Manuscript 315, Hunterian Library, Glasgow University.
51 James Barry to William Hunter, n.d. Hunter-Baillie Papers, vol. 1, fol. 10.
52 James Barry, *Works*, 2 vols. (London, 1809), II, pp. 330, 347.
53 George Fordyce, 'An examination of various ores in the museum of Dr. William Hunter', *Philosophical Transactions* 69 (1779), 527–36.
54 Trustees' Catalogue of Minerals. Hunterian Museum Records 23. Hunterian Library.
55 Minutes of meeting of the Trustees of the Hunterian Museum. 27 October 1809. Hunterian Museum Records 49. Hunterian Library.
56 John Bedford to William Hunter, 29 September 1782. Hunter Papers H 195.
57 Charles Combe, *Nummorum veterum populorum et urbium qui in museo Gulielmi Hunter asservantur, descriptio* (London, 1782).

was 'shown to the inquisitive and learned of every nation with the
utmost affability and condescension'.[58]

Thus, whether or not he derived real happiness from the support of
his sister and her family, or merely satisfaction in a duty performed,
undoubtedly, as he himself stated, he got great happiness from making his fortune. The pleasures that his collecting gave him were many
and various. There was the excitement of the chase, but financial
prudence probably controlled his desires. Then there was the pride of
possession: No other private museum in Britain could compare with
his, and this gave him an international status. By making his collections available to the use of the public he achieved a reputation for
scholastic benevolence. But I do not think that these were the only
pleasures he derived from his riches and collections.

His medical practice brought him in contact with the men of power
whose wives he attended. His collecting furthered his acquaintance
with such men, for many of them like Bute, Sandwich, Shelburne and
Rockingham were also collectors with whom he was in contact. As he
moved amongst these men of power he was often able to use them to
further his own interests.

He got medical appointments in the army for his favourite pupils.[59]
He obtained a scholarship for Matthew Baillie through his acquaintance with the archbishop of Canterbury. He canvassed the duke of
Argyll to get William Cullen appointed professor of chemistry at
Edinburgh[60] and then canvassed Lord Bute to get him the chair of the
practice of physic when Dr Rutherford retired, but Rutherford opposed the appointment.[61] William used Bute again to get his brother-
in-law, James Baillie, appointed professor of divinity at Glasgow,
which was achieved against opposition.[62] He may have used Bute on
other occasions as well, for Bute's brother described William as 'most
reasonable in any request he makes'.[63]

58   Peter Clare, *A New and Easy Method of Airing the lues venerea by the Introduction of
Mercury into the System* (London, 1780).
59   Thomas Reid to William Hunter, 6 May 1778. Hunter-Baillie Papers vol. 1, fol.
74 (refers to Hunter's obtaining appointment as a hospital mate for Reid's son
George).
60   William Hunter to William Cullen, 3 August 1754 and 13 December 1755. J.
Thomson, *William Cullen.*
61   William Hunter to William Cullen, 1 April 1765. J. Thomson, *William Cullen.*
62   W. Mure, *Selections from the Family Papers Preserved at Caldwell* (Glasgow, 1854).
James Stuart Mackenzie (brother to Lord Bute) 15 February 1763: 'I should be
mighty glad to do something upon this occasion for Mr. Baillie, brother-in-law to
my little friend Dr. Hunter, who has my brother's promise and who has had mine
repeatedly that he should be taken care of the first opportunity.' (This was with
reference to the Chair of Divinity at Glasgow.)
63   W. Mure, *Selections from Family Papers.*

It was probably through William's direct and indirect influence with the Lords of the Admiralty that Lieut James Cook, in 1768, was advised, on his voyage round the world, to use wort in the prevention and treatment of scurvy,[64] as suggested by David McBride, rather than James Lind's proven treatment with citrus fruits. It was to William that McBride's ideas were sent and who, with the help of Henry Tom, one of the commissioners for taking care of sick and wounded seamen, arranged trials of wort both at sea and at the naval hospitals of Portsmouth and Plymouth;[65] at sea, at least, it appeared to be useful.[66] This advice might have been disastrous for Cook if he had not insisted on fresh fruit and vegetables being eaten whenever available and had managed to get the crew to eat sauerkraut, which contains some vitamin C (wort contains none). As it was, scurvy was not a problem on his voyages.

William's friends used him to forward their interests. On behalf of Samuel Johnson, he presented to the king a copy of Johnson's *Journey to the Western Isles of Scotland* (1775) for Johnson was too nervous to do it himself.[67] Dr John Fothergill, through William, requested Lord Hertford, at that time Lord Chancellor, to have Samuel Foote's play *Devil on Two Sticks* suppressed for he was ridiculed in it.[68] Robert Barclay, William's Scottish lawyer, asked William to intercede through the queen on behalf of the son of a poor Glasgow widow who was condemned to death. But William would not act for the king had reviewed the case and the sentence stood. All William could do was commiserate with the poor widow in having a worthless son.[69] John Millar requested Lord Shelburne, through William, to allow him to

---

64   Admiralty Secretary to Mr James Cook, 30 July: 'There being great reason to believe from what Dr. McBride has recommended in his book Experimental Essays on the Scurvy (copies enclosed) that Malt made into wort may be of great benefit to seamen in scorbutic and other putrid diseases, experiments with it are to be made in the present intended voyage.' Quoted from J. C. Beaglehole, ed., *The Voyage of the Endeavour* (Cambridge, 1955), app. VI, p. 610. Though rob of oranges and lemons, made by boiling the fruit till it was reduced to a paste thus destroying all vitamin C, was ordered to be taken on the voyage, no reference was made to James Lind's work at Haslar Hospital. James Lind, *An Essay on the Most Effectual Means of Preserving the Health of Seamen in the Royal Navy* (London, 1757). (Nor does Cook appear ever to have heard of it.)
65   David McBride, *Experimental Essays in Medical and Philosophical Subjects*, 2d ed. (London, 1767).
66   James Badenoch's case reports on the treatment of scurvy at sea in David McBride, *An Historical Account of a New Method of Treating Scurvy at Sea, Contained in Ten Cases* (London, 1767).
67   Samuel Johnson to William Hunter, n.d. Hunter-Baillie Papers, vol. 1, fol. 53.
68   John Fothergill to William Hunter, n.d. Hunter-Baillie Papers, vol. 1, fol. 53.
69   William Hunter to Robert Barclay, 20 March 1782. Royal College of Physicians and Surgeons, Glasgow.

dedicate to him his *Management of the Diseases of the Army* (1783).[70] Even
the queen asked him to try and obtain for her from Dr Fothergill one of
the tea plants she heard he had just received.[71]

Obviously people believed that William was influential. James
Trail, bishop of Down and Connor, wrote begging him to use his
influence with David Hume to dissuade him from taking up an appointment as secretary to Lord Hertford in Ireland where Hume's
character 'as a Philosopher is an object of Universal disgust not to say
detestation and his historical Character, especially where Ireland and
the Stuarts are concerned, is excessively disliked'.[72] Whether William
conveyed this message to Hume is not known, for Hume for his own
reasons declined to go to Ireland.

Of course it was by no means all one way. The powerful found the
wealthy useful to them. When Alexander Wedderburn, Lord Lough-
borough, had not the money to buy the stock he wanted he asked
William to lend him £1,200 which William was pleased to do at 4
percent interest.[73] When Sandwich was short of money, William
agreed to buy his coin collection from him.[74] Lady Hertford, a patient
of William's for whom he seems to have had great affection (he had a
portrait of her by Alexander Rosslin), employed him to look after her
affairs and run messages for her, dispatching wallpaper to France,[75]
buying for her government stock and taking out a power of attorney
to act on her behalf while she was abroad.[76]

Lord North, whose wife was another patient of William's, when he
was chancellor of the exchequer, asked William in 1769 to go and vote
in his suggested compromise between the government and the East
India Company.[77] Perhaps William pleaded an urgent case to excuse
him from voting for he had friends in both camps.

---

70 William Hunter to Lord Shelburne, 28 December 1782. By permission of the
Trustees of the Bowood Manuscripts.
71 Mrs Schellenberg to William Hunter, 11 September 1769. Hunter-Baillie Papers,
vol. 1, fol. 83. (asking William Hunter on behalf of the Queen to 'make interest with
Doct. Fothergill to get her only one of them [tea plants] for her Majesty's own
garden'.
72 James Trail to William Hunter, 14 November 1765. Hunter-Baillie Papers, vol. 1,
fol. 100.
73 Alexander Wedderburn to William Hunter, n.d. Hunter-Baillie Papers, vol. 1,
fol. 108.
74 Sir George Macdonald, *Catalogue of Greek coins in the Hunterian Collection in the
University of Glasgow*, 3 vols. Glasgow 1899, vol. 1. Promissory note William Hunter
to Lord Sandwich 16 July 1777. Hunter Papers H 387.
75 *The Yale edition of Horace Walpole's Correspondence*, ed. W. S. Lewis, 39 vol.
(Oxford, 1937–74), vol. 39, p. 35.
76 William Hunter's bank account.
77 Lord North to William Hunter, 9 February 1769. Hunter-Baillie Papers, vol. 1,
fol. 63.

Initially William's sympathies were with the Whigs, but as his friendship with the royal family developed this was an embarrassment and he went over to the court party, going so far as to advertise his allegiance in his lectures. According to Horace Walpole:

Dr. Hunter, the Scotch night man, had the impudence t'other day to pour out at his anatomic lecture a more outrageous Smeltiad than Smelt himself, and imputed all our disgrace and ruin to the opposition. Burke was present and said he had heard of political arithmetic but never before of political anatomy.[78]

William, as he lay dying, must have looked back with satisfaction over his progress from a modest Scottish farm through hard work, economy and good fortune, to wealth, fame and influence. Happiness there certainly was in his possessions and in the position that he had achieved in the world of medicine and in society. His influence would die with him. His medical achievement well might be long remembered, but only within a limited circle. But his wealth had ensured his immortality. By leaving all his collections to Glasgow University, to be preserved for ever, for the improvement of students and the use of the public,[79] he had set up a lasting memorial to himself. Perhaps this, for him, was the greatest happiness of all.

Acknowledgements

I am grateful to the President and Council of the Royal College of Surgeons of England and to the University Court of the University of Glasgow for permission to quote from manuscript material in their possession. I also thank the Bank of England, Messrs Drummonds, Branch of the Royal Bank of Scotland plc., London, and the India Office Library for permission to use material from their records in the appendix to this chapter.

Appendix: William Hunter's bank account

William Hunter's account with Drummond's Bank, Charing Cross (opened in 1755) was for its first three years of existence a very modest affair (Table 2.1, Fig. 2.1), and at the end of 1757 he closed his account. It was re-opened in 1759 and sufficient money was deposited to allow him to make on 28 April a third payment of £200 on £2,000 (nominal) government stock, the purchase of which he completed in October, leaving him with some £560 in hand. The

---

78 *Horace Walpole's Correspondence*, vol. 29, p. 86.
79 *Deeds Instituting Bursaries, Scholarships and Other Foundations in the College and University of Glasgow* (Glasgow, 1850).

Table 2.1. *William Hunter's bank accounts (reported in £.s.d)*

	Credit								Debit					
	Balance	Carried over	Cash received	Bills	Government stock	Lottery	East India Co. stock	Interest	Payments	Withdrawals	Government stock	Lottery stock	East India Co. stock	Carried forward
Drummond's bank														
1755	230. 0. 0	—	230. 0. 0	—					377. 0. 0	230. 0.0				—
1756	1,000. 0. 0	—	1,000. 0. 0	—					—	—				—
1757	1,148. 0. 0	623. 0. 0	525. 0. 0	—					—	1,148. 0.0				623. 0. 0
1758														
1759	2,222. 8. 0	562. 8. 0	800. 0. 0	1,422. 8. 0		356.10.0			—	50. 0.0		1,610.0.0		562. 8. 0
1760	3,142. 8. 0	780. 0. 0	2,223.10. 0	—					100. 0. 0	12. 8.0		2,250.0.0		780. 0. 0
1761	17,608. 8. 7	3,410.10. 0	3,811. 8. 8	2,077. 5. 3	750.13.4	10,163. 8.0		25.12.4	609. 0. 0	3,000. 0.0	4,418. 5.3	6,170.0.0		3,410.10. 0
1762	32,026.13. 3	382. 8. 3	7,067. 7. 6	3,418.15. 0	17,282.10.0	847.10.9			974. 5. 0	1,820. 0.0	28,850. 0.0			382. 8. 3
1763	20,115. 8. 9	—	1,899. 0. 6	300. 0. 0	15,556. 5.0	1,977.15.0			920. 0. 0	—	17,397. 8.9	1,798.0.0		—
1764	1,420.12. 0	17. 7. 0	1,420.12. 0	—					898. 0. 0	58. 0.0	464. 5.0			17. 7. 0
1765	2,121. 5. 6	187. 3. 0	2,003.18. 6	100. 0. 0					1,054.15. 0	225. 0.0	654. 7.6			187. 3. 0
1766	17,378.11. 3	45. 0. 5	4,380. 8. 3	100. 0. 0	12,711. 0.0				4,412. 9. 7	706. 0.0	942.11.3		11,272.10.0	45. 0. 5
1767	28,266. 4. 8	490.16. 4	2,045. 9. 3	460. 0. 0	14,195. 0.0		11,520.15.0		2,639.18. 4	333. 0.0	10,695. 0.0		14,107.10.0	490.16. 4
1768	3,766. 5. 0	547. 4. 0	3,205. 8. 8	70. 0. 0					3,069. 1. 0	150. 0.0				547. 4. 0
1769	4,563. 5. 0	869.13. 3	3,966. 1. 0	50. 0. 0					2,817. 6. 9	—	876. 5.0			869.13. 3
1770	19,835. 8. 9	14,374.15. 1	6,965.15. 6	12,000.					4,866. 8. 8	—	597. 5.0			14,371.15. 1
1771	31,127. 5. 1	136. 4. 8	4,466. 9. 0	12,286. 1. 0					30,991. 0. 5	—				136. 4. 8
1772	2,556.14. 8	619.15. 9	2,390.10. 0	30. 0.10					1,861.18.11	75. 0.0				619.15. 9
1773	3,130. 3. 1	177.15. 7	2,459. 6. 6	51. 0.10					2,952. 7. 6	—				177.15. 7
1774	4,028. 2. 7	843.17. 7	3,746.17. 0	103.10. 0					2,572.15. 0	611.10.0				843.17. 7
1775	4,192. 6. 7	730.13. 3	3,273. 1. 3	75. 7. 9					3,161.13. 4	300. 0.0				730.13. 3
1776	6,263. 4. 1	257.16. 9	5,450.14. 0	81.16.10					5,928.10.10	76.16.6				257.16. 9
1777	8,479.18. 1	—	7,023. 5. 4	666.10. 0	532. 6.0				6,767.13.10	1,182. 0.0	530. 5.0			-16.11.11
1778	5,261. 0. 7	711. 9.10	3,756. 2. 7	1,504.18. 0					3,864.10. 3	685. 0.6				711. 9.10
1779	4,344.14. 0	273. 8. 5	2,449.11.10	1,183.12. 4					3,603. 5. 7	468. 0.0				273. 8. 5
1780	3,874. 6. 6	21.13. 9	2,161.16. 1	1,439. 2. 0					2,840.12. 9	1,012. 0.0				21.13. 4
1781	6,532.14.11	60.17.11	2,735. 7. 0	3,775.14. 2					5,983. 2. 0	488.15.0				60.17.11
1782	4,324.14. 5	217.18.10	3,603.16. 6	660. 0. 0					4,036.15. 7	70. 0.0				217.18.10
1783	1,207. 0.11	—	420. 0. 1	569. 2. 0					350. 9. 6	—				856.11. 5
Bank of England														
1764	11,158.15. 3	—	11,158.15. 3						11,125.19. 3					32.16. 0
1765	3,993. 4. 0	32.16. 0	3,960. 8. 0						3,919. 7. 9					73.16. 3
1766	73.16. 3	73.16. 3							73.16. 3					—

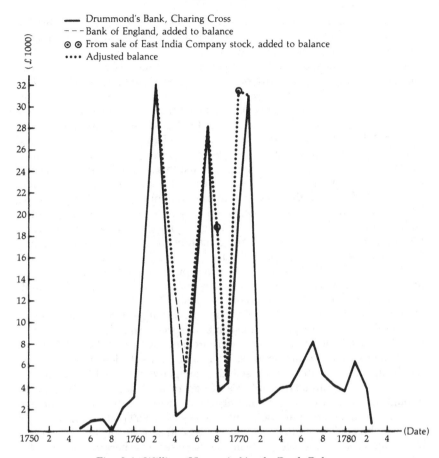

— Drummond's Bank, Charing Cross
- - - Bank of England, added to balance
⊙ ⊙ From sale of East India Company stock, added to balance
•••• Adjusted balance

Fig. 2.1. William Hunter's Yearly Bank Balance

money available for this purchase probably came from his medical practice in sums of about £100 paid into his account as cash.

The purchase of government script was a speculation in the 1759 state lottery. (For the purposes and conditions of the annual lotteries see Cecil L. Ewen, *Lotteries and Sweepstakes* [London, 1932].) Generally each £100 of script purchased entitled the purchaser to one lottery ticket. Tickets could also be bought separately. Prizes were in the form of allotments of government stock. Between 1759 and 1763, except 1762 when there was no lottery, Hunter invested most of his money held at the bank in the lotteries. During these years his bank balance leapt from £2,222 in 1759 to £32,000 in 1762, suggesting the winning of a large prize, but this cannot be identified as such in his bank account. Unfortunately no prize lists survive. Always buying script in instalments, he often sold off part of his allotment to friends and some of his tickets, even before the draw, which generally took place in November. Indeed, from what is recorded in his bank account he appears to have lost on his lottery speculations (Table 2.2) but it is difficult to believe he would have persisted in this activity if this was so.

After 1763 he abandoned the lotteries and speculated instead in government stock, rarely holding any of his purchases for more than a year. Between 1762 and 1767 he bought £67,300 of stock for £58,378 and sold it for £58,837, not a very lucrative speculation. He continued buying small amounts of stock until 1770, but the sale of this did not pass through his bank.

A Dr William Hunter held an account at the Bank of England from June 1764 to January 1766. It is not possible to be certain of the identity of this William Hunter, but during the two years that this account existed, Hunter's account with Drummond's Bank was much reduced. Nor, except payments to 'Hunter', do any of the payees from this account correspond to people to whom Hunter was making payments from his Drummond account. But John Hunter, to whom William was making payments, received none from William's Drummond's account during this time. So it has been assumed that these Dr William Hunters are identical.

By 1765 he must have embarked on the purchase and adaptation of his premises in Great Windmill Street, where he started lecturing in 1767 and took up residence in 1768. Between 1766 and 1770 payments to solicitors, carpenters, cabinet-makers, upholsterers, etc. are suggested by names in the account that may correspond with such tradespeople in Kent's London Directories 1754–1780 and in 1770 he paid his architect, Robert Mylne, £1,500.

But the expenses of his house still left him with sufficient money to get caught up in speculations in East India Company stock in 1766. Only his purchases in 1766 and 1767 and sale of part of his holding in 1767 passed through his bank account. Though at first he made a reasonable profit, he held on too long and finally sold out at a loss of £2,000 (Tables 2.1, 2.3).

In 1771 he paid out to Robert Barclay, his Scottish solicitor, £14,000, possibly to hold till some suitable mortgate (heritable security) became available. In 1774 a mortgage on the lands of Orr of Barrowfield was purchased for £14,000. Further mortgages were added subsequently, some redeemed, so that at his death in 1783 he held £16,000 in mortgages. These were good investments paying interest at 5 per cent. He also received approximately £70 a year from the rent of land around Long Calderwood. Part only of this income was sent to Hunter in London, the rest was held in Scotland and from it was paid an annuity of £100 to Hunter's sister, Dorothea Baillie, and the expenses of maintaining and managing his property. At his death some £600 was on deposit in Scotland.

From 1762 onwards payments to book sellers and auctioneers occurred in the account, but it was not until 1770 that they exceeded £1,000 a year. At his death identifiable expenditure on his collections exceeded £26,000. Receipts for many of his purchases of minerals and a record of what he spent on his coin collection are in the Hunterian Library, Glasgow University, but some of these payments did not pass through the bank. Nor are all his purchases of books, pictures, natural history specimens and anatomical preparations iden-

Table 2.2. *William Hunter's dealings in the state lotteries 1761–2 from his account with Drummond's bank*

Date	Bought	Paid (£)	Date	Sold	Received (£)
1761					
Jan. 3	15% of £10,000 script 1761	1,500.0.0	Jan. ?	15% of £500 script[a]	
Feb. 28	2nd payment 15% of £9,500	1,425.0.0	Feb. 27	15% of £4,750 script but Hunter	
Apr. 14	3rd payment 10% of £4,750	475.0.0		had paid 30% on this	712.10.0
May–August	4th–7th payments of 10% of £4,750	1,900.0.0	Sept. 10	£1,520 script	883.10.0
				£3,230 script	1,877. 8.0
Total		5,300.0.0	Total	(£4,650)	3,473. 8.0
Apr. 18	16% on £2,000 script	320.0.0	May	£2,000 script	612. 0.0
	3rd payment 10% £2,000 script	200.0.0	Total		612. 0.0
Total		520.0.0			
March	2nd payment 25% on 50 tickets	125.0.0	June	55% on 25 tickets	137. 0.0
April	30% on 50 tickets	150.0.0	Total		137. 0.0
June	30% on 25 tickets	75.0.0	Jan. 14	£90 prizes + 17 blanks (1759)	137. 0.0
Total		350.0.0	Feb. 5	£2,100 3% consols (1759 lottery)	146. 7.6
				(for which he paid £2,000)	
			Sept. 8	£100 long annuity (? prize)	1,529. 2.6
			Sept. 8	£2,000 4% annuity (1760 lottery)	2,379. 0.0
				(for which he paid £2,000)	
			Total		1,867.10.0
					5,840. 0.0
1762	No lottery		**1762**		
			Feb. 19	£200 long annuity (? prize)	801. 0.0.
			Apr. 21	£68 blanks prizes[b]	46.10.9.
			Total		847.10.9.

[a]Sale not recorded in bank account.

[b]For each lottery it was decided how many tickets would be for sale and how many would carry prizes; the rest would be 'blanks'. In some lotteries, however, e.g., in the 1761 lottery, each £10 blank ticket was worth £6 in government stock.

C. Helen Brock

Table 2.3. *William Hunter's dealings in East India Company stock*

Bought			Sold		
Date	Stock (£)	Paid (£)	Date	Stock (£)	Received (£)
2 Oct. 1766	2,500	5,610.12.6			
4 Oct. 1766	2,500	5,661.17.6			
			21 Feb. 1767	5,000	11,520.15.0
7 Mar. 1767	6,000	14,107.10.0			
			3 Oct. 1768	5,500	15,125. 0.0ᵃ
27 Oct. 1768	1,500	4,125. 0.0ᵃ			
15 April 1769	4,000	10,960. 0.0ᵃ			
			16 Oct. 1770	6,000	11,598. 0.0ᵃ
Total		40,465. 0.0	Total		38,243.15.0

Note: The buying and selling prices have been calculated from the market price of stock on the relevant day.
ᵃThese transactions did not pass through Drummond's Bank.

tifiable. Incidental expenses of his museum are suggested by payments to possible glass merchants, chemists, picture framers and bookbinders.

From 1766 onwards regular payments to domestic staff occur, but what his other household expenses were is not deducible. Payments to his assistants are also recorded, but neither the expenses of running his anatomy lectures nor his fees from students can be determined. A few of the costs of producing his *Anatomy of the Human Gravid Uterus* (1774) are reflected in his bank account.

That he continued to speculate is suggested by payments exceeding £19,000 between 1771 and 1781 to J. Maddison, almost certainly a stockbroker of Charing Cross. He received between 1770 and 1776 over £25,000 from Wilson and Co. – possibly a firm of stockbrokers with whom Maddison was associated – but the nature of many of his payments and receipts remains a mystery.

His bank account is therefore interesting, yet it is impossible to deduce from it how much of his wealth came from his medical practice, how much from teaching anatomy and how much from his other activities. If the bank accounts of some of his patients, particularly aristocratic ones like the Hertfords, the Chathams, the Suffolks, Lord Sandwich and the Hollands can be located, then perhaps it will be possible to determine how, when and how much he was paid by them for his services. At present there is evidence that William Hunter's account with Drummond's Bank is not a full account of his financial activities.

PART II. MEDICAL EDUCATION

3

The role of apprenticeship in eighteenth-century medical education in England

JOAN LANE

WANTED

An Apprentice to a SURGEON and APOTHECARY in full Practice, at North-ampton, where there are great Opportunities of improvement.

Coventry Mercury, 22 March 1784.

Apprenticeship as a form of technical training in England has early medieval origins, generally thought to be a sequel to the Norman Conquest, its rules and organisation spreading outwards from London to the great provincial trading centres and eventually reaching even the smallest communities. From the early period apprenticeship was well recorded, since it was illegal to practise an occupation without having served an apprenticeship and proof of apprentice status was essential to a man's livelihood. Sources for the study of apprenticeship consist of individual indentures and enrolment registers, often kept in Latin until about 1700, held by such important trading and administrative centres as York, Norwich, Coventry or Bristol, but also by ancient boroughs such as Kendal, where apprenticeship had important social and economic significance. At this early period, of course, the medical practitioners' apprentices were bound to barber-surgeons and apothecaries, quite separate occupations, taking their place amongst the other crafts and trades of a community. The early eighteenth century saw the gradual disappearance of the barber-surgeon (although surviving longer in remote, traditional areas like Kendal) and the emergence of the surgeon-apothecary, separate from the apothecary, who continued to sell and dispense drugs as he had always done. Physicians, without exception, were university men and not apprenticed, although a minority had begun their medical careers as surgeon-apothecaries before seeking the physician's status. This survey will concentrate on surgeon-apothecaries, their apprenticeship and training (since the apprenticing of apothecaries has already been described in great detail)[1] during the period of William Hunter's lifetime (1718–83), but refer to the so-called long eighteenth century (the late seventeenth century to the early nineteenth century) when necessary.

In the modern period apprenticeship has been frequently under attack, criticised both as a philosophy (by Adam Smith, for example) and as a practice, its image undoubtedly tarnished by the nineteenth-century's abuses, when the word 'apprentice' was applied to children in the notorious sweated trades, in factories and sweeping chimneys. Yet these unfortunate adolescents technically were apprentices, even if in name only, an indication of how the letter of apprenticeship could be followed and its spirit abused. Boys indentured to surgeon-apothecaries were never in this category of apprentices, their quite substantial premiums alone securing them at least humane treatment, with parents or guardians to whom they might complain and masters whose own poverty did not cause them to overwork the apprentices brutally. The surgeon-apothecary is one of the eighteenth century's most interesting examples of personal and professional upward social mobility and of steadily enhanced status, not only in London, where the 'surgeon-princes' had always prospered, but also in the English provinces, where their houses, marriages and affluence were worthy of contemporary comment. This was in contrast to other honourable, ancient crafts that fell in public esteem and profitablity in the decades of William Hunter's lifetime, pushed downwards by changing fashions (the staymaker), by mass-production methods (the metal and leather trades) or even by an altered international situation (the gunsmith).

The laws governing apprenticeship required that a written indenture was essential; an oral agreement would not suffice (Appendix 1). The master could not dismiss the apprentice during the term unless the boy broke one or more of the indenture's conditions repeatedly; the apprentice was obliged to live in the master's house, his primary duty 'duly and truly to serve'. The apprentice was also contracted to keep his master's trade secrets, an especially important consideration to the surgeon-apothecary, and not to waste or lend his master's goods. He was forbidden to 'commit fornication', marry or gamble during the term and was not to enter taverns or theatres. There were

---

1   J. G. L. Burnby, 'Apprenticeship Records,' *Transactions British Society for the History of Pharmacy* (London, 1977), I, part 4; Burnby, *A Study of the English Apothecary from 1660 to 1760*, supp. 3 (1983) to *Medical History*. The surgeon-apothecary was a well-known hybrid in Edinburgh by the early eighteenth century. See C. H. Creswell, *The Royal College of Surgeons of Edinburgh* (Edinburgh, 1926).

important practical reasons for such wide-ranging proscriptions, since the apprentice had unsupervised access to his master's property and many opportunities for dishonesty. Marriage was simply impracticable, since the master's house would at best have had only dormitory or garret-type accommodation for the apprentice, who, in any case, had not money wages with which to keep a wife and family. 'Fornication' meant that the apprentice risked fatherhood and a paternity order he could not pay. Gambling of all kinds was, according to contemporary comment, a particular vice of apprentices, from the most sophisticated city youth to the rural craftsman's pupil, and, lacking cash, wagering a master's goods or money was a constant temptation. Apart from the unacceptable company to be found in inns and playhouses, unfitting for a Christian boy, masters were particularly opposed to such gatherings of apprentices, who might reveal trade secrets and compare their conditions of service. Early records of the Surgeons' Company[2] illustrate the frequency with which these rules were infringed, and general control of apprentices by the eighteenth century had so deteriorated that they made frequent appearances at Quarter Sessions.

The master was entitled to behave as if he were a parent, to exercise 'moderate' physical correction of the apprentice, and although cases of masters being extremely cruel to their apprentices were fairly common in the eighteenth-century courts, the surgeon-apothecary's pupil was generally not treated so badly that legal proceedings ensued. The most noteworthy feature of the apprenticeship indenture remained the child's security from dismissal, unlike the hired worker. Numerous legal suits suggest that even deliberate absence, staying out at night, theft, sexual misdemeanours or occasional drunkenness were not necessarily grounds for dismissal, even if the apprentice deliberately erred in order to be able to leave his apprenticeship. His only means of escape was to abscond, and the frequency of newspaper advertisements for runaway apprentices in the eighteenth century indicates that many boys (but fewer girls) chose to do so. The basic conditions of apprenticeship, laid down in 1563 in the Statute of Artificers,[3] were not amended until its repeal 250 years later in 1814, to which a substantial proportion of contemporary opinion was opposed. In the same period, guild control over apprenticeship as a whole slowly weakened, so that, for example, masters increasingly took several apprentices simultaneously, although specifically forbid-

2 Sidney Young, *Annals of the Barber-Surgeons* (London, 1890), cites many interesting examples of apprentices and masters infringing the rules.
3 5 Eliz. I, c.4.

den by many craft guilds from doing so, and fines were no longer
regularly enforced for such offences.

An important event for the history of nonpauper apprentices and
invaluable to historians was the 1709 Stamp Act,[4] which fixed a tax
scale (6d. in every £1 on premiums less than £50, 1s. in every £1 for
larger sums, plus 6d. stamp duty) on premiums paid to the master.
Although the act was originally intended to operate for only five
years, it proved so lucrative a source of regular income that it was not
repealed until the nineteenth century and in its first year alone the
Stamp Act produced an income of £3,792 10s., in spite of evasions and
some careful arranging of premiums so that they came below £50 and
therefore in a lower tax band. Apprenticeships were to be entered in
registers kept in London, stating the essential details of child, master
and premium. In 1777 the Stamp Duty on apprenticeship indentures
was so valuable an income for the government that it was increased
by Act of Parliament to 5s. 3d.

Fortunately for historians, these great apprenticeship registers
have survived in the Public Record Office.[5] The returns were gathered locally and then entered in the registers county by county,
chronologically. There were a few administrative muddles, so that,
for example, two counties' returns were sometimes mixed (as were
those for Northamptonshire and Warwickshire for some years), making modern research unduly slow. Even allowing for underregistra-
tion, which cannot be assessed, these registers are an incredibly rich
source for the historian, although their quality deteriorates seriously
after 1760, with certain essential details, especially the child's home
and the master's occupation, erratically omitted. A practical disadvantage of these splendid volumes is their size and weight, over five
hundred pages each, measuring twenty inches by fourteen and a half
inches and some three or four inches thick.

The middle decades of the century saw the enactment of four statutes that further controlled apprentices and their masters, which suggests that certain aspects of apprenticeship were being abused by one
side or the other, especially with weakened guild control. In 1747 an
act was passed to permit any apprentice, pauper or non-poor, whose
premium was less than £5, to complain to two local justices 'concerning any Misusage, Refusal of necessary Provision, Cruelty or Ill-Treat-
ment'.[6] If the accusation were proved, the child was to be discharged
from his apprenticeship and return home, but the master was not to

4   8 Anne, c.9.
5   Public Record Office (hereafter P.R.O.), I.R.1.
6   20 Geo. II, c.19.

be punished and was to retain the premium. By setting the limit as low as £5 the act in practice covered most parish apprentices and the lower but respectable trades; of the 265 occupational premiums listed for London by Campbell in the same year the act was passed, only 27 were in this category, and surgeon-apothecaries were certainly not.[7] As the master could himself complain of the child's behaviour, the act could easily be misused by the unscrupulous or unsuccessful master to rid himself of an unwanted apprentice. A decade later, in 1757, indentures ceased to be legally necessary but were replaced by a stamped deed, and increasingly by a printed one, with specific limitations on the apprentice's leisure activities, as well as reaffirming his duties and tasks.[8] Apprentices had already been forbidden to hunt in 1693,[9] but from 1757 they were also not allowed to play various games of hazard, especially in public houses.

During the Seven Years War opportunities for apprentices to abscond and enlist were greatly increased, and the frequency of advertisements by masters indicated this trend. So commonplace was the absconding apprentice that an act of 1766 specified that when a runaway boy was caught, the length of time he was missing from his master's service should be added on to the original term of the contract, so that the master should not be deprived of the child's labour nor the apprentice lack part of his training.[10] An act of 1768 shortened the term by three years, so that a male apprentice completed his term when he was twenty-one instead of twenty-four, an age that was frequently required in the poorer trades.[11]

The considerable benefits of apprenticeship must account for its vigorous survival, in spite of criticism, but many of its advantages applied to a stable economy and static social order, so that even if economic change, fashion or war necessitated more or fewer workers, greater or reduced output, even different products, apprenticeship was inflexible, a brake and hindrance to change. To all occupations the advantages of apprenticeship were both economic and social. Primarily, it guaranteed a level of competence in the qualified adult and controlled entry of new recruits, thus preventing overstocking with too many skilled men. This in its turn maintained the qualified man's income and reduced competition, as well as reassuring the customer or client. It was illegal to practise a trade or craft (including that of the surgeon-apothecary) without having first been appren-

7   R. Campbell, *The London Tradesman* (London, 1747).
8   30 Geo. II, c.24.
9   4–5 Wm. and Mary, c.23.
10   6 Geo. III, c.25.
11   8 Geo. III, c.28.

62   *Joan Lane*

ticed, and the numbers of cases in Quarter Sessions in the eighteenth
century for this offence indicate that those who did so were promptly
punished. Apprenticeship brought certain acknowledged social benefits; if an apprentice became a freeman he had specific rights in the
community. An important privilege was that of franchise and the
right to vote in parliamentary elections that could either be exercised
or sold. A freeman and his family also had access to local privileges,
of sending his children to certain schools, of help from special charities and a share in common land rights. Participating in freemen's
activities (dinners, processions and other celebrations) was a further
privilege for the formally apprenticed. In purely personal terms,
many contemporaries held the view that children were better brought
up and trained in other people's houses, dwelling amongst strangers
and acquiring the social skills and acquaintance of their future career
rather than living at home. Lawrence Stone has also suggested that
apprenticeship helped avoid incest in the overcrowded family
home.[12] Foreign visitors frequently commented on the 'want of affection' manifested by the English towards their children, of which apprenticeship was an example. In spite of different levels of prosperity,
the characteristics of apprenticeship were common to all occupations.
As well as learning his master's style of life, the child was firmly
committed, by virtue of his parents' choice, to a career that might last
for thirty years or more, which in its turn influenced his income,
status and environment, even his choice of spouse.

Throughout this survey male apprentices only are considered. Girls
were not prevented from becoming apprentices, but their range of
occupations was of necessity limited to the decorative fashion skills
(millinery and mantua-making), domestic or agricultural work and
the sweated trades. They were not apprenticed to surgeon-apothecaries, although there were rare instances of widows or daughters as
masters, managing the apprentices and practices of their late husband or father, generally with the help of a qualified assistant. Such
arrangements were often formal, legal partnerships,[13] occasionally
made permanent by marriage between the parties. Unapprenticed
and unqualified women certainly advertised medical services in the
eighteenth-century press, but not as surgeon-apothecaries. They
were usually anxious to emphasise that they used the 'methods and

12 Lawrence Stone, *The Family, Sex and Marriage in England, 1500–1800* (London,
1977), p. 108.
13 Warwick County Record Office, CR 1596/Box 90 (itemised in Appendix 5);
Thomas Cooper died two years after the partnership was dissolved. See also A. L.
Wyman, 'The Surgeoness: The Female Practitioner of Surgery, 1400–1800', *Medical
History*, XXVIII (1984), pp. 22–41.

medicines' of their late husband, father or brother; thus the widowed Lady Read in 1719 claimed to use Sir William's techniques of couching for cataract,[14] and Mary Turberville, sister of the noted West Country oculist, Daubeney Turberville, MD (1612–96), practised in London in the early eighteenth century 'with good reputation and success. She has all her brother's receipts, and having seen his practice during many years, knows how to use them.'[15] By the period of Hunter's lifetime, however, qualified surgeon-apothecaries and their apprentices were male, and women remained as fringe practitioners.

In the eighteenth century apprenticeship undoubtedly came under attack but survived successfully into the nineteenth century as a form of technical training, although finally doomed by educational changes and increased industrialisation to become craft instruction for those traditional skills whose quality work (the saddler, silversmith or cabinet-maker) could not satisfactorily be produced by machinery. All these changes affected the surgeon-apothecary and his apprentice. In William Hunter's lifetime the number of practitioners grew very considerably, the population who were their patients nearly doubled, their premiums increased markedly, the range of surgical techniques and medicines at their command expanded, as did outlets for their employment as the Industrial Revolution progressed. Practitioners' social standing rose, along with their incomes, and by the end of the eighteenth century a new breed of prosperous, senior professional men, especially in the provinces, can be discerned, reflected in their social life and community status (their houses, marriages and public appointments), far removed from the traditional barber-surgeons still practising when Hunter was born.

The first problem for the apprentice, or his parents, and the master was one of matching the two parties of the proposed arrangement, and it is apparent that the few ways of child and master finding each other were common to most occupations. Thus personal recommendation must have been the most frequent way of contact and in some occupations, for example the London printing trade, complex networks of acquaintance and patronage have been traced.[16] Since many apprentices and masters shared the same surname, a family connection seems probable; equally, a master might have the same occupation as the child's parent or other relative. Thus in 1756 Edward

14 Cited in Ivy Pinchbeck, *Women Workers and the Industrial Revolution, 1750–1850* (reprint; London, 1969), p. 302.
15 Richard Colt Hoare, *A History of Modern Wiltshire*, 6 vols. (London, 1843), VI, p. 467.
16 Paul Morgan, *Warwickshire Apprentices in the Stationers' Company of London, 1563–1700* (Dugdale Society, 1978).

Pennell, a surgeon in the Bull Ring, Birmingham, took Charles Pennell as an apprentice for five years with the substantial premium of
£80; the master was presumably the apprentice's uncle or brother.[17]
Religious links could also account for apprenticeship choices, as in
the case of William Lucas, a Quaker apprentice to a London chemist
of the same faith in the early nineteenth century.[18] Sometimes quite
remote associations secured an apprentice for a master, so that, for
example, James Yonge, a Plymouth surgeon, noted in 1672 how 'May
the 14th was bound an apprentice to me Thomas Read, the son of one
Mr Read of Havant in Hampshire, whose father being dead was
under the care of his uncle Coll. Crooke (son to Judge Crooke), who
lived at Oxford and by means of my Brother Samuel was sent to me.'

A few years later, in 1679, Yonge took another apprentice, William
Wyat, 'recommended by my friend, Dr Waterhouse'.[19] If personal
sponsorship were impossible or unsuccessful the usual alternative
was to advertise, and notices by masters requiring apprentices and by
parents or guardians seeking places for children were regularly inserted in local newspapers, which, in the eighteenth century, had a
wide regional circulation. By the later eighteenth century, when truly
local newspapers were established, advertising about apprenticeships was commonplace, and a reasonable proportion of these
were for surgeon-apothecaries, suggesting the entry of boys new to a
medical career who lacked a family network of recommendations.
The essential facts a master included in his notice were his occupation, the optimum age and social background of the child ('honest
parents', 'respectable family') and the apprentice's requisite moral or
physical qualities ('of liberal education', 'a steady, healthy boy'). The
more prosperous master also advertised that the apprentice would be
well treated and live 'in every respect as one of the family'. The
premium was the most variable element in all the advertisements;
very few stated the sum required, which was negotiable according to
the master's assessment of the parents' wealth and his willingness to
take the child. Some masters mentioned in their advertisements that
they would need a 'substantial' or 'adequate' premium, deliberately
indefinite to discourage all but the serious applicant, while other men
simply stated that a premium would be required. However, as masters were also businessmen, selling products or services to the readers, many also used the advertisement for an apprentice to promote

17 P.R.O., I.R.1./52.
18 *A Quaker Journal*, ed. Gilbert E. Bryan and George P. Baker, 2 vols. (London,
1934).
19 *The Journal of James Yonge [1647–1721], Plymouth Surgeon*, ed. F. N. L. Poynter
(London, 1963), pp. 142, 161.

their firm or practice. Where one surgeon-apothecary referred to his 'extensive practice', another master added that the 'apprentice's opportunities of improvement will be great'. Thus typical surgeon-apothecaries' advertisements for apprentices would require 'one who has had a good education and can be well recommended' or 'a young man of good classical Education'. Only a minority of surgeon-apothecary masters included their name in such advertisements:

AN APPRENTICE wanted, by a SURGEON and APOTHE-CARY in good Business. A Youth, properly educated, may meet with a Situation, attended with peculiar Advantages. He will be treated as one of the Family. An adequate Premium will therefore be expected.[20]

Since the period of apprenticeship did not begin for most occupations, including that of surgeon-apothecary, until the age of fourteen, the problem of the child's education was not the master's but the parents' concern. Clearly educational levels and requirements varied enormously from the poorest crafts, through the prosperous trades to the professions, but no indenture normally specified that the apprentice would be taught anything more than the master's 'art and mystery', in the sense of craft rather than any secret of the trade. However, a literate and numerate apprentice in medicine was clearly essential, and in 1727 the Barber-Surgeons' Company required that 'apprentices shall be called in and examined by themselves touching their skill in ye Latin tongue'. As knowledge of Latin for their apprentices had been one of the Company's orders 170 years earlier, the need to reiterate it suggests that Latinity had been declining amongst entrants.[21] In 1747 Campbell considered that the way 'most likely to produce a good surgeon' was to instruct a boy for seven years after he had learned both Greek and Latin. The apprentice should begin his term at fifteen or sixteen and spend five years with 'an honest judicious Surgeon, who has a tolerable Share of Practice', followed by a year at Edinburgh (for anatomy and materia medica classes), as well as at Paris (for midwifery). Campbell's views on medical education in general, still a topical subject only two years after the Barbers and Surgeons had separated from each other, often bordered on the waspish:

A sordid Cramped Education proves a dead Weight upon the best Natural Genius on Earth, and produces but a bungling ignorant Quack; but if liberal, and attended with Natural Talents and due Application, there are none of the Liberal

20 *Aris's Birmingham Gazette,* 26 Jan. 1795.
21 Young, *Annals,* p. 354.

Arts more likely to procure a Livelihood than this. An ingenious Surgeon, let him be cast on any Corner of the Earth,
with but his Case of Instruments in his Pocket, he may live
where most other Professions would starve.[22]

Information about a surgeon's formal education is particularly difficult to obtain for the eighteenth century, although many boys were
undoubtedly pupils at the excellent local grammar schools that most
counties could boast, such as those founded by King Edward VI.
Thus in Birmingham, for example, a number of surgeons' sons were
pupils and held exhibitions at this period at the town's grammar
school before becoming medical apprentices. An early example of a
surgeon's formal education was that given to James Yonge, himself a
Plymouth surgeon's son, who, by the age of nine had 'learnt to read
and write well. My father placed me to the Latin School . . . where in
two years, I went through the forms of Cato. fables, and was newly
into Ovid.'[23] A far less prosperous boy, George Crabbe, was educated
at a dame school and then by 'a skilful mathematician', Richard Had-
don, at Stowmarket; even as a young child Crabbe was always a
voracious reader and had at least a basic grasp of Latin.[24]

As the master was in law and popular concept in loco parentis to his
apprentice, religious instruction was also necessary. Thus from the
sixteenth century onwards the candidate for Anglican confirmation
was required to have learned the catechism, for which 'Fathers,
Mothers, Masters and Dames' were to prepare their 'children, servants and apprentices'. By the eighteenth century, however, it was
necessary for Samuel Richardson to devote over a third of his Vade
Mecum, a tome of advice to apprentices, against 'the Scepticism and
Infidelity of the present Age', describing the 'Essential Principles' of
Christianity in detail for young apprentices to follow,[25] suggesting
that earlier standards were not being maintained and that boys new
to apprenticeship required such guidance. Apart from religious instruction, the actual indenture set out requirements of honesty, so-
briety and obedience for the apprentice towards his master and the
master's family.

Education was, of course, closely linked to the apprentice's own
social background; in the eighteenth century the surgeon-apothecary's origins are of considerable interest, and source material for this
aspect of apprenticeship is reasonably full and nearly always reliable.
Of the surgeon-apothecaries' and surgeons' apprentices listed in the

22 Campbell, Tradesman, p. 57.
23 James Yonge, p. 27.
24 George Crabbe, The Life of George Crabbe by his Son (London, 1947), p. 15.
25 Samuel Richardson, The Apprentice's Vade Mecum (London, 1734), p. 55.

London registers (1710–60), the names of boys and masters from four English counties (Surrey, Sussex, Warwickshire and Wiltshire) have been extracted. Even though the occupation or status of the surgeon-apothecaries' apprentices' fathers was not always stated, the size of the premiums alone indicates prosperity, although some of these must have been the ambitious parents condemned by Campbell, motivated by pride or avarice, anxious for social advancement, to suit their own 'notions of grandeur' rather than the child's aptitude.

In the aforementioned counties, a total of 11,138 apprenticeships was recorded in the half century between 1710 and 1760; of these, 124 referred to surgeon-apothecaries, who formed 1.11 per cent of all the apprentices registered. Of the 124 boys, 17 were fatherless (13.6 per cent), but with mothers prosperous enough to pay premiums ranging from 45 to 100 guineas; occasionally, however, money was bequeathed for an apprenticeship premium in a man's or woman's will. The others' fathers were described as gentlemen (seven), clerics (five), substantial traders (two maltsters, a currier, vintner and mercer) and other medical practitioners (a physician, an apothecary and a surgeon). There were also two fathers of apparently humble origins but nevertheless able to pay a £50 premium each, a blacksmith and a parkkeeper, but the terminology may disguise a large-scale metalworker and the agent of an estate. Just as the later seventeenth century had seen a tendency of gentry families, impoverished by the Civil War or the Restoration, to become 'the most zealous partisans of commerce' and put their sons to trade,[26] so in the eighteenth century youths entered law and medicine, as well as the nascent professions such as architecture. Attracting boys of good family as apprentices to medicine encouraged others to follow them and, freed from their ancient links with the barbers, eighteenth-century surgeon-apothecaries made noticeable social advances.

Apart from proscribing the apprentice's personal behaviour and listing the activities he was to avoid (gambling, women, the theatre) as well as the qualities he should cultivate (obedience, honesty and loyalty to his master) the indenture also specified his premium and term (the length of service as an apprentice). The premium is perhaps the best yardstick of occupational status, prosperity and esteem in the materialistic eighteenth century. A premium was paid by the apprentice's parents or guardian to cover the master's expense of keeping the child for seven years; it covered food, accommodation and tuition. Usually the premium also obliged the master to provide clothes, but in certain cases clothes and shoes were bought by the apprentice's

26   J. W. von Archenholz, *A Picture of England*, 2 vols. (London, 1791), II, p. 138.

family, so that, for example, three of James Yonge's apprentices were clothed by their parents rather than by Yonge. Although the eighteenth century was well beyond the medieval sumptuary laws, the prosperous apprentice, especially in London, who dressed ostentatiously beyond his rank was a constant annoyance to the more sober citizens of a community and was condemned by Richardson, for example, as 'Sir Fashioner'. Medical attention was also a rare provision in an apprenticeship indenture, either for the master or the parents to provide, but not mentioned in the surgeon-apothecary's apprentice's conditions since the master would automatically cover this just as the cordwainer provided his apprentice with a leather apron or shoes – his own products – free.

As well as covering the child's instruction, board and lodging, the premium also recompensed the master for the materials the apprentice might spoil or for the customers and clients he might offend, especially in the early years. The custom of paying a premium arose, according to Defoe, in the seventeenth century from the optional gift the child brought to his new master's wife, 'to take motherly care of him', and this was gradually converted to cash.[27] Writing in 1724 Defoe considered that in the 1660s and 1670s the highest premium ever paid to 'eminent Turkey merchants' in London was £200, very rarely £300, although by the 1720s they were accepting £1,000 with an apprentice.[28] The widespread use of premiums can be assessed by the introduction of the 1709 Stamp Act and the sale of printed indentures at law stationers with a space left blank for the premium to be inserted. Big premiums were increasingly expected by men who took 'new' boys as apprentices, to enter an occupation without the personal connections that might prove influential and profitable. Defoe noted the difficulties of controlling apprentices with large premiums; their masters were obliged to treat them as lucrative pupils, 'too high for reproof or correction' and unwilling to perform such humble tasks as opening the shop windows, delivering medicines or sweeping the premises.[29] High premiums of several hundred pounds, even in the provinces, were normal in trades dealing with valuable raw materials, in the fashion trades with a wealthy clientele and also in risk industries or those with substantial capital tied up in stock and plant. In all these categories a large premium enabled a child to enter a very profitable occupation for life and expect a 'genteel' existence.

In 1747 Campbell indicated a range of premiums for occupations in

27 Daniel Defoe, *The Complete English Tradesman*, 4th edn. (London, 1738), p. 127.
28 Daniel Defoe, *The Great Law of Subordination Consider'd* (London, 1724), pp. 10–11.
29 Daniel Defoe, *The Family Instructor*, 2 vols. (London, 1715), II, p. 261.

Table 3.1. *High premiums in London trades, 1747*

Range of premiums	Trades
£50 to £300	Banker, all kinds of merchants
£50 to £200	Brewer, mercer, scrivener, woollen draper
£50 to £100	Artist, coachmaker, conveyancer, coal factor, insurer, laceman, notary public, sugar baker, timber merchant, wool stapler
£30 to £100	Ironmonger, tobacconist
£20 to £200	Apothecary, attorney, hosier, jeweller
£20 to £100	Bookseller, box maker, butcher, calico printer, chaser, chemist, druggist, grocer, linen draper, silkman, surgeon
£20 to £50	Distiller, goldsmith, leather seller, mathematical and optical instrument maker, upholsterer
£10 to £50	Card maker

London as a guide to parents seeking a career for their children, and the amount of literature on apprenticeship at this period, particularly instructions to apprentices about personal behaviour, suggests that many potential readers required such guidance, whereas at an earlier period this advice would have been superfluous. For the surgeon in London Campbell noted a premium of between £20 and £100, a much wider range than for many other occupations, which placed the surgeon alongside other substantial traders but below the attorney, the apothecary and the city merchant[30] (Table 3.1). However, a master of repute could always attract considerably more than these sums, so that, for example, Caesar Hawkins took £200 with a Lancashire gentleman's son, William Hewitt, in 1736,[31] and William Cheselden received £150, £210 and £350 respectively with three apprentices in the years 1712–30.[32] At most periods premiums outside London fluctuated far less, especially before provincial hospitals were established. Thus in Surrey, Sussex, Warwickshire and Wiltshire premiums of £20 to 80 guineas were paid, with £60 or guineas (£63) the commonest sum of all (25.7 per cent) (Table 3.2).

Surgeon-apothecaries apprenticing their own sons, did not, of course, pay premiums, although an indenture was normally prepared as legal proof that a term had been served. A reduced premium

30 Campbell, *Tradesman*, pp. 331–40.
31 Cited in G. C. Peachey, *A Memoir of William and John Hunter* (Plymouth, 1924), p. 39.
32 Burnby, *Records*, p. 159.

Table 3.2. *Apprenticeship premiums*
to provincial surgeon-apothecaries,
1710–60

Premium (£)	Number recorded	Per centage
210	2	1.5
140–150	2	1.5
100–107	17	12.8
86–90	2	1.5
70–84	18	13.6
60–63	34	25.7
50–55	23	17.4
40–48	13	9.8
20–35	17	12.8
1–12	4	3.0

was usually paid for an apprentice bound to an uncle or other relative as well as for a shorter term, usually because a boy had been partly trained and transferred from another master. Thus Bradford Wilmer, a Coventry surgeon, took four apprentices in the years 1773–95; a man of local repute and large practice, his premiums increased considerably during two decades. With his first apprentice he received £130 for a seven-year term; with another boy in 1792 the premium was £120 for only three years (he was presumably assigned from another master), but with his last apprentice in 1795 Wilmer took 200 guineas (£210) for only a five-year term.[33] Although the inflation of the late eighteenth century accounts for a proportion of these increased premiums, the master's reputation and the standing of the medical profession as a whole were also vital factors. In contrast the century's earlier decades were relatively stable, so that premiums changed little and masters took similar sums with apprentices several years apart, often little different from their own premiums ten years earlier. In Sussex Thomas Frewen of Rye received £50 with each of his two apprentices, bound in 1743 and in 1749, and Richard Drinkwater of Chichester had £100 or guineas (£105) with each of his three apprentices in the years 1739, 1743, and 1749.[34] The relationship between the term and the premium may be seen in the two apprentices

33 P.R.O., I.R.1./58, 66, 67.
34 *Sussex Apprentices and their Masters, 1710–52,* ed. R. Garraway Rice (Sussex Record Society, XXVIII, 1922), pp. 13, 158, 121.

taken by John Smith of Chichester; with the first, Francis Tourner in 1721, he received £50 for three years and with the next boy, John Clark in 1725, the premium was double, £100 for seven years.[35] A further variation for a master, himself newly out of his time, was to take a smaller premium than his own had been, for the sake of the boy's labour and the value of some cash as capital to a newly established practice. Such a man was Henry Manning, an orphan in 1716 when bound with £100 premium to Richard Russell of Lewes for seven years. Out of his time by 1723 and practising in Lewes, in 1724 he indentured William Rickwood for seven years with a premium of only £60. In 1730, with John Mower, the son of a Cranleigh mercer, the premium had risen to 80 guineas (£84) for seven years.[36]

The provincial surgeon-apothecaries who took £100 or more with their apprentices are an interesting group, far removed from the rural practitioner described by George Crabbe, whose premium of a few guineas placed him on a level with other respectable tradesmen rather than with the attorney, merchant or manufacturer. The provincial surgeon-apothecaries who could attract substantial premiums had certain factors in common, but their places of practice seem crucial. Such men were likely to practise in an administrative or trading centre (Lewes, Birmingham, Coventry or Devizes), or be situated near the house of a great family (Petworth); cathedral cities always attracted men of substance as practitioners.

Practitioners in cathedral cities such as Salisbury were likely to find a hospital built in their community by the late eighteenth century, and the men in these cities with hospital appointments attracted the highest premiums of all outside London. Their established clientele, including the clergy, were substantial patients, as the physician Claver Morris had noted in Wells early in the eighteenth century.[37] Thus in Salisbury Edward Goldwire took 200 guineas (£210) in 1753 with John Sketchley for six years and again the same sum in 1759 with John Pearce for a year more. In the same city in 1753, 'Thos Tatum and Co.', presumably several practitioners in partnership, received £140 with James Ford, bound for six years.[38] The Salisbury Infirmary was built in 1767 and both Goldwire and Tatum held appointments there, important men at the head of a city's medical community. In 1760 Tatum sought an MD degree at St Andrew's, invited, he said, by 'the principal inhabitants of the Neighbourhood to practise Physic

35 Ibid., pp. 190, 40.
36 Ibid., pp. 120, 159, 133.
37 *The Diary of a West Country Physician, AD 1684–1726*, ed. Edmund Hobhouse (Rochester, 1934).
38 P.R.O., I.R.1./51, 53, 51.

only'.[39] In Birmingham the men who received the high premiums were to form the staff of the General Hospital when it opened in 1779. The apprentices of men with hospital appointments were frequently able to benefit from their former masters' patronage in securing posts in hospitals, dispensaries and practices, which later critics considered an obvious abuse of the apprenticeship system but of which such eminent men as Sir George Brodie openly boasted. Not all parents, however, were prepared to accept a large premium, so that, for example, when in 1692 James Yonge proposed placing his son with George Horsnel, 'an eminent surgeon in Hatton Garden', he did not proceed with the apprenticeship because he considered the 'price would be too high'.[40] The premium was presumably well over £100, since he himself took sums of up to £90 with his apprentices in Plymouth.

The other aspect of apprenticeship, the term, was always stated even when the premium was not recorded. It varied very little; 'seven long years' was normal and traditional for most occupations throughout the eighteenth century, irrespective of the skill involved and including that of the surgeon-apothecary. Of all aspects of apprenticeship it was the one to which supporters of the system clung most tenaciously, citing custom, practice and usage of great antiquity whenever proposals for change were made. Of the surgeon-apothecary's apprentices in Surrey, Sussex, Warwickshire and Wiltshire, the seven-year term predominated (Table 3.3).

The surgeon-apothecary's apprentice was likely to be fourteen years old when beginning his term, and Campbell commented tartly that children indentured younger than this were bound 'more for the Advantage of the Master than any thing they can learn of the Trade in such infant years'.[41] The importance of the seven-year term may be seen in the number of by-laws enacted by the ancient trading companies in its support. The value of the term to the master was that he was sure of the apprentice's unpaid service for a number of years, and in the last part of his term the apprentice was a source of profit to his master, capable of most work unsupervised. The injured tone of advertisements placed in the press by masters whose apprentices had absconded in their last year indicates how valuable their labour was. A major disadvantage of the term was that, should a master's circumstances decline and he wished to give up his trade or be rid of the expense of keeping the apprentice, he could not do so except by absconding himself or by brutalising the child into becoming a

39 Roll of St Andrew's graduates, testimonials, 1746–60.
40 *James Yonge*, p. 204.
41 Campbell, *Tradesman*, p. 260.

Table 3.3. *Apprenticeship terms*
to provincial surgeon-apothecaries,
1710–60

Term in years	Percentage of apprentices
8	2.5
7	64.7
6	7.6
5	12.6
4	4.2
3	1.6
2	.8
Record faulty	5.8

runaway. However, in the prosperous occupations, such as that of the surgeon-apothecary, absconding masters and apprentices were few indeed. The importance of having served a term with a master of repute can hardly be overestimated and is illustrated in the number of surgeon-apothecaries advertising their services in local newspapers who state the name of the man to whom they had been bound. At the end of his term the apprentice usually celebrated, although surgeon-apothecaries do not appear to have had the complex rituals of 'coming out' associated with many traditional skills, for example the printers or the coopers. Parson Woodforde recalled how he 'danced the whole night and part of the morning till 4 o'clock on account of Mr Jas Clarke's apprenticeship being expired'. They had a 'very good band' and 'a great deal of company';[42] in 1783, sixteen years later, James Clarke was still practising in Ansford, Somerset.

The distance an apprentice travelled to find a master varied greatly in different occupations and decades, but evidence suggests that the most and least prosperous children travelled furthest from home. Thus, although the majority of apprentices travelled only twenty-five or thirty miles to find a master, those bound to surgeon-apothecaries journeyed considerably further. Obviously, parental participation was essential in the expense and trouble of sending a child far from home. Even though surgeon-apothecaries' apprentices were literate, poor transport and communications meant that contact with home and family during their apprenticeship was for many boys minimal.

42 *The Diary of a Country Parson: The Rev. James Woodforde, 1758–1802*, ed. John Beresford (Oxford, 1978), p. 40.

Of the fifteen Surrey boys bound to surgeon-apothecaries five remained within the county, two left it for Kent and Sussex respectively
and six boys were apprenticed from Cambridgeshire, Denbighshire,
Hampshire, Lancashire, Middlesex and Norfolk; two boys' homes
were not recorded. Of the fifty-nine apprentices for Sussex (1710–60),
twenty (33.8 per cent) remained in the county, one boy from Lydd
(Kent) went to a master in Rye and eleven boys (18.6 per cent) left
Sussex to find masters in Kent (three to Sevenoaks, one to Cranbrook
and one to Tenterden), Hampshire (two to Eastbourne), Middlesex
(Holbourne and Westminster) and Surrey (Farnham and Southwark);
the homes of twenty-seven boys were not recorded. Later in the
century, of the twelve boys bound to Coventry surgeon-apothecaries
(1781–1806) six came from the city (two of whom served their own
fathers), two came from other Warwickshire towns (Birmingham and
Bedworth) and four came from adjacent counties (Gloucestershire,
Leicestershire and Northamptonshire); the home of one boy was not
given.[43] Living in the master's house and lacking contact with his
parents was an important aspect of apprenticeship for the child, who
was likely to be more malleable and obedient when dependent on the
master's daily goodwill.

Having found a master, signed an indenture, paid a premium and
travelled to a master's home, the apprentice began his seven years of
technical training, about which relatively little first-hand information
can be discerned. Letters and diaries kept by adolescents have survived only rarely or, because of low literacy, long hours and lack of
privacy, were never kept at all. Even the occasional apprentice who
did so (for example John Coggs, indentured to a London printer early
in the eighteenth century) used code and shorthand for fear of others
reading his diary. Much more is known about the apprenticeships of
less prosperous children, although written by outsiders, for their
lives were occasionally described in some detail when, abused or
neglected, the child died and criminal proceedings resulted. Although the personal apprenticeship experiences of most surgeon-
apothecaries will never be known, a small number wrote diaries,
memoirs, poetry and letters describing aspects of their apprenticeship, usually in a critical, even hostile, way.

One of the indenture's main conditions was that the master should
teach and instruct the apprentice in 'the same Art which he now
useth, by the best means that he can'. In the early part of his term,
especially if senior apprentices were kept, the newcomer was ex-

43 *Coventry Apprentices and their Masters, 1781–1806*, ed. Joan Lane (Dugdale
Society, XXXIII, 1983).

pected to undertake such menial tasks as cleaning the master's equipment, preparing the work-space, sweeping the floor, trimming the lamps and opening the windows and shutters. Delivering goods and running errands were generally resented by the prosperous apprentice, as were all similar tasks he presumably had never done at home; boys appear to have particularly objected to menial domestic work normally done by household servants. As late as 1834 the Select Committee on Medical Education heard how the duties of a surgeon-apothecary's apprentice were to answer the door, receive messages and make up medicines. In all occupations, the most disagreeable and repetitive jobs were always given to the apprentice, and the prospective surgeon-apothecary was no exception. Thus James Yonge, apprenticed to a ship's surgeon, outlined his first duties as 'slavery . . . but such as usually chyrurgeon's mates were obliged to perform in the navy: For boiling gruel, barley water fomentations, washing rollers, and making lint, spreading plaisters and fitting the dresses, was wholly on my hands, besides often emptying the buckets they went to stool in, a nasty and mean employment.'[44] Although masters rationalised such treatment of apprentices as the only means of ensuring that they knew their occupation in all respects and could therefore supervise others in the future, it is obvious that much of the philosophy of apprenticeship was to subdue the new entrant by humiliation, hence the significance of initiation ceremonies. The novice then might slowly be accepted by his fellow workers and finally come to enjoy all the privileges of craft brotherhood, including the right to humiliate newcomers.

As an indication of the tasks the apprentice might perform, the hero of *Roderick Random*, by Tobias Smollett (1721–71), who had himself served a surgeon's apprenticeship, assured his would-be master, Launcelot Crab, that his skills included being able to 'bleed and give a clyster, spread a plaister and prepare a potion'.[45] One Bolton practitioner's apprentice set out in great detail the tasks he performed, and detested, in the first six months of his term:

> I studied hard; learned the Linnean names and doses of drugs; attended seven surgical operations; worked from nine to nine daily, Sundays included; made mercury ointment in the old style by turning a pestle in a mortar for three days in succession, to amalgamate the quicksilver with the pig's grease; made up what the doctor called his 'Cathartic acid bitter mixture', as a sort of fill-up for every purgative bottle,

44 *James Yonge*, p. 42.
45 Tobias Smollett, *Roderick Random* (London, 1979), p. 27.

and almost every disease that 'flesh is heir to'; made up
boluses of a teaspoonful of preserve with half-a-grain of
opium, as a sedative; drew a tooth for 6d; and took 4d if the
sufferer had no more; and did many things during that six
months which gave me a distaste for the practice of medicine,
and made me desirous of other employment.[46]
His wish was granted, and he left his apprenticeship in medicine for
the law, but his early training must have been of use in the office of
coroner he subsequently held.

At the beginning of the nineteenth century another provincial apprentice surgeon's tasks were to roll pills and paint bottles in the
dispensary before 'progressing to tooth extraction'.[47] Watching post-
mortem examinations was also part of the surgeon's training; Barclay
Fox, a West Country Quaker diarist, described such an examination
of a family pet, a dog suspected of having rabies. Fox noted in his
journal that 'the two apprentices, Dr Fox and Surgeon Williamson &
self were in attendance', but fortunately the animal showed no signs
of hydrophobia.[48]

Even in a rising profession, there remained humble and relatively
poor practitioners whose apprentices paid smaller premiums and
who could expect their status in the community to remain equal with
the upper craftsmen likely to be their patients, rather than any fashionable clientele. Symbolic of such men, George Crabbe wrote
movingly of his experiences as a village surgeon in an unprosperous
parish in the later eighteenth century. Even allowing for poetic li-
cence, his descriptions of the life of the labouring poor, the village
midwife and the parish surgeon depict a society of desperate poverty.
His more lurid accounts, however, are not entirely supported by an
examination of local records for the period. The details of his life are
of considerable interest; Crabbe was indentured to Mr Smith at Wick-
hambrook (Suffolk) in 1768 at the age of fourteen. His premium is not
recorded, but it cannot have been large as his father held the ill-paid
post of collector of salt duties. Crabbe was obliged to help his master
on the farm and became 'the bedfellow and companion' of the
plough-boy, whom he envied because the lad was hired by the year
whereas Crabbe had to serve out his seven-year apprenticeship. During his time with Smith, he delivered medicines on foot to Cheveley,
some seven miles away. His leisure time was spent 'reading ro-
mances' and with his fellow adolescents, mostly farm boys, with

46 John Taylor, *The Autobiography of a Lancashire Lawyer* (Bolton, 1883), p. 22.
47 V. Mary Crosse, *A Surgeon in the Early Nineteenth Century: The Life and Times of John Green Crosse* (Edinburgh, 1968), pp. 14–15.
48 *Barclay Fox's Journal*, ed. R. L. Brett (London, 1977), p. 94.

whom he once watched a travelling conjuror perform. He did, however, learn to bleed from Mr Smith, before returning to the family home at Aldeburgh. In 1772 he was reindentured to John Page, surgeon-apothecary at Woodbridge, one of the four practitioners listed there in 1783. With his second master Crabbe experienced more enlightened treatment; he joined a local supper and discussion club and, aged eighteen, had time to begin writing, including his poem, 'Inebriety', based on his observations of life in rural Suffolk. He also developed an interest in botany, characteristic of many eighteenth-century practitioners, that was to last all his life.[49]

As apprenticeship was essentially a practical training, the pupil normally watched and listened and, when possible, accompanied his master. Thus one Nottinghamshire parish surgeon took his nineteen-year-old apprentice with him 'on his rounds to the poor and Poor House to visit the sick'. This particular apprentice, Henry Jephson, wrote home in delight:

> I can with just pleasure add that he behaved like a Gent and has promised to let me visit them alone. I assure you it has happened exactly right in my last year, as I can visit them more than I did before, indeed he advised me to pay attention to the various diseases I see, and you may depend upon my taking it.[50]

There is no suggestion that the practitioner encouraged his apprentice to be equally attentive to his non-poor patients in the area. However, even a physician as eminent as John Coakley Lettsom began his career as an apprentice and in the 1760s recalled how he took charge of the practice and visited patients 'often . . . when [his] master was out of town or engaged in midwifery'. He was refreshingly honest about his own incompetence, 'never having heard a lecture or seen any anatomical figure, except a skeleton'.[51]

The most detailed account of a surgeon-apothecary's life at this period is that of Richard Kay, indentured to his father, a surgeon at Baldingstone, near Bury (Lancashire).[52] It is also one of the rare written accounts that is not extremely critical of the training and treatment the apprentice received, which is not surprising, since Kay regularly handed his diary to his parents to read. Most diarists appear to wish to unburden themselves of resentment, even of a sense of in-

49   Crabbe, *Life*, p. 26.
50   Warwick County Record Office (W.C.R.O.), Z 574.
51   Cited in Arthur Raistrick, *Quakers in Science and Industry* (Newton Abbot, 1968), p. 279.
52   *The Diary of Richard Kay of Baldingstone, near Bury, 1716–51*, ed. W. Brockbank and F. Kenworthy (Chetham Society, 1968).

justice, in their writings, but Richard Kay seems, after more than two centuries, to have been enthralled with medicine as a career, anxious to do well, a highly motivated apprentice any master would have been pleased to teach. Apart from his father's instruction, Kay also went, towards the end of his term, to hear public scientific lectures on mathematics, optics and geography that were held locally. He was able to attend exclusively medical lectures and watch operations in Lancashire while still an apprentice, the kind of demonstrations commonly held in London and Oxford in the first half of the eighteenth century but thought to have been a very rare occurrence elsewhere. Thus, on 18 March 1742 he went to Manchester, his expenses defrayed by his cousin, a local physician, to an 'anatomical Lecture which represented a Woman big with Child, with several other Anatomical Preparations'. A month later he travelled to Bury and was 'something of an assistant while Mr Richard Holt a young Surgeon from Hallifax in Yorkshire amputated or took off a young Woman's Leg from that Countrey'. In June 1742 he watched several operations performed in Manchester by 'the famous occulist', Dr Taylor from London, and a year later he attended a lecture, also in Manchester, where 'they have dissected an Eye and lectured to us upon it'. Later, when Kay had returned to practise in Lancashire after his year's training in London, he himself was watched by his father, brother, the local schoolmaster, two clerics and 'Mr Nightingale', who was apprenticed to a Bolton surgeon-apothecary named Clough, when he (Kay) amputated a woman's leg.[53] Such exchanges clearly broadened the range of cases that any one master might show his own apprentice, although they were, of course, never to equal the variety offered in a medical school.

When nearly qualified, Kay, like Lettsom, often attended patients in the surgery while his master undertook domiciliary visits, frequently many miles from home. In 1737, at the age of twenty-one, Kay noted that he had attended many 'different Kinds of Disorders . . . wounds, Bruises, and Broken Bones' as well as 'difficult Parts of Chirurgery'. He occasionally listed all the cases he had seen on one day and they indicate the wide range of skills the provincial surgeon-apothecary required in the middle decades of the century. Kay's father always expected an account of his son's activities when he returned from his round and commented on the young man's treatments and advice. When his father was absent, Kay also spent time 'in his Closet, [and] endeavoured to get better Knowledge in his

Drugs', piously adding the prayer, 'Lord, give me a Genius for the study of Medicine'. Even the newly qualified man could make potentially fatal errors; Kay recorded his distress at prescribing too large a dose of calomel, for which his father 'blamed [him] very much', adding, 'I am no little uneasy about it, but I hope it will be a Means to make me very careful for the future.'[54] The patient's response was not recorded. Although his apprenticeship left him little leisure time in Lancashire, Richard Kay helped with the harvest, joined in hare coursing, worked in the family garden, attended the theatre (at Whitehaven) and watched the Jacobites march in 1745. His social life in London was far fuller.

A seven-year term was all the training most surgeon-apothecaries ever had to cover a very wide range of medical tasks. However, other means of expanding their medical education were available, both abroad and in Britain, and during Hunter's lifetime further training opportunities increased enormously. Although substantial sources exist for the study of apprenticeship it has been relatively ignored while, paradoxically, post-apprenticeship medical training, often noticeably short of source material, has occupied medical historians' interest for decades. However, apprenticeship was compulsory, whereas later training remained entirely voluntary and, by its expense, available only to young men from prosperous families. At the end of the term the English surgeon-apothecary could, in both London and the provinces, be taught by the mid-eighteenth century in hospitals by eminent practitioners, attend courses of lectures and demonstrations and enter private medical schools, as well as join the increasing numbers of medical and scientific societies that were being formed.

As several researchers have shown, even in the decades before William Hunter was born, eminent surgeons gave lectures and demonstrations, especially in London, often open to the general public as well as to medical practitioners. In 1692, for example, when James Yonge was visiting London to indenture his son, he attended a 'publique dissection at the Surgeons' Hall 3 days, where I heard Dr Tyson read'.[55] However, with twenty-six new English civilian provincial hospitals founded in Hunter's lifetime (Table 3.4), many more training facilities were available for post-apprenticeship instruction. London, by 1783, was exceptionally well provided with hospital and dispensary appointments for all categories of practitioners and many

54 Ibid., pp. 16, 22, 38.
55 *James Yonge*, p. 204.

Table 3.4. Provincial medical practitioners in England in 1783

County	Surgeon-apothecaries	Physicians	Surgeons only	Apothecaries only
Bedfordshire	17	2		
Berkshire	44	11(2)[b]	1	
Buckinghamshire	27	3		
Cambridgeshire[a]	20	3	4	
Cheshire[a]	48	5	5	1
Cornwall	71	6		
Cumberland	60	11 (1)[b]		
Derbyshire	35	6		
Devonshire[a]	117	11	8 (1)[b]	17
Dorset	59	9	1	
Durham	52	8		
Essex	112	13 (1)[b]		
Gloucestershire[a]	60	6	2	
Hampshire[a]	86	6		
Herefordshire[a]	33	5	3	1
Hertfordshire	37	7		
Huntingdonshire	17	4		
Kent	161 (1)[b]	12 (1)[b]		
Lancashire[a]	102	26	14 (1)[b]	6
Leicestershire[a]	43	6		
Lincolnshire[a]	94	18	1	2

Middlesex	68	3		1
Norfolk[a]	129	14	1	1
Northamptonshire[a]	46	9	1	
Northumberland[a]	66	13		2
Nottinghamshire[a]	38	5		
Oxfordshire[a]	54	9	4	1
Rutland	5	1		
Shropshire[a]	84	4		1
Somerset[a]	93	29	18	53 [+ 2 men-midwives]
Staffordshire[a]	70	7		1
Suffolk	70 (1)[b]	10	2	
Surrey	63	8		
Sussex	81	5	3	3
Warwickshire[a]	54	9	10	4
Westmorland	13	2		
Wiltshire[a]	78	9	3	1
Worcestershire[a]	67	5		
Yorkshire[a]	233	42	8	11
Totals	2,607	363	89	105 [+ 2]
Percentage	82.3	11.4	2.8	3.3

[a] Hospital being built or in existence in 1783 (two in the case of Lancashire and three each in Somerset and Yorkshire).

[b] Retired practitioner(s) included in total.

Source: The Medical Register, 1783.

apprenticeship opportunities with the 600 apothecaries and 220 surgeons practising in the city at this time.[56] One of the hospital surgeon's privileges was to take apprentices and pupils, in a personal
capacity, and few men did not do so, for the young men's fees were
often considerable and a useful source of income in a lump sum to
men holding honorary posts. Pupils, however, were a different category from the traditional apprentices, for they received instruction
from the eminent hospital surgeon after their adolescent apprenticeship had been served, but gained experience by watching and
assisting in a hospital, a distinction noted by Sir Astley Cooper.
Cooper set out a scale of fees for the different categories of young
men to be taught in a hospital. The apprentice, who should lodge and
board in the surgeon's house, would pay between £500 and £600 for
the six- or seven-year term, but only £300 or £400 if he were not
boarded. The 'perpetual' pupil paid £26 5s. for twelve months,
whereas the dresser paid £50 for a year's instruction, for which he
was also allowed to 'dress' the master's patients in hospital.[57] Sir
Anthony Carlisle recalled, in 1834, that he had had only one apprentice personally, who had served five years, boarded in the family
home and had a premium of 300 guineas (£315); Carlisle had himself
been apprenticed in 1784 to a surgeon at Durham and therefore presumably understood how the system worked in the later eighteenth
century.[58]

Generally, the more senior the surgeon in a hospital, the more
apprentices he was permitted to take, but that the considerable fees
involved could cause professional dissent and disharmony may be
seen from John Hunter's quarrels with his colleagues and the governors of St George's hospital in the 1790s.[59] Other eminent London
surgeons with hospital appointments also took apprentices and
pupils, of whom, fortunately for historians, Richard Kay was one, for
he described his training in London during twelve months in 1743–4
in considerable detail.[60] It was Kay's father who first suggested he
should go to London at the end of his apprenticeship 'to spend some
time for my Improvement in the Hospitals there'. Although his absence would be inconvenient to 'the Business and Concerns of the
Family' his parents were willing to 'deny themselves' that he might
go. His cousin, a Manchester physician, made the arrangements,

56 See W. F. Bynum, chap. 4, this volume.
57 Select Committee on the Education and Practice of the Medical Profession in the
United Kingdom (hereafter S.C.M.E.), Parliamentary Papers 1834 (XIII), pp. 96–7.
58 Ibid., pp. 148, 150.
59 Discussed by Toby Gelfand, chap. 5, this volume.
60 *Kay, Diary*, pp. 66–89.

writing to Benjamin Steade, apothecary to Guy's Hospital, to secure Richard Kay's entry. Steade, one of whose duties was the supervision of pupils, replied that he had a vacancy in June 1743, and required a master's certificate before training began. When Dr Kay was tardy in replying, Steade wrote to remind him that he was keeping another 'young Gentleman in Suspense'. The tuition fee was paid by Dr Kay in advance to Steade. Richard Kay left Lancashire on 1 August 1743 to spend a year in London where he was taught by John Girle, William Smellie, Thomas Baker, John Belchier and Samuel Sharp, whose lectures William Hunter had attended three years earlier. Kay also benefited from Mr Steade's overall direction of his studies and his personal companionship.

From Kay's diary it is possible to reconstruct how he spent his time as a pupil. The theoretical part of his training consisted of lectures by Sharp and Girle (analysed in Appendix 2); he also attended Surgeons' Hall to hear four lectures, including two on 'dead bodies', in February 1744. As practical training he watched operations in the hospital, not all of which he named; these obviously impressed him greatly and included various amputations (one of which was a thigh), two operations for the stone and one for hare-lip. His training was even busier from 7 May 1744, when he began Smellie's first midwifery course. Between 7 May and 14 July, as well as two more lectures from Sharp and two from Girle, Kay attended seventeen lectures by Smellie, divided into two courses, the second of which began on 27 June, chiefly comprising evening lectures. On 3 July he 'attended a Birth with Mr Smelly [sic]', piously adding in his diary, 'Lord, Thou knowest what thou art designing to do with me in Life, qualify me for it, and then mercifully call me forth unto it.' A week later, on 12 July, he noted, 'This Last Night I attended a poor Woman in Labour, she was deliver'd this morning about 11 o'th'clock.' On the next night Kay again 'attended a Poor Woman in Labour', but Smellie himself delivered her at 11 p.m., 'it being proeternatural', but accompanied on this occasion by Benjamin Steade. A fortnight later Smellie 'sent' for Kay to deliver yet another poor patient, the last labour of the four he attended in London. Although so much of his time was spent on midwifery training, Kay attended a further handful of lectures by Girle and Sharp in August before being given his attendance certificate signed by Sharp.

While training in London, Kay made the acquaintance of other young men intended for a medical career and shared his social life quite extensively with Benjamin Steade (five breakfasts, four evenings, including Kay's twenty-eighth birthday, two dinners, one supper, a sermon and two visits to the theatre). He also enjoyed the city's free sights, visiting Bedlam twice, St James's Palace, the Old Bailey and the Tower, as well as watching an execution, the Lord Mayor's Show and Commodore Anson's treasure wagons pass through London. A regular worshipper, he usually sought out fine preachers to hear on Sundays.

One aspect of training, the financial cost of being a London medical student at this period, is little recorded, except for apprenticeship premiums and pupil fees. However, in 1812 a Yorkshire diarist accidentally provided some information on this aspect of medical training while intending to comment on the longevity of the practitioner and on inflation: 'Mr Dawson (of Sedburgh) now 75 . . . went to London to study Medicine, he lived at the rate of 8d per day; . . . he took £60 with him which maintained him for one year and a half, paying for lodging, attending lectures, ec.'[61] The practitioner who lived so frugally was John Dawson, born in 1737, presumably apprenticed to a surgeon-apothecary in about 1751 and therefore training in London in about 1758. Dawson was listed in the 1783 *Medical Register* in practice at Sedburgh and this contemporary estimate of the cost of a London medical training is at least a useful yardstick. For the really poor young man, however, anxious to receive London training, prospects were difficult and again George Crabbe may be symbolic. After finishing his apprenticeship term in 1775, he practised briefly at Aldburgh, where

> . . . having some conscientious scruples [he] began to study also: [he] read much, collected extracts and translated Latin books of physic with a view of double improvement: [he] studied the *materia medica* and made some progress in botany. [He] dissected dogs and fancied [himself] an anatomist, quitting entirely poetry, novels and books of entertainment.

After a year, with enough money saved, he went to London, to 'pick up a little surgical knowledge as cheaply as he could'. He lived economically in lodgings with a wig-maker; when desperate for cash he pawned his surgical instruments for 8s., noting, 'It's the vilest thing in the world to have but one coat.'[62] Although he attended lectures and was even suspected of body-snatching, most of Crabbe's energies seem to have been devoted to literature rather than medicine and to the search for patronage, in which he was finally successful, enabling him to leave medical practice for the church.

Not all former apprentices could aspire immediately to be taught by

61 *The Diaries and Correspondence of James Losh, 1811–23*, ed. Edward Hughes (Surtees Society, 171, 1956), I, p. 17.
62 Crabbe, *Life*, pp. 57–8.

leading practitioners for large fees. In the early nineteenth century the newly qualified Henry Jephson, apprenticed in Nottinghamshire, wrote to his brother that, on finishing his apprenticeship, he thought his 'seeming inexperience' would be overcome by having trained further in London, where he hoped to meet distinguished practitioners. After he had spent some years in practice in Warwickshire, he was able to be taught by MacMichael and Brodie in London before going to Glasgow for a year to obtain his MD and eventually becoming a leading physician in Leamington Spa.[63]

However, although London hospitals had the majority of pupils in the early eighteenth century, after about 1740, with more provincial infirmaries opening every decade, post-apprenticeship training and hospital apprenticeships for surgeon-apothecaries became available outside the capital. The 1740s were the decade when most such foundations (seven) opened, both to serve large communities and in county towns (Bath, Exeter, Liverpool, Northampton, Shrewsbury, Worcester and York). In many of these eighteenth-century foundations local surgeon-apothecaries played an important part, raising funds, donating money themselves, serving on the management committee and holding honorary appointments, as well as taking apprentices and pupils. Liverpool Infirmary, established in 1749, is typical, with James Bromfield, a local surgeon, contributing £32 6s, to the building fund, one of its largest donations, as well as giving an annual subscription of two guineas. He was also involved in helping the trustees to secure a site for the infirmary. He was elected senior surgeon when the hospital opened, a post he held until 1763, the year before his death. As he already had a substantial local reputation and practice, he was able to influence his wealthy patients, such as the Blundell family of Little Crosby Hall, to support the hospital. He and the two other surgeons at Liverpool, Thomas Antrobus and William Pickering, were allowed two pupils each at the infirmary and could keep the tuition fees.[64]

In the same decade (1743), Northampton General Hospital was founded, modelled in some respects on the Winchester Infirmary, but the medical initiative there came from Dr James Stonhouse, a midland physician of repute. With this, as with many other charitable ventures, an unedifying quarrel between the participants marred its establishment. The first surgeons there were Charles Lyon and Edward Litchfield; Lyon's apprentice and pupils were to be permitted to at-

63   E. G. Baxter, *Dr Jephson of Leamington Spa* (Warwick, 1980), pp. 6–7.
64   George McLoughlin, *A Short History of the First Liverpool Infirmary, 1749–1824* (Chichester, 1978), pp. 13–4, 36–7.

tend the hospital and see patients' dressings changed. They were also
to watch and assist at operations, an arrangement to which Litchfield,
in 1764, objected, according to the terse hospital committee
minutes.[65]

At other midland infirmaries, where there had been similar medical
participation in founding the institution, different restrictions were
applied to pupils and apprentices. At Hereford General Hospital,
founded in 1776, each surgeon was allowed two pupils at any time,
for which he was to receive a 'satisfactory gratuity for their instruction'; neither pupil nor apprentice might perform an operation, but
had 'liberty to dress a patient under the direction of his master'.[66] At
Birmingham, established three years later, the statutes allowed each
surgeon three pupils 'to attend the hospital for instructions, but no
pupil or apprentice [was to] be permitted to perform any operation'.[67]
Occasionally a pupil found himself unavoidably carrying out his master's duties if the surgeon were unavailable. At the London Hospital,
one of George Harrison's pupils, named Wood, was obliged to set a
compound fracture when Harrison was out of London visiting a patient. Wood had served his apprenticeship and had spent almost a
year at the hospital; although the patient died, Wood was exonerated
and Harrison criticised, perhaps because he was already under attack
by a faction within the newly founded hospital.[68]

As a reflection of the increased demand for medical training, towards the end of the eighteenth century some hospitals insisted that
no pupil would be admitted unless he had already served a satisfactory apprenticeship. At Manchester Infirmary by 1790 the apprenticeship premium was 100 guineas (£105), but additional restrictions
were applied to exclude the unsuitable applicant. Thus at Manchester
the apprentice was obliged to apply two months in advance of beginning his term so that 'enquiries' might be made about his character,
and if reports were favourable, he would be taken on three months'
trial. In addition to an interesting change in the operation of apprenticeship as an institution, these conditions also suggest that medical
apprentices were no longer personally known to their intended mas-

65   F. F. Waddy, *A History of Northampton General Hospital, 1743–1948*
(Northampton, 1974), pp. 19–20.
66   A. W. Langford, 'The History of Hereford General Hospital', *Woolhope Natu-
ralists' Field Club Transactions*, XXVIII (1959), pp. 149–60.
67   *The Statutes and Rules for the Government of the General Hospital, near Birmingham*
(Birmingham, 1779), p. 16.
68   A. E. Clark-Kennedy, *London Pride, the Story of a London Voluntary Hospital*
(London, 1979), pp. 48–9.

ter and that the original network of influence and family in arranging apprenticeships was considerably weakened by this period.[69]

The contemporary charitable impulse to build hospitals in eighteenth-century England incidentally provided unprecedented and expanded opportunities for medical training, especially in the provinces. When Addenbrooke's Hospital was opened in Cambridge in 1771, Dr Samuel Hallifax, later bishop of Gloucester, commented that charitable hospitals might deflect contemporary criticisms against English universities, where only theoretical medical instruction was given, obliging many young men to seek training outside England.[70] This view was endorsed in a sermon on behalf of the Shrewsbury Infirmary in 1777, when the Reverend Dr William Adams declared that charitable hospitals were 'now considered the best schools in physic and surgery, attendance at which is reckoned as the finishing part of the doctor's education which crowns the rest'.[71] For all the later criticisms of eighteenth-century hospitals as 'gateways to death', foreign visitors viewed and commented favourably on the movement, even if erroneously in some details: 'A great number of hospitals, which are the *ne plus ultra* of that kind of establishments, by their order, their arrangement, and their cleanliness, are open to the sick of all nations and religions, whom they entertain by means of annual subscriptions.'[72] Prosperous young men who sought further training in the European medical schools were primarily physicians. James Yonge's son, for example, was to have gone to Leiden for training until it was discovered that he had secretly married and Yonge was obliged to change his plans for his son.[73] Certain European medical schools were also an obvious choice for young Roman Catholic practitioners, newly out of their term. Thus, as late as 1830, Henry Peart, later to practise in Worcestershire, spent three months in Paris, where he attended lectures and dissections, having already taken part in two winter courses in London medical schools.[74]

Attending dissections formed an important part of pupil and apprentice training, although the difficulty of securing corpses was noted by one foreign visitor in the late eighteenth century.

69 E. M. Brockbank, *The Foundation of Provincial Medical Education in England* (Manchester, 1936), p. 58.
70 S. Hallifax, *A Sermon for the Governors of Addenbrooke's Hospital* (Cambridge, 1771); see also Keel, chap. 8, this volume.
71 W. Adams, *Sermons and Tracts* (Shrewsbury, 1777).
72 Archenholz, *Picture*, II, p. 75.
73 *James Yonge*, p. 204.
74 W.C.R.O. CR 1840.

The aversion of the English to anatomical dissections, is another of the prejudices which characterize that nation. The surgeons have great difficulty in procuring dead bodies; they are obliged to pay large sums for them, and are forced to carry them to their houses with utmost secrecy. If the people hear of it, they assemble in crowds around the house, and break the windows.

What greatly augments the general aversion to so useful a science, is, that the sextons are oftentimes induced, by the certainty of a reward, to dig up corpses from the church-yards.[75]

Other apprenticeship experiences in dissection were recalled in the early nineteenth century by Joseph Hodgson, the first provincial surgeon to become president of the Royal College of Surgeons, who, with his friend, James Russell, both apprentices in Birmingham, practised dissection and injection on 'pieces' that Russell's master, the surgeon John Blount, brought them from the workhouse, where he held an appointment. To extend their social life and education, they formed a 'little society' that met in the house of Hodgson's master, John Freer, a surgeon at Birmingham Hospital, and at which they read papers to each other.[76]

Occasionally, condemned criminals sold their own bodies for dissection, as did one James Brooke, who made this offer in 1736, writing to Edward Goldwire at Salisbury as 'the only surgeon in this city or county that anatomises men'.[77] Provincial newspapers often announced dissections to be held in a local practitioner's house. The difficulty of securing corpses was an original and inventive excuse for an attempted robbery at the house of William Hunter shortly after his death, reported on the front page of at least one provincial news-paper:

During the thunder-storm on Sunday night, four or five men came to the house of the late Dr Hunter, in Windmill street, seemingly labouring under a heavy load; they told the house-keeper they had brought a corpse according to order, and desired admittance. The maid told them she had no orders about it from her master, and she should not open the doors at that time. They pressed hard to have the door opened, but in vain. They swore than they must throw it into the area. This making no impression on the resolution of the servant,

75 Archenholz, *Picture*, II, pp. 154–5.
76 R. E. Franklin, 'Medical Education and the Rise of the General Practitioner, 1760–1860' (PhD thesis, University of Birmingham, 1950), pp. 67–8.
77 Cited in Peachey, *Memoir*, pp. 42–3.

they at last threw down their load, which lay there for some time; but by and by, when the watchman came to examine the body, the dead man took to his heels.[78]

Apart from dissection, theoretical instruction was available for the surgeon-apothecary after finishing an apprenticeship at various private medical schools, by attending short lecture courses or even by membership of the increasing numbers of medical and scientific societies that were founded in the eighteenth century. London, of course, was well provided with medical lectures. In the year of Hunter's death the *Medical Register* could publish a list of eleven topics available in the metropolis, many given by extremely eminent men (physic and materia medica, clinical paediatrics, animation, chemistry, natural history, anatomy, midwifery, surgery, dentistry and natural philosophy).[79] The growing number of dispensaries by the later eighteenth century were, as Sir Zachary Cope has shown, to play a significant part in practical medical training.[80]

Less famous teachers also ran private lecture courses, for example Thomas Tomlinson at Birmingham in the 1760s or Edward Grairiger (1797–1824), who epitomised the expansionist outlook of contemporary medicine. Although Tomlinson is a fairly shadowy figure in the eighteenth century and of only local influence, he saw the importance of provincial medical education and had himself a wide clinical experience in practice, at the workhouse infirmary and in the Birmingham Hospital. He had been workhouse surgeon for nine years when he published his *Medical Miscellany*,[81] which went into a second edition in 1774; he had already published on variolation in 1767. When moves to establish the Birmingham Hospital were made in 1765, Tomlinson was one of the town's nine surgeons who each donated five guineas and subscribed two guineas annually; he served there as a surgeon into the early nineteenth century.[82] As well as practising as a surgeon-apothecary, he was also one of the three male midwives in Birmingham, listed as such in two trade directories of 1767[83] and 1770; by 1791,[84] however, he was described only as a surgeon and by that year had moved to one of the best addresses in the town, Temple Row, where two other surgeons and two physicians were his neigh-

78 *Jopson's Coventry Mercury*, 8 Sept. 1783.
79 *The Medical Register for the Year 1783* (London, 1783), p. 50.
80 Sir Zachary Cope, 'The Influence of Free Dispensaries upon Medical Education in Britain', *Medical History*, XIII (1969), pp. 29–36.
81 Thomas Tomlinson, *Medical Miscellany* (Birmingham, 1769).
82 W.C.R.O. CR 764/270.
83 *Sketchley's Birmingham, Walsall and Wolverhampton Directory* (Birmingham, 1767), pp. 2–3.
84 *Sketchley's Birmingham . . . Directory* (Birmingham, 1770).

bours.[85] Tomlinson expounded his views on medication, diseases of the poor and occupational health of the area in his writings, which have a direct and pithy tone. He did not set out the topics he taught in his series of twenty-eight weekly lectures, but claimed that he expounded 'a familiar view and description of different parts of the body' and recommended 'proper authors'; he insisted that his course was only introductory and that others might expand his teaching.

Although little is known about Tomlinson's own training, he dedicated his *Medical Miscellany* in admiration to Caesar Hawkins; as a teacher himself he must have been successful since, in 1782, one of his pupils, Richard Pearson, won a gold medal for a dissertation on putrefaction in competition with 'men of long practice and experience'.[86] Much more is known about another midland man, Edward Grainger; educated at King Edward's School, Birmingham, the second son of a surgeon in the town, he went as a student of anatomy to St Thomas's and Guy's hospitals, and was 'noticed' by Sir Astley Cooper, who 'received him as a dresser without the usual fee'. Having 'distinguished himself highly' in this capacity, Grainger founded the Webb Street School of Anatomy in 1821. He had previously given lectures in a private house and his lectures were so popular that he was obliged

> . . . to deliver the same lecture twice daily, a circumstance, it is believed, hitherto unknown in the annals of this department of teaching; in fact, his tide of success, impelled by talents and acquisitions of the highest order, knew no reflux. As a Surgeon and Anatomist, with many competitors of very high reputation, [he] obtained an eminence almost unparalleled, and exceeding even his most sanguine hopes and expectations.[87]

Grainger died at the age of twenty-six, and his pupils subscribed for a bust of him by Peter Hollins as a mark of their regard. He was succeeded at Webb Street by his younger brother, Richard, who was later appointed to St Thomas's and found fame for his share in the second parliamentary report on children's employment in 1843.[88]

85 *The Universal Trade Directory* (London, 1791), pp. 207–8.
86 *Coventry Mercury*, 11 Nov. 1782.
87 John Merridew, *Catalogue of Engraved Portraits of the Nobility, Gentry, Clergymen and Others* . . . (Coventry, 1848), pp. 27–8.
88 Peter Hollins (1800–86) was the eldest son of a Birmingham architect; he sculpted other works of medical interest, a statue of Henry Jephson, MD, and a bust of Gabriel Jean Marie de Lys, MD, the founder of the Birmingham Deaf and Dumb Institute, whose monument is in St Bartholomew's Church, Edgbaston, on the outskirts of Birmingham. The bust of Edward Grainger, classical and handsome, is one of a series placed above the staircase at the Royal College of Surgeons of England; Hollins also sculpted a bust of Percivall Pott.

The growth of provincial scientific societies in the eighteenth century is one of the period's well-researched phenomena, and a large medical membership was commonplace. Although only a minority, as at Colchester, were actually called medical societies, others, including literary and philosophical societies, had a large number of practitioners as members. Thus the Derby Philosophical Society, founded in the year Hunter died, had fifty-six members in the first two decades of its existence, of whom eleven were definitely surgeons and fifteen were other medical members, including physicians.[89] The Manchester and Leeds societies were similarly dominated by a medical membership, and local practitioners regularly held posts and served on the committees. The most famous of such groups, the Lunar Society of Birmingham, had only fourteen members, of whom three were physicians (Darwin, Small and Withering); it was clearly not a meeting-place for the more junior practitioners, although its interests were strongly medical. Even if such organisations were influential in disseminating new ideas in science, they appear to have been equally important as social occasions, and it would be optimistic to suppose that the young, newly qualified man participated, although enabling his master to attend.

Once a young surgeon-apothecary had finished his apprenticeship and any further training he was able to secure, he faced the prospect of earning his living from medicine. In this respect, the young man who had had hospital experience and had been taught by a senior man within an infirmary had greater prospects of employment by patronage and of having prominent families as patients. In Wiltshire the men apprenticed to Salisbury Infirmary surgeons obtained posts that reflected their training and justified the large premiums their parents had paid to secure their future. Although criticised by some practitioners in the nineteenth century, the eminent men who wielded such influence were swift to defend its virtues; Astley Cooper was convinced that hospital posts were best filled by former apprentices because their characters were already known, and he stoutly resisted a charge of nepotism in his own appointees, although obliged to admit that one was a relation and two had married into his family.[90]

Patronage and influence, however, may have been less important in the expanded employment prospects that the eighteenth century offered the surgeon-apothecary in more parish work, in dispensaries and in public institutions such as gaols and workhouses, as well as

89 Derby Public Library (local history section); cash ledger, catalogue and loan register of the Society's library.
90 S.C.M.E., p. 98.

extended inoculation and vaccination opportunities. Industrialisation in its turn provided new posts in workers' health schemes (for example those arranged by Josiah Wedgwood at Etruria and by Matthew Boulton at Soho, Birmingham) as well as in appointing surgeons to examine poor children intended for factory apprenticeships and to serve as visitors to the factories themselves. As the eighteenth century was a period of almost continuous warfare for England, more military appointments existed for the surgeon, while inspection of recruits was also an expanding aspect of the practitioner's work, as was the provision of private madhouses run by surgeon-apothecaries.

Birmingham is a good example of the increase in the numbers of medical practitioners at this period, as a community particularly affected by industrial growth. In 1767, as well as three physicians, there were twenty surgeon-apothecaries in the town, of whom three were also man-midwives.[91] In 1791, twelve years after the General Hospital was founded, their number had increased to eight physicians and to thirty-seven surgeons.[92] The town's population at this period expanded considerably from 23,688 in 1750, to 42,250 in 1778, to 52,250 in 1785 and to 73,670 by the first census in 1801.[93] In the year of Hunter's death the *Medical Register* suggested that of the 3,166 men practising in the English counties the surgeon-apothecaries overwhelmingly predominated (2,607 or 82.3 per cent). They were at first sight distributed fairly erratically round the provinces, but on closer examination it is apparent that the sparsely populated (Herefordshire) or very small (Huntingdonshire) counties predictably had fewer men in practice, while those counties with large industrial and trading centres were well supplied with practitioners (Table 3.4).

Establishing himself in practice was of critical importance for the young man, either by setting up for himself, by outright purchase of goodwill or by partnership. In setting up in practice on his own account, premises were important, often with goodwill attached if long established for medical occupation, so that, for example, Smollett moved into John Douglas's house in Downing Street, London, in 1744,[94] and John Blount practised in the 1780s from a house in Temple Row, Birmingham, where 'Chesshire the surgeon used to live'.[95] In 1710, when Dr John Cawood, 'the Oculist from Dublin', proposed practising in Liverpool he was helped to find consulting rooms there

91   *Sketchley* (1767), pp. 2–3.
92   *Universal Trade Directory*, pp. 207–8.
93   *Victoria County History of Warwickshire* (Oxford, 1964), VII, p. 8.
94   Peachey, *Memoir*, p. 78.
95   Franklin, 'Education', p. 67.

by one of his patients, a local squire, who noted how he went with 'Dr Cawood to assist him in geting Acquaintance and to procure a Chamber for him where his Pasients may come to him'.[96] For practical reasons the surgeon-apothecary needed a workspace, not just a consulting room, and the term 'shop' was regularly used for this room. James Yonge recorded how he fitted up his own shop in 1671 and also how he 'furnisht' a shop for his son twenty years later,[97] and Richard Kay referred to his father's shop as a room in the family house in 1743. The term shop was widely used, especially in the provinces, throughout the eighteenth century. Thus when William Bouchier Lennard, a surgeon and man-midwife, advertised his newly established practice at Leeds in 1781, he described his premises as a 'Shop four Doors below the New King's Arms in Briggate'.[98] In the same year when a Warwick surgeon, George Weale, died, the inventory of his goods used the same term. However, apart from the shop and its contents, Weale also had a room on the ground floor called the surgery, whose contents were 'a slate table, shelves, glass case, cupboards etc' (Appendix 3).[99] As in the partnership agreement of 1777 (Appendix 4) this use of the word 'surgery' as a place is seventy years earlier than that cited in *The Oxford English Dictionary*. To acquaint prospective patients with available medical services in the area the newly arrived practitioner frequently distributed handbills, an English phenomenon noted with surprise by one foreign visitor in the late eighteenth century. Although of use only to patients who were literate, these were presumably the citizens whom a surgeon-apothecary wished to attract:

> One person informs you that his MAD-HOUSE is at your service; a second keeps a boarding-house for idiots; a good natured man-midwife pays the utmost attention to ladies in certain situations, and promises to use the most scrupulous secrecy. Physicians offer to cure you of all manner of disorders, for a mere trifle.[100]

Not only dubious services such as these were advertised in this way and handbills continued to flourish in the nineteenth century; the impeccably respectable young Henry Jephson, for example, proposed to use them on his return to Nottinghamshire to publicise his recent training in London.[101] More competition in medical practice, with

96   *The Great Diurnal of Nicholas Blundell*, ed. J. J. Bagley (Lancashire and Cheshire Record Society, vol. 114, 1968), part I, p. 258.
97   *James Yonge*, pp. 141, 205.
98   *Leeds Mercury*, 24 July 1781.
99   W.C.R.O. CR 1596/Box 30.
100 Archenholz, *Picture*, II, p. 156.
101 W.C.R.O. Z 574.

increased numbers of practitioners not necessarily in proportion to the population growth, meant that some men were prepared to undercut contract rates for certain work, such as parish surgeon appointments or institutional posts, for example as gaol surgeons.

The costs of setting up in practice could, of course, be considerable, and early in the century the acerbic Mandeville deplored the ambitious parent, able to find an apprenticeship premium beyond his true means, for

> . . . a Man that gives Three or Four Hundred Pounds with his Son to a great Merchant, and has not Two or Three Thousand Pounds to spare against he is out of his Time to begin the World is much to blame not to have brought his child up to something that might be follow'd with less money.[102]

A practitioner might begin his professional life by setting up in practice on his own account or by buying a partnership with an established surgeon-apothecary, although, as the 1783 *Medical Register* makes clear, only a minority were in partnerships.[103] As early as 1747 Campbell reminded his readers of the hazards of establishing a new practice in an area and insisted that the young man should have an independent income or parental support to live on during the early years when he was unknown, with few patients and small repute.[104] By 1761 it was still necessary to give the same warning to newly qualified men:

> But though it requires no great sum to buy a set of instruments, &c yet the youth should have a fortune sufficient to support him like a gentleman, till he becomes known, and renders his merit conspicuous; and he may hasten this knowledge by freely and generously giving relief to those who are unable to pay him.[105]

A share in the practice might be purchased when entering into partnership by paying a lump sum (again, usually with family help for the young man), which of course provided a share in the practice profits rather than a fixed salary.

For the less prosperous young man, or as a concession to a former assistant, a partnership or practice might be sold for either a lower sum or for several instalments spread across a period of years; for example, Gideon Mantell, a former assistant, paid his master £95 a

102 Bernard Mandeville, *The Fable of the Bees*, 2 vols. (London, 1714), I, pp. 58–9.
103 Joan Lane, 'The Medical Practitioners of Provincial England in 1783', *Medical History*, XXVIII (1984), pp. 353–71.
104 Campbell, *Tradesman*, p. 57.
105 Joseph Collyer, *The Parent's and Guardian's Directory and the Youth's Guide* (London, 1761), p. 270.

year for seven years to purchase a practice outright in Lewes (Sussex) in the early years of the nineteenth century.[106] Personal recommendation in finding an assistantship in practice was the most common method, although occasionally such notices can be found in the press:

To the FACULTY

WANTED immediately; – an Assistant that is properly Qualified in Surgery and Pharmacy: – Any Person that can bring Testimonial of his real Qualifications, &c may be informed of an advantageous Place by applying to the Printer of this Paper.

N.B. None need apply whose character will not bear the most strict Examination.[107]

An apprentice newly out of his time might also marry his former master's widow and take over the practice by this means, although a degree of public disapproval can be discerned towards marriages, however expedient, where there was a great age discrepancy. Even into the nineteenth century such unions were not uncommon, and marriage with a former apprentice ensured the practice would continue and gave the master's widow a more secure future than if she had simply sold it. Sometimes the widow and former apprentice or assistant entered into a legal partnership, but not always harmoniously or permanently (Appendix 5).

It was, of course, possible for a surgeon-apothecary to establish himself in practice by inheritance, by family links or by marriage. In the early medieval period the first Master of the Barber-Surgeons' Company, Richard le Barber, left his former apprentice his shop in Bread Street, London, in 1310.[108] Family links, however, were a more common means of acquiring a practice for a surgeon-apothecary (Appendix 4), in descent from father to son or from uncle to nephew. A family practice was clearly an excellent opportunity for an erstwhile apprentice, saving him the cost of equipment, stock, premises and instruments, although Richard Kay, for example, bought his own new set of instruments in London before returning home to practise in Lancashire, as well as a supply of drugs. Such a young man also benefited from his father's goodwill, reputation and a ready-made clientele, and on his father's death would expect to inherit the practice. Marriage to his former master's daughter was a further well-tried means of establishing a practice or business, with Dick Whittington and Hogarth's Frank Goodchild as exemplary models. The advan-

---

106 *The Journal of Gideon [Algernon] Mantell, Surgeon and Geologist, 1818–52,* ed. E. Cecil Curwen (Oxford, 1940), p. 1.
107 *Coventry Mercury,* 29 Nov. 1784.
108 Young, *Annals,* p. 25.

tages for an apprentice of marrying his master's daughter were obvious; he had a ready-made living, no setting-up expenses, needed no assistance from his own parents, acquired a clientele and excellent prospects of ultimately taking over the whole practice. In addition, he would also have known his future wife for a long time, unlike some arranged marriages in which the participants were almost strangers. For the master too such a marriage could be advantageous. He gained a young partner, trained in his ways, who would be able to keep the practice profitable when his own health began to fail, one who would protect professional secrets, especially remedies, and who would not, when out of his time, become a rival's assistant or set up in practice for himself, taking valued patients with him. A smaller dowry for his daughter might be a further benefit, but the arrangement was unlikely to bring the master a substantial payment for goodwill, often a welcome injection of capital for the smaller practitioner. Attaining a practice by marriage was generally publicly approved, mentioned, for example, in obituary notices of practitioners. A surgeon-apothecary's daughter was also likely to prove a suitable bride for a practitioner, well experienced in the demands and requirements of medical practice.

The establishment of medical families lasting for several generations is a noticeable aspect of the eighteenth century.[109] Not only famous London surgeons, such as the Hawkins family, formed 'dynastic chains'; in the English provinces too, medical families were being established that were to last for a century or more, some until the present day, often remaining in the same area. The Brees of Warwickshire exemplify this trend; in 1676 a gentleman's son from Kenilworth, Thomas Bree, was bound to a London barber-surgeon, Edward Cockayne, for seven years (Fig. 3.1). By the eighteenth century Robert Bree, MD, held appointments at Leicester and Northampton infirmaries,[110] and another member of the family was a surgeon-apothecary at Solihull (Warwickshire).[111] In the same county there were also the Burman, Kimball and Welchman families, each with nearly two centuries of practitioners.[112] Some men displayed impressive social mobility within medicine at this period, moving from rural surgeon-apothecary to city physician, but others remained as country practitioners from one generation to another; the Taylors

109 Geoffrey Holmes, *Augustan England, Professions, State and Society, 1680–1730* (London, 1982); chap. 7 outlines the rise of important medical families for this period. Other examples are cited by Burnby, *English Apothecary.*
110 Waddy, *Northampton*, p. 158 and *Medical Register . . . 1783*, p. 92.
111 *Med. Reg.*, p. 115.
112 Joan Lane, 'The Parish Surgeon and His Services to the Poor, 1750–1800', *Bulletin of the Society for the Social History of Medicine*, 28 (1981), pp. 10–14.

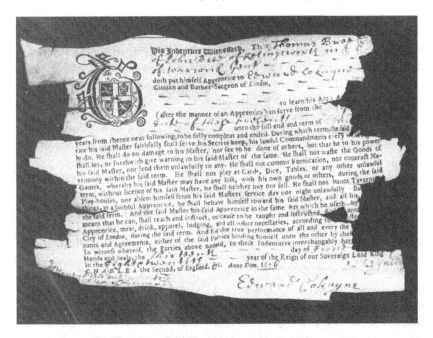

Fig. 3.1. An apprenticeship to a London barber-surgeon, 1676 (Warwick County Record Office, CR 1279/16 by kind permission of S. E. M. Twist, Esq.)

of Whitworth (Lancashire) were an interesting example of such professional mobility.[113] Some families retained a long-standing connection with their county infirmary; thus in Hereford the general hospital was served by several generations of the Cam family from the 1780s until the late nineteenth century. One member of this family held a hospital appointment for forty-seven years, and in 1783 three others were practising in the city, one physician and two surgeons.[114]

The prosperity of the surgeon-apothecary was always extremely varied, depending on where he practised as much as any other factors. Since they had a fairly small stock of goods, with low-risk capital, surgeon-apothecaries (unlike apothecaries, who regularly featured amongst the frequent bankruptcies of the period) were rarely forced out of practice for financial reasons. Although practitioners often waited a year or more to be paid, such delays were not serious in a stable economy and were significant only when inflation began to rise. London had always provided a prosperous livelihood for the

113 John L. West, *The Taylors of Lancashire* (Manchester, 1977).
114 Langford, 'Hereford General Hospital', p. 157.

most senior men, with aristocrats and country gentry as their patients, but even in the provinces a surgeon such as James Yonge, his
only income from fees, could give a dowry of £450 when his younger
daughter married.[115] In the next century a Gosport (Hampshire) surgeon, Rowland Frogmore, was able to leave £500 in his will towards
the founding of Worcester Infirmary,[116] and other county hospitals
were recipients of similar bequests.

Although income was an important measure of a practitioner's success, there were other marks of achievement based on his standing
within the community and accorded by his fellow citizens. These
include public offices or honorary appointments held, and the social
circle within which he moved was perhaps a more reliable guide than
the printed obituary notice or the carved church memorial. Eighteenth-century public offices were of enormous variety, with every
local charity choosing trustees and with many parish, borough or city
posts to be filled every year. Surgeon-apothecaries appear consistently in all these categories. Thus, for example, in 1780 when four
new governors were elected for King Edward's School in Birmingham, one was a local surgeon, Francis Parrott, and the other
three were all merchants; seven years later Parrott was elected bailiff,
an office of great honour.[117] Surgeon-apothecaries regularly became
mayors of their towns, for example William Dawson in Leeds in
1770[118] or Edward Harper in Coventry in 1778. Harper was also a
magistrate and sheriff twice, as well as acting as executor to a patient's will;[119] like attorneys and clerics, surgeon-apothecaries were
also beneficiaries in wills, an interesting yardstick of their status at
this period. There is ample contemporary evidence that eighteenth-
century surgeon-apothecaries lived a full social and sporting life with
their neighbours, often including the gentry, into whose ranks, by
purchasing estates, some successfully moved. In 1785 Mrs Lybbe
Powys felt it worthy of comment in her diary that a retired surgeon
had recently bought a large estate near her own,[120] as if exemplifying
the view of foreign travellers who frequently asserted from such superficial evidence that England was virtually a classless society in the

---

115 *James Yonge*, p. 206.
116 William Henry McMenemey, *A History of the Worcester Royal Infirmary* (London,
1947), p. 67.
117 *The Records of King Edward's School, Birmingham*, ed. Philip B. Chatwin (Dugdale
Society, XXV, 1963), p. 36.
118 *Leeds Mercury*, 2 Oct. 1770.
119 Coventry City Record Office, 101/9/7, 391/4.
120 *Passages from the Diary of Mrs Philip Lybbe Powys of Hardwicke House, 1756–1808*,
ed. Emily J. Climenson (London, 1899), p. 221.

eighteenth century. (In this case, the surgeon was Richard Davenport, recently in practice in Essex Street, London.)[121]

During the eighteenth century apprenticeship remained the essential means of training an English surgeon-apothecary for an adult career, its basic characteristics of the term, the premium and living in the master's house unchanged. Even by 1791, it has been calculated that only 40 per cent of the surgeon-apothecaries listed in a contemporary trade directory in Lincolnshire and Essex had had training in London hospitals.[122] It is to be expected that a much lower proportion than this would be found in an earlier period and in counties farther from the capital. However, contemporary pressures, which included inflation, warfare, population growth and disease patterns, apart from any relevant scientific advances, affected the eighteenth-century surgeon-apothecary in many respects. His widened employment prospects and the numerical increase of the whole medical profession in this period were crucial. The stabilising effect of the emergence of medical dynasties and a discernible change of status of the individual practitioner in the eyes of his contemporaries were also significant factors for the surgeon-apothecary, although affecting only the more prosperous apprentices at first. The value of apprenticeship for the surgeon-apothecary was more than simply acquiring professional skills. Particularly important to the boy whose own family was not a medical one, the surgeon-apothecary's resident apprentice learned his master's way of life. In the practice he had the older apprentice, the qualified assistant and his master as role models. His master's prosperous house, carriage and way of life were an incentive to the apprentice that one day he might attain such status himself. The apprentice learned too of the demands made by practice – the erratic work-hours and how to respond to patients. He acquired the techniques of running a practice in the eighteenth century, how to keep case-notes, how to judge the urgency of calls and plan his round of visits and transport accordingly. He watched his master buy and control his stock of drugs as well as render annual accounts to patients. Such necessary chores were an essential part of practice, and a Sussex practitioner noted that at the end of one year he sent out nearly seven hundred bills to patients.[123] The apprentice learned how to estimate a scale of fees appropriate to the patient's purse or to negotiate an annual parish contract with the Overseers of the Poor,

121 *Medical Register . . . 1783*, p. 19.
122 Joseph F. Kett, 'Provincial Medical Practice in England, 1730–1815', *Journal of the History of Medicine*, XIX (1964), p. 19.
123 *Journal . . . Mantell*, p. 3.

an increasingly important aspect of practice in the eighteenth century. These were all essential skills in running an eighteenth-century medical practice successfully, as was supervising the apprentice himself and employing unqualified staff, such as a groom, coachman or servant.

The critics of apprenticeship focused on its great expense and its lack of a systematic curriculum, as well as inflexible, out-of-date masters and a narrow range of medical conditions to study in most practices. However, even critics of the 1834 Select Committee on Medical Education, many of them, such as Guthrie, apprenticed men themselves, admitted that the ratio of one-to-one, master to apprentice, could not be bettered in medical schools. In addition the existence of some outstanding provincial practitioners in the eighteenth century suggests that innovative masters with a wide range of skills could provide excellent instruction for the apprentice. Before the establishment of county hospitals in the provinces apprentices undoubtedly saw a wide range of cases, as Richard Kay recorded, that would in future decades automatically be consigned to a hospital and out of the surgeon-apothecary's care. The importance of apprenticeship can hardly be overestimated in a young man's career since for the majority of surgeon-apothecaries in the eighteenth century it was their only means of technical training before becoming practitioners in their own right.

Appendix 1: An apprenticeship indenture to a surgeon, 1705

John Beale of Woolscot in the county of Warwick puts himself apprentice to William Edwards surgeon of Kenilworth to learn his art and with him after the manner of an apprentice to serve for four years from this date. During the term the apprentice shall faithfully serve his master, his secrets keep, his lawful commandments gladly obey; the apprentice neither to do damage to his master nor see it done; the apprentice not to waste his master's goods nor lend them unlawfully. The apprentice not to commit fornication nor contract matrimony during the term; the apprentice not to play at cards or dice or any unlawful game that may cause his master loss. The apprentice not to haunt taverns nor ale-houses nor be absent unlawfully day or night from his master's service but in all things behave as a good and faithful apprentice towards his master.

William Edwards, in consideration of the sum of £53 16s, shall teach the apprentice all the art he uses by the best means he can. William Edwards shall find the apprentice in meat, drink, washing and lodging during the term.

   1 May 1705   signatures of John Beale, William Edwards and two witnesses. (Warwick County Record Office, CR 556/364)

Appendix 2: Lectures attended in London by Richard Kay, 1743–4

Lectures given by Samuel Sharp August to December 1743
Anatomy
Vertebrae and ribs
Bones
Corpse
Coats and humour of eye
Vision
Outer ear
Dead bodies (two)

Lectures given by John Girle August to December 1743
Anatomy
Aliment through body
Slink calf [an aborted foetus]
Eye
Ear
Amputation of a leg
Cranium
Teeth and bones of lower cranium
Anatomy

January to April 1744
Heart and lungs
Circulation of the blood
Topic unspecified
Bones
Skull
Midwifery

January to April 1744
Dead bodies (three)
Five lectures: topics unspecified
Bandages
Dead body
Two lectures: topics unspecified
Lacteals of the dog [lymphatics]

Appendix 3: Inventory of George Weale, surgeon, of Warwick, 1781

Rooms downstairs: Best parlour, little parlour, kitchen, brewhouse.
The shop: Mortars, weights (three sets), scales, infusion pots, pewter basons, porringers, serches etc., thralls in cellars, two plaister pans, spatelas, knives, bolus stones etc.
Surgery: Slate table, shelves, glass case, cupboards, etc.
Rooms upstairs: Back room, dining room, little room [a bedroom], back, west, middle, red and end garretts.
(Warwick County Record Office, CR 1596/Box 30)

Appendix 4: Partnership agreement between George Weale, surgeon-apothecary of Warwick, and Edward Weale, surgeon, apothecary and man-midwife of Warwick, May 1777

1. The partnership is to last for seven years from 16 April last.
2. Edward Weale to pay his father for half the drugs in the shop and surgery.
3. Edward Weale to pay £60 to enter the partnership.
4. Future drugs etc to be bought jointly.
5. Work to be done only on behalf of the partnership.

6. George Weale to retain his personal appointment as county gaol surgeon and keep the fees from the appointment.
7. Edward Weale to practise midwifery and to keep the fees.
8. Neither to pay for drugs used in the above [numbers 6 and 7] or in treating their own families.
9. Accounts to be kept relating to drugs, visits and attendances. Profits and debts to be shared equally.
10. Each partner to provide and keep one horse at his own expense.
11. A servant to be paid jointly by the partners to look after the horse, attend the shop and other necessary tasks.
12. Edward Weale to pay George Weale £3 a year as half the rent of the shop and surgery and for the use of drawers, counters, shelves, mortars, stills, stillhorse, instruments and articles.
13. If either partner should die, his share is to belong to his executors.

(Warwick County Record Office CR 1596/Box 90)

Appendix 5: Partnership agreement between Sarah Bradford of Warwick, widow and relict of John Bradford, surgeon-apothecary, and Thomas Cooper, surgeon-apothecary of Warwick, 24 May 1777

1. Sarah Bradford and Thomas Cooper to share the profits equally.
2. The partnership to last for six years.
3. Thomas Cooper to pay Sarah Bradford half the value of the drugs now in Sarah Bradford's shop at the valued price, within one month.
4. Thomas Cooper to pay Sarah Bradford £6 a year for his half share of the use of the shop, warehouse, utensils of trade and the stable.
5. Thomas Cooper to pay £5 a year towards the maintenance of a servant boy.
6. Thomas Cooper to pay Sarah Bradford 6s 6d weekly for his board and lodging.
7. No other trade to be carried on by either nor the work of a surgeon-apothecary for individual benefit.
8. Sarah Bradford and Thomas Cooper to share the ground rent for the area occupied by the horse and servant boy.
9. Accounts were to be kept, to which both parties were to have free access. Monies were to be rendered every three months or more often if needed.
10. If either should die during the partnership, the survivor to render a final financial account to the deceased's executors.

The partnership was dissolved in June 1782 under the following terms:
1. The stock of drugs on the premises was to be divided equally between the partners; if the quantity were too small it was to be set aside and divided by two indifferent [impartial] persons of the Faculty. If the partners disagreed about sharing the drugs, they were to cast lots.

2. Whatever fixtures, utensils etc Thomas Cooper brought into the shop he was to remove.
3. Whatever fixtures etc were in the shop when the partnership began to belong to Sarah Bradford.
4. An account to be made of the finances and the profits divided; the account books to be given to two senior tradesmen in Warwick.

(Warwick County Record Office, CR 1596/Box 90)

4

Physicians, hospitals and career structures in eighteenth-century London

W. F. BYNUM

I

The year 1983 marked another bicentennial. Some six months after William Hunter's death on 30 March 1783, Samuel Foart Simmons, Hunter's biographer, penned the preface to the third, most complete and accurate, but, unfortunately, final edition of his *Medical Register*.[1] Its existence is a reminder both of eighteenth-century enterprise and of the visibility of medical men exactly seventy-five years before the Medical Act made the annual publication of a medical register a legal matter. This third edition bore testimony to the continued enthusiasm of Simmons and his collaborators and, if the preface is to be believed, to the public spirit of Joseph Johnson, its publisher, who had defrayed the expenses of preparing the work. For the historian of late eighteenth-century British medicine, the *Medical Register* is a godsend, for despite its gaps and unofficial status, it offers an accessible geographical profile of ordinary and élite practitioners, identified by the traditional labels of physicians, surgeons and apothecaries, along with hospitals, infirmaries, dispensaries and medical charities, court and royal appointments, medical members of the Royal Society and other learned societies, and a wonderful sprinkling of foreign doctors, mostly professors at Continental universities or medical members of national academies.

Simmons's *Register* is not complete, as he himself recognised, for he listed in italics the towns where 'the editors believe [the lists] to be accurate', and places like Wells and Walthamstow, Aldborough and Lowestoff, stubbornly appear in Roman type. Almost a year elapsed between the printing of the first sheets and the publication of the work, creating inaccuracies only partially rectified by an appendix.

1 [Samuel Foart Simmons], *The Medical Register for the Year 1783* (London, 1783). The first two editions appeared in 1779 and 1780.

Although Simmons was based in London, and its medical corporations helped make practice and practitioners more visible in the capital than in the provinces, even the London listings are incomplete.
Simmons knew this: The first fifty pages of this book, the index of
which starts on page 227, are taken up with London matters. Since
the work begins with a description of the Royal College of Physicians,
it is not immediately apparent what Simmons thought of the quality
of his London material. But in the 'provinces', under 'Middlesex',
where we find such familiar London names as Hampstead, Islington,
Highgate and Hammersmith, we also find the following terse entry:
'London. See page 1.' Unlike the other Middlesex names, London is
Romanised. A simple measure of the gaps in this unofficial register
can be seen by comparing it with the 1784 edition of *The Royal Kalendar*, a kind of annual 'Who's Who' for Georgian England. The
Kalendar provided listings of such individuals as Members of Parliament (both Commons and Lords), the court, officers in the army and
Royal Navy and holders of various other public offices, including the
universities and hospitals and other medical establishments. The
points at which the *Register* and *Kalendar* agree far outweigh the individuals and establishments listed by only one of these sources, and,
on the whole, the *Register* provides a marginally more complete picture of the medical terrain. Nevertheless, the *Royal Kalendar* lists ten
or so medical men as holding appointments at various medical establishments, and although the men (with one possible exception) themselves may be found in the *Register*, the appointments are not noted.
There are a slightly larger number of 'public' men, and five dispensaries, recorded in Simmons but not in the *Kalendar*. The *Kalendar* did
not list medical men without some form of institutional affiliation.[2]
    The last edition of Simmons's *Medical Register* has been recently
analysed for provincial England by Joan Lane, and I have found his
section on London doctors of immense value, partly, I should con-
fess, because it has confirmed the conclusions I had formed from
other approaches.[3] Although this essay is limited primarily to physicians, my conclusions can be anticipated by the discerning reader
when I give the bald, uncorrected figures that Simmons's *Medical
Register* and the *Royal Kalendar* allow us to derive for the structure of
medical practice in London, 200 years ago. First, there were a *lot* of
doctors in London, some 960 physicians, surgeons and apothecaries
serving a population of about 800,000 – a ratio of about 1 doctor to 850
individuals, somewhat in excess of the general ratio of 1 to 950 or so,

2 *The Court and City Kalendar* began publication in 1745 and went through various
changes in name, usually called *The Royal Kalendar* after 1767.
3 Joan Lane, 'The Medical Practitioners of Provincial England in 1783', *Medical
History*, XXVIII (1984), 353–71; and Ch. 3 of this volume.

reckoned about right in present-day Britain. Second, and even more significantly, Simmons identified 148 physicians, about 220 surgeons and about 600 apothecaries practising in London. These figures, with the ratio of about one physician for every one and a half surgeons and every four apothecaries, are more weighted towards the élites – physicians and pure surgeons – than was the case in the provinces, where apothecaries and surgeon-apothecaries were more in evidence. Thus, in Derbyshire, five physicians, no 'pure' surgeons and thirty-four surgeon-apothecaries were identified in Simmons's register, a ratio of élites to ordinary practitioners of about 1:7. Not surprisingly, physicians clustered in prosperous market towns, and locations with hospitals or infirmaries, whereas surgeon-apothecaries were more evenly dispersed throughout the country. For London, however, the other operative figure is the ratio of each of the medical orders to the number of hospital, infirmary or dispensary posts available. For the 148 physician and physician-midwives had at their disposal eighty-six posts in these medical institutions, a ratio of one post for each 1.7 physicians. The 220 surgeons had sixty-two posts, about one for each 3.5 surgeons, while of the 600 apothecaries, only 44 (ratio of 1 to 14) were occupied in hospital, dispensary or medical charity service.[4] The figures 1:1.7, 1:3.5 and 1:14 should be borne in mind as we look at our primary question, What was the relationship between London physicians and hospitals in the eighteenth-century metropolis?

II

It is generally accepted that hospitals, by which I mean all formal medical institutions, with their three primary functions of patient care, teaching and research, have played a central role in the rise of the modern medical profession. Through the work of Michel Foucault, E. H. Ackerknecht and others, the 'birth of the clinic' or the development of 'hospital medicine', as these historians have called it, has been established as an epoch – indeed *the* crucial epoch – in modern medical history.[5] This phenomenon was largely French in

4 I have not attempted to use my fuller figures here, since they are still changing; they will modify but not substantially alter the general picture that can be derived from Simmons's *Medical Register.*
5 Michel Foucault, *The Birth of the Clinic,* trans. A. M. Sheridan Smith (London, 1973); E. H. Ackerknecht, *Medicine at the Paris Hospital, 1794–1848* (Baltimore, 1967); R. H. Shryock, *The Development of Modern Medicine* (London, 1948); David M. Vess, *Medical Revolution in France, 1789–1796* (Gainesville, Fla., 1975); W. F. Bynum, 'Health, Disease and Medical Care', in G. S. Rousseau and Roy Porter, eds., *The Ferment of Knowledge: Studies in the Historiography of Eighteenth-Century Science* (Cambridge, 1980).

origin and coalesced around the reorganisation of the Paris medical
school in 1794. Its consequences for medical knowledge were large,
for this hospital-based medical education unified medicine and surgery, taught doctors to think in terms of local lesions, to use the
techniques of careful, systematic physical diagnosis, to correlate
whenever possible the signs and symptoms observed during the patient's life with the changes in his body discoverable at post-mortem
examination, and to make use of the large medical experience available through hospitals in more accurate disease descriptions and
more careful therapeutic evaluations. Both Foucault and Ivan Waddington have stressed the importance of the power structure within
this new medical milieu.[6] In the hospitals, doctors were kings and in
the atmosphere of professional dominance and autonomy, diagnosis
(satisfying the doctor's curiosity) could take precedence over therapeutics (making the patient feel better).

Now, there can be no doubt about the main outlines or importance
of this story, just as there can be no doubt, following Toby Gelfand's
researches on the Paris College of Surgeons in the eighteenth century, and Othmar Keel's more general work on clinical teaching
throughout eighteenth-century Europe, that what Foucault calls the
'clinic' had a gestation as well as a birth and that many of the professional attitudes and educational patterns had been widely effected
before more systematic adoption in France during the Revolutionary
period.[7] Furthermore, it is well known that, particularly after the
close of the French wars, the impact of these French medical and
educational ideals on the British scene was considerable. The Dublin
school of Robert Graves and William Stokes; the 'Great Men of Guy's'
– Thomas Hodgkin, Thomas Addison and Richard Bright; James
Hope at St George's and William Jenner at University College Hospital – these and other high priests of Victorian hospital medicine explicitly acknowledged their debts to France, and Jeanne Peterson's
study, *The Medical Profession in Mid-Victorian London*, has reinforced
the extent to which the formation of the professional élite in the 1840s
and 1850s was bound up with the holding of an official post of physician or surgeon in one of the large general voluntary hospitals.[8] So
necessary was the consultancy post for medical positions of high

6 Ivan Waddington, 'The Role of the Hospital in the Development of Modern
Medicine: A Sociological Analysis', *Sociology*, VII (1973), 211–24; Michel Foucault,
Birth of the Clinic.
7 Toby Gelfand, *Professionalizing Modern Medicine: Paris Surgeons and Medical Science
and Institutions in the 18th Century* (Westport and London, 1980); Gelfand, 'Gestation
of the Clinic', *Medical History*, XXV (1981), 169–80; and chap. 5, this volume.
8 Jeanne Peterson, *The Medical Profession in Mid-Victorian London* (Berkeley, Calif.,
1978).

status and income that many ambitious young doctors, unable to make the breakthrough within the general voluntary hospitals, started their own smaller, specialist hospitals as alternative routes to the possible professional, social and financial heights that medicine offered to a few. By the mid-Victorian period, in London, at least, Peterson could find fairly precise divisions of doctors into those with and those without hospital appointments: between consultants and general practitioners, a separation still perpetuated within the NHS. Indeed, Waddington has suggested that outside London this consultant–general practitioner distinction was emerging during the late eighteenth century and for provincial England was more significant than the more conventional division of medical men into physicians, surgeons and apothecaries, a suggestion compatible with a close reading of Simmons's *Register*.[9]

If we can accept that hospitals did come to symbolise for British doctors much that was characteristic of French hospital medicine – particularly the power and prestige that were reflected in the new professional dominance they came to enjoy with their clients outside the hospitals – we must remember that the organisation of medical services in Britain meant that 'pure' hospital medicine was never so encapsulated here. For the possibility of salaried, full-time medical teaching and research, present for a few at least since 1794 in France, was not a British adaptation.[10] The voluntary hospitals worked as they did essentially because consultant physicians and surgeons were prepared to donate their hospital services gratuitously. The fringe benefits, of course, were considerable: The prestige of the hospital appointment made it easy to attract rich patients, access to the hospital's governors was often to the cream of local élites, it could be good for business to be seen to be charitable, and for many doctors, medical teaching could also be lucrative. But British hospital physicians and surgeons almost always had at least one eye on their private consulting rooms, for it was here that the wealth that spelled professional success was to be had.

All of this may seem somewhat remote from William Hunter's London. But I originally conceived the study on which I am currently

9 Ivan Waddington, 'General Practitioners and Consultants in Early Nineteenth-Century England: The Sociology of an Intraprofessional Conflict', in John Woodward and David Richards, eds., *Health Care and Popular Medicine in Nineteenth Century England* (London, 1977); cf. Joan Lane, 'Medical Practitioners', and I. S. L. Loudon, 'Provincial Medical Practice in Eighteenth-Century England', *Medical History*, XXIX (1985), 1–32.
10 To the references cited in n. 5 can be added George Weisz, 'Reform and Conflict in French Medical Education, 1870–1914', in R. Fox and G. Weisz, eds., *The Organization of Science and Technology in France, 1808–1914* (Cambridge, 1980).

engaged as a means of examining the background to the situation that Peterson described for the mid-Victorian period. My work has been thrown into sharper focus by the recent book by Geoffrey Holmes, *Augustan England*, which argues that both for the traditional learned professions (the church, the law, medicine), as well as for a number of nascent professional groups – schoolmasters, architects, landscape gardeners, musicians perhaps – the period from 1680 to 1730 was crucial in the expansion of demand for the services of these groups and hence for their rising social and economic expectations. Medicine is for Holmes a particularly telling case in point: The first of his two long chapters on the subject, entitled 'The Coming of the Doctor', contains the fullest statement so far offered on the recruitment to and the rewards of medicine in Augustan England. He admits that London and the provinces are different cases, partly because of the greater concentration of people and wealth in the capital, partly because of the existence in London of the medical corporations with certain legal rights in the regulation of medical practice. Nevertheless, Holmes believes that the differences between London and the provinces are less significant than the fact that throughout the country, doctors during the period increased markedly, in numbers, in public visibility, in income, in education and even, he sometimes suggests, in diagnostic and therapeutic acumen. As he summarised his description of the characteristics of Augustan medical men:

> However the 'doctor' of 1730 was formally labelled, he was by and large far more versatile than his predecessor two generations back, less hidebound by the old circumscriptions and the prejudices and more responsive to change. He was likely to be more receptive to the virtues of what we now call 'preventive medicine'; and he was furnished with laudanum, with specifics such as mercuric oxide, cinchona ('Jesuit's bark', a close relative of quinine), calomel and ipecacuanha, and, if not equipped with then often backed by, surgical skills of no mean order. If he was a trained surgeon or surgeon-apothecary even the instruments he used were better, more sophisticated and varied than those of sixty years before, and provincial as well as London craftsmen had begun to produce them.[11]

Sometimes, it must be admitted, Holmes stretches his temporal limits, dragging material from the 1740s, 1750s and sometimes 1760s, to support a thesis that has an official cut-off date of 1730. Thus, for

11   Geoffrey Holmes, *Augustan England: Professions, State and Society, 1680–1730* (London, 1982), 205.

instance, the diary of Richard Kay, a young Lancashire doctor who studied in London in 1743–4, is cited as evidence of the extent of medical education available in the London hospitals, even though the situation fifteen years earlier was rather different. Nevertheless, since Holmes is attempting to push back the vocabulary of professionalism by a whole century, a few decades do not seriously disturb the thrust of his claims. Furthermore, Holmes is not particularly interested in sociological definitions of a 'profession', or in a profession's legal status, but in the mutual identity of its members. For him, an Augustan profession seems to be a collection of middle-class men, entitled to prefix their names with 'Mr', earning a living in roughly the same way. Whether such a use of the word 'profession' would satisfy a modern sociologist, it could be argued, is beside the point: Holmes uses it in its eighteenth-century sense (profession to Samuel Johnson was 'known employment'[12]), and we should not be surprised that twentieth-century professionalism did not exist two centuries ago.

The question I wish to pose, however, is this: If eighteenth-century doctors achieved a far greater degree of visbility, income, prestige and social status than the traditional picture, which viewed the medical corporations as quintessential instances of Old Corruption, and doctors as generally 'unprofessional' in their behaviour, fractious, ill-educated and unregulated, what role might hospitals and other medical institutions have played in this former process? Did these institutions confer on those medical men associated with them the professional clout that historians of the nineteenth-century profession have asserted to be the case for that period? Like many historical questions, the verdict can probably be delivered as yes, no, or it all depends. I am in the process of collecting prosopographical data that I hope will provide some kind of more substantial answer. In particular I am trying to assess the social roots, education and careers of the doctors–physicians and surgeons – who held appointments in eighteenth-century London medical institutions. Eventually I hope to extend this to apothecaries, as well, for apothecaries, even though generally full-time resident employees while engaged by the hospitals, also seem sometimes to have used these appointments as stepping-stones in their careers. But the apothecaries are frequently relatively obscure men, visible during their hospital stays but disappearing from view afterwards. The surgeons, too, present difficulties as a group, for although the records of the Company of Surgeons give some sense of their internal professional hierarchies and networks, even the barest

---

12   Samuel Johnson, *A Dictionary of the English Language,* facsimile reprint of 1755 edition (London, 1983), entry 'profession'.

biographical information is not easily available for many of the hospital surgeons of eighteenth-century London. Given Gelfand's and Keel's work, the obvious use surgeons made of hospitals for training opportunities and pupils, and the extent to which surgical thinking was bound up with the hospital medicine of the 1790s, London surgeons clearly deserve a more systematic analysis than I have yet been able to do.[13] At this stage of my research, and in what follows, I must confine myself primarily to the physicians.

Now, a brief point of method: I have included not just hospitals *per se*, but also dispensaries and charities with a substantial medical brief. Since many of the dispensaries and medical charities were small, did not survive, and have disappeared from historical view, my list is still growing from its present size of about 570 physicians and surgeons holding more than 700 separate appointments during the century. I have a card for each, summarising their education, publications, appointments and other pertinent biographical facts. One unexpected benefit of looking systematically at the London medical scene in this way has been to discover the sheer extent of eighteenth-century institutional activity. The four 'hospitals' of 1700 appointing physicians – St Bartholomew's, St Thomas's, Bethlem and Christ's – had grown to something like forty public institutions (plus another twenty or so that had come and gone) and more than a dozen private ones by the first decade of the nineteenth century. To the two general hospitals had been added five more – Westminster, Guy's, St George's, the Middlesex, the London.[14] St Luke's now provided alternative hospitalisation for the insane and numerous private madhouses vied for a share in the growing and lucrative 'trade in lunacy'.[15] Other specialist hospitals and medical charities included the Lock, two Misericordia, the Magdalen and Smallpox hospitals for venereal disease, penitent prostitutes and smallpox, and at least ten lying-in hospitals and maternity charities. The French Protestants and

13 See Owsei Temkin, 'The Role of Surgery in the Rise of Modern Medical Thought', in his selected essays, *The Double Face of Janus* (Baltimore and London, 1977); and the essays by Gelfand and Keel, chaps. 5 and 8 this volume.
14 Individual hospitals have not in general attracted systematic analysis by professional historians, and the quality of existing hospital histories varies considerably. Of the genre dealing with London hospitals, the best examples are probably A. E. Clark Kennedy, *The London: A study of the Voluntary Hospital System*, 2 vols. (London, 1962), and A. C. Cameron, *Mr. Guy's Hospital, 1726–1948* (London, 1954). There is a useful short discussion in David Owen, *English Philanthropy 1660–1940* (Cambridge, Mass., 1965).
15 W. L. Parry-Jones, *The Trade in Lunacy* (London, 1972) is a pioneering study of the private psychiatric sector. From his book can be pieced together references to at least thirteen private madhouses in London and the adjacent counties during the eighteenth century.

Portuguese and Spanish Jews each maintained hospitals, some of the functions of the latter, however, not being strictly medical. There were foundlings in Captain Coram's institution, sick and decaying soldiers at Chelsea, old salts at Greenwich. Some dozen and a half dispensaries offered out-patient services, home visits and home deliveries to the worthy poor all over London. The National Truss Society had since 1786 offered free advice and trusses to the ruptured poor. Clearly, by the end of the eighteenth century, medical charity was alive and well in London. Anthony Highmore's pious 1810 description of London's multitude of charities runs just shy of 1,000 pages.[16] The number of hospital beds in London could not match that in Paris – estimated on the eve of the Revolution as holding 6,326 persons plus 14,105 people in hospicelike accommodations – but the range was impressive nonetheless, and the figure sometimes given, of 3,000 patients and 4,000 hospital beds in all of England in 1801, is palpably an understatement.[17] The Appendix lists the London medical charities I have uncovered to date, with brief details of their medical functions and the institutional opportunities they offered to medical men.

III

It is now appropriate to ask who were the physicians to these dozens of medical establishments, and how did the group who held appointments differ from their colleagues without commitments in the formal charitable sphere? There are two ways of tackling the problem: first, via the prosopographical material on the hospital physicians themselves, and second, via the larger group of physicians attached either as Fellows or licentiates of the College of Physicians.

What, first, of the educational backgrounds of eighteenth-century London hospital physicians? Did they need to come from Oxford or

16 Anthony Highmore, *Pietas Londinensis* (London, 1814), and Patrick Colquhoun, *Police of the Metropolis* (London, 1797), contain the fullest contemporary listings of London charities, including medical ones. For modern discussions of some aspects of these specialised medical institutions, see, *inter alia*, Dorothy George, *London Life in the Eighteenth Century* (Harmondsworth, 1966 [first published in 1925]); Betsy Rodgers, *Cloak of Charity* (London, 1949); Ford K. Brown, *Fathers of the Victorians* (Cambridge, 1961); Ruth McClure, *Coram's Children* (New Haven, Conn., and London, 1981); I. S. L. Loudon, 'The Origins and Growth of the Dispensary Movement in England', *Bulletin of the History of Medicine*, LV (1981), 322–42. The copy of Highmore in the Wellcome Institute Library is dated 1814, although the preface and most copies are dated 1810.
17 The Paris figures, taken from Jacques Tenon's survey, are discussed in Ackerknecht, *Medicine at the Paris Hospital*, pp. 15ff; the English figures, from the first census, are used by Brian Abel-Smith, *The Hospitals, 1800–1914* (London, 1964).

Cambridge – and thus be eligible to Fellowships in the College of
Physicians – before they could expect to obtain a hospital appointment? Not surprisingly, the answer is that it depends on which part
of the century and which hospital. In 1700, the answer was yes:
Except for Caleb Coatsworth at Thomas's, all the physicians at the
four ancient establishments were Oxbridge Fellows of the College. St
Bartholomew's, which stayed High Church and Tory, continued to
prefer the safety of the ancient universities, only once in the entire
century daring to appoint someone from outside that orbit. This was
in 1752 when Robert Pate, a licentiate of the College with an Aberdeen medical degree, was appointed physician. I do not know why
Pate was chosen, since there is nothing obvious about his career: He
published nothing and seems not to have left a mark on his time. At
any rate, when Pate died in 1762 he was replaced by Richard Tyson
(MD Oxford), nephew of another Richard Tyson, physician to Bartholomew's, and grandnephew of the comparative anatomist.[18] The
other hospital that kept a perfect track record with the ancient universities was Bethlem, where Edward Tyson and his successor Richard
Hale were succeeded by the dynasty of Oxford-trained Monros.

St Thomas's, though, was Whig in politics and more eclectic in its
appointment policies. Coatsworth was a disenfranchised surgeon created doctor of medicine by the archbishop of Canterbury, and during
the century physicians with medical degrees from Leiden, Glasgow,
Aberdeen, St Andrew's and Edinburgh served along with representa-
tives from Oxford and Cambridge. There is no particular pattern in
the sequence of appointments.[19] Across the street, Guy's Hospital
was somewhat more prone to Oxbridge graduates, although Leiden,
in the first half of the century, and Edinburgh in the second half,
contributed significant numbers of medical sons to Guy's staff.[20]
Westminster and St George's both favoured Oxbridge slightly more
often than not, whereas the Middlesex chose Oxbridge less than half
the time, and only five of seventeen physicians at the London Hospital were from Oxford or Cambridge.[21] I have not quantified these
figures because, in the mid decades of the century, it was not infrequent for Cambridge degrees to be given out by royal mandate to
medical graduates of other universities, thus complicating the university background somewhat.

Looked at from the perspective of the Royal College of Physicians,

18 See V. C. Medvei and J. L. Thornton, eds., *The Royal Hospital of Saint
Bartholomew, 1123–1973* (London, 1974).
19 F. G. Parsons, *The History of St. Thomas's Hospital*, 3 vols. (London, 1932–6).
20 See Cameron, *Mr. Guy's Hospital.*
21 J. G. Humble and P. Hansell, *Westminster Hospital, 1716–1966* (London, 1966);
G. S. Peachey, [The History of St. George's Hospital] (London, 1910–14); H. A. St
G. Saunders, *The Middlesex Hospital, 1745–1948* (London, 1949).

however, a slightly different pattern emerges, for before mid-century, Fellows stood a much better chance of obtaining a hospital appointment than did the more lowly licentiates. Indeed, no licentiate made the grade until David Ross and Daniel Cox, elected licentiates in 1749, were appointed physicians to St George's and the Middlesex respectively. However, no fewer than sixteen medical graduates from other universities – mostly Leiden and Rheims – became Fellows through mandated Cambridge medical degrees. Thus, none of the 47 licentiates elected between 1700 and 1748 obtained a hospital appointment, whereas 42 of 111 Fellows did. After mid-century, however, the situation changed, for 84 of the 205 licentiates elected between 1749 and 1800 are known to have held London hospital or dispensary appointments. The figures for the Fellows are 64 of 99: 40 per cent versus 65 per cent, a big difference but not one that suggests the licentiates were finding it impossible to find institutional appointments.[22]

These figures demonstrate that hospital appointments were not very difficult to come by in eighteenth-century London, at least for those attached to the College of Physicians. A few on my list were not affiliated with the College – the College did virtually nothing during the century towards exercising its monopoly over medical practice in London – but most of my men can be found in the annals of the College, for none of the major hospitals appointed from outside the College's ranks (although sometimes election to the licentiate or fellowship followed appointment to the hospital by a year or two).

The second half of the century saw the Scottish universities replace the Continental ones – largely Leiden and Rheims – as the dominant non-Oxbridge universities; it also witnessed the attempt, essentially unsuccessful in the short run, by licentiates such as William Hunter to liberalise the policy of election to fellowships to include others besides those from Oxford and Cambridge. This episode has already been analysed by Clark, Stevenson and Waddington and I shall not add anything to it here.[23] Now, the activities of many of the Scottish-

22   These figures are based on William Munk, *The Roll of the Royal College of Physicians of London*, 7 vols. (London, 1878–1984). Volume II covers the period 1701 to 1800. Although Munk is not always a completely reliable guide, the instances in which I have discovered that he has failed to note an institutional affiliation do not seriously disturb the general thrust of these figures. The licentiates will be under-represented, since their appointments were more often to obscure and short-lived institutions than was the case for Fellows. A figure of 50 per cent for the licentiates will probably eventually be shown to be nearer the mark.
23   Sir George Clark, *History of the Royal College of Physicians of London*, 2 vols. (Oxford, 1964–6); Lloyd G. Stevenson, 'The Siege of Warwick Lane: Together with a Brief History of the Society of Collegiate Physicians (1767–1798)', *Journal of the History of Medicine and Allied Sciences*, VII (1952), 105–21; Ivan Waddington, 'The Struggle to Reform the Royal College of Physicians, 1767–1771: A Sociological Analysis', *Medical History*, XVII (1973), 107–26.

trained men are highlighted by the range of institutional appointments they held. The active involvement of Scottish graduates is
perceptible in the profusion of smaller, specialised institutions founded after mid-century: The dispensaries bear a distinctive Scottish flavour and the Oxbridge élites did not generally deliver babies.[24] The
latter, however, was often an extremely lucrative business, for a
number of fortunes were made in eighteenth-century London by
physician-*accoucheurs*. Early in the century, Sir David Hamilton lost
£80,000 of midwifery earnings in the South Sea Bubble.[25] William
Smellie was successful both at delivering babies and teaching others
how to do so. William Hunter did well off obstetrics, James Ford
made a large fortune in only a decade or so of fashionable practice.
Thomas Denman took a little longer, but was so rich by the age of fifty
that he took only the occasional consultation, otherwise preferring to
spend his time in promoting charity.[26] The range and variety of lying-
in hospitals and maternity charities deserve more systematic examination.[27]

So do the dispensaries, although Irvine Loudon's researches are
helping to illuminate this relatively neglected aspect of the history of
medical care. The General Dispensary, London Dispensary, Western
Dispensary, Bloomsbury Dispensary, Marylebone Dispensary, Surrey Dispensary, Finsbury Dispensary, New Finsbury Dispensary,
Public Dispensary, London Electrical Dispensary – and undoubtedly
others – were by 1800 vying with the hospitals for charitable pounds.
Since they could be run on much smaller budgets, yet still reach large
numbers of patients, they claimed to offer more cost-effective ways of
spending pious money. As Anthony Highmore summarised the situation in 1810, '50,000 were relieved for £5,000 [at the dispensaries], a
sum not exceeding one third of a single hospital which relieves
scarcely 6,000 a year.'[28] For our purposes, even more significantly,
they were initially not simply advocated as philanthropic enterprises

---

24   Frank Nicholls (1699–1778), an Oxford MD and FRCP with a strong interest
in midwifery, could be argued as an exception to the general pattern for male
midwives. On the other hand, Nicholls was not a typical 'élite' figure, and
according to Munk, his relations with the College were not happy.
25   P. Roberts, ed., *The Diary of Sir David Hamilton, 1709–1714* (Oxford, 1975).
26   In addition to the essays on obstetrics in this volume, see Jean Donnison,
Midwives and Medical Men (London, 1977); and Audrey Eccles, *Obstetrics and
Gynaecology in Tudor and Stuart England* (London, 1982).
27   See the works cited in n. 26; S. A. Seligman, 'The Royal Maternity Charity: The
First Hundred Years', *Medical History*, XXIV (1980), 403–18; Margaret Versluysen,
'Midwives, Medical Men and "Poor Women Labouring of Child": Lying-in Hospi-
tals in Eighteenth-Century London', in Helen Roberts, ed., *Women, Health and
Reproduction* (London, 1981), pp. 18–49.
28   Highmore, as quoted by Loudon, 'Dispensary Movement in England', 339.

but as means of advancing medical knowledge. John Coakley Lettsom was definite that the wider experience offered to doctors through contact with large numbers of the sick poor would ultimately benefit medical knowledge. Lettsom and many of his colleagues – often active in the Medical Society of London, which Lettsom himself had founded in 1773 – stressed what Tröhler has called the 'quantification of experience' – the increased use of multiple case reporting, and the call for all medical institutions to improve medical record-keeping and to publish detailed annual results.[29] Their banner was a reformist one, and not surprisingly, those who took up the call were mostly Scottish graduates, many with military experience, where there was some direct relevance to keeping a check on large numbers of individuals and where reporting to one's superiors was routine. The work of Sir Gilbert Blane and Sir James McGrigor in the reform of the military medical services along these lines is well known, and Blane put some of his military ideas into civilian practice during his twelve years as physician at St. Thomas's.[30]

By the 1780s, then, an articulate group of physicians was insisting that hospitals had other than simply philanthropic functions, and although the sentiment was not novel, the ways it was put into practice have some claims to innovation. But most physicians to the general eighteenth-century London hospitals do not seem to have made much use of the wider medical experiences such appointments offered them. Most of course never wrote any books, and two especially popular topics among those who did were smallpox and fevers, with patients suffering from the former always, and the latter generally, excluded from admission to the great voluntary hospitals. The position is less clear for the specialist institutions, for male midwifes like John Leake and Robert Bromfield made much explicit use of their hospital cases in their published writings, as did William Woodville at the Smallpox Hospital. But the Lock and Misericordia hospital physicians never published anything on venereal disease, Woodville's predecessors at the Smallpox were completely silent about their own hospital experiences, and only John Monro's defence of his father's memory emerged from the eighteenth-century Bethlem physicians. Samuel Foart Simmons, physician to St Luke's and the keeper of a successful private lunatic asylum, published a life of William

29 Ulrich Tröhler, 'Quantification in British Medicine and Surgery 1750–1830, with Special Reference to its Introduction into Therapeutics' (PhD thesis, University of London, 1978); Thomas Hunt, ed., *The Medical Society of London 1773–1973* (London, 1972); J. J. Abraham, *Lettsom: His Life, Times, Friends and Descendants* (London, 1933).
30 In addition to Tröhler, 'Quantification in British Medicine', see Christopher Lloyd, ed., *The Health of Seamen* (London, 1965), and Richard L. Blanco, *Wellington's Surgeon General: Sir James McGrigor* (Durham, N.C., 1974).

Hunter and books on gonorrhoea, anatomy and consumption, but nothing on insanity. There were, of course, some exceptions, but most eighteenth-century London physicians apparently saw posts in hospitals as (1) ways of being publicly and visibly charitable; and (2) aids to their own private practices. Such an appointment was usually sought early in one's career or not at all. For instance, George Baker, newly come to London (1761) and with his baronetcy, royal appointment and presidency of the Royal College of Physicians still before him, contemplated accepting posts at both St Thomas's and Guy's, but decided they were too far from his residence. St Bartholomew's was a more attractive proposition, but he failed to secure a position there. 'A Hospital, for the sake of a number of diseases, would . . . be very acceptable for a year or two, if it was within a reasonable distance', he wrote to a friend.[31] In the end, the success of his private practice was such that he never got around to joining the staff of any hospital.

Even after obtaining a hospital appointment, the really successful often resigned after a few years, when the private practice itself was well established. Thus, Richard Mead resigned from St Thomas's in 1714, when his practice grew large. So did Richard Warren, Sir Lucas Pepys, Sir Richard Jebb, Matthew Baillie and a number of others, in a pattern too common to mean anything but that most physicians saw private practice rather than hospital work as the primary preoccupation of their careers. They saw hospitals as a means to a successful private practice rather than private practice as a burden necessary to support the more interesting hospital work. In that sense, hospitals did not have for eighteenth-century doctors the same significance that they did for their nineteenth-century colleagues. Doctors would often maintain contact with their old hospitals as governors, or, towards the end of the century, be elevated to the honorary post of consultant physician. But hospitals were means to ends, rather than ends in themselves. Incidentally, this is not the case for surgeons, who were much more likely to die in office or to retire simultaneously from hospital and practice than were physicians, the obvious difference being the much greater use that surgeons made of hospitals in the training of apprentices, dressers and pupils. Furthermore, there were simply many more surgeons around to vie for the available hospital appointments, the possession of which increased dramatically the apprenticeship premiums a surgeon could command.[32] A

31 Baker to Garthshore, quoted by H. A. Waldron, 'On the Life of Sir George Baker', *Medical History* (in press).
32 See T. Gelfand, chap. 5, this volume, and the forthcoming PhD thesis of Susan Lawrence, University of Toronto.

striking indication of this greater use surgeons made of hospitals for educational purposes can be found at the Middlesex, where 'Surgeons' Pupils' were registered from 1763 and 'Physicians' Pupils' from 1766. Between then and 1800 forty-seven physicians' pupils and 146 surgical pupils were enrolled there. In addition, there were 'House Surgeons' in residence at the Middlesex at least as early as 1763.[33] We should recall here the figures extracted from Simmons's 1783 *Medical Register:* More than half the physicians but less than a third of the surgeons could expect to hold an institutional appointment. Competition for such posts simply was not so keen amongst the physicians.

Physicians thus had less need of permanent hospital affiliations to obtain professional success, and sufficient eighteenth-century London physicians achieved eminence and wealth without *any* hospital appointment to suggest that such appointments, while desirable, were hardly necessary. Peter Shaw and John Fothergill are two examples of success stories achieved outside the hospital; William Hunter is another, though as Porter has reminded us, a special instance. Sir John Pringle is a fourth.[34] Pringle's case, however, reminds us of an alternative road to medical riches: the armed forces. It is well known that the Scots kept the British armed forces manned during the eighteenth century; their medical needs were often looked after by Scottish physicians and surgeons, with a liberal sprinkling of the Irish. Surgeons' mates of course used the navy as a means of setting up civilian surgical practice without fear of prosecution from the Company of Surgeons. An alternative for ex-military surgeons was to purchase a Scottish medical degree and set up as a physician or as an obstetrician. Such, for instance, was the path chosen by Maxwell Garthshore (1732–1812), who after army service, practised for a while in Uppingham. There he was befriended by Sir George Baker, already a London success, who encouraged him to move to London, for which purposes an Edinburgh degree was deemed necessary.

Garthshore's case illustrates a final ingredient for getting on in Georgian London: There can be no doubt about the value of patronage in the medical world of the eighteenth century. Richard Mead's famous father, the Nonconformist divine Matthew Mead, used his

---

33 These figures are taken from the two manuscript volumes of 'Middlesex Hospital Pupils' still in possession of the hospital. The volumes are described in H. C. Thomson, *The Story of the Middlesex Hospital Medical School* (London, 1935), 15.

34 In fact, Pringle did have a dispensary appointment, as *consultant* physician to the Dispensary for the Infant Poor in the 1770s, but such appointments seem to have been used primarily as a way for eminent physicians and surgeons to patronise institutions, or to maintain formal contact with a hospital with which they had been long been associated.

120   W. F. Bynum

pulpit to advance his son's medical career. Richard Warren was started on his meteoric rise to fortune when Sir Edward Wilmot, looking
towards retirement, recommended Warren as his assistant in being
physician to George II's daughter, Princess Amelia. (Warren left his
own family £150,000.) Sir William Duncan's patronage helped John
Eliot, also later knighted, to a practice worth £5,000 per year. The wife
of Lord Burlington was so pleased with the care given her husband by
Dr Robert Taylor that she made her own carriage available to transport patients to his consulting rooms. Further, she sought out invalids, on all of whom she forced her favourite physician.[35]

The ultimate patron, of course, was the king. An appointment to
the medical establishment of the royal household was a coveted mark
of recognition that could only have been socially and financially bene-
ficial. Nor was such an appointment an impossible dream. Between
1762 and 1800, some fifty physicians and thirty-five surgeons held
royal appointments.[36] Furthermore, such testimonies extended further down the medical ranks. In 1783, for instance, there were not
only eight physicians and six surgeons with official responsibilities
toward the royal person, but also four apothecaries, a chemist, an
oculist, an aurist and two dentists with their own particular specialist
functions. There was even an 'anatomist to the household'. The
queen and the Prince of Wales had their own, smaller medical establishments. The role of royal patronage in eighteenth-century England
deserves more systematic examination, but some indication of its
importance can be seen from the fact that the strongest correlation
with professional success, measured either by income or the acquisition of a knighthood or baronetcy, is linked not to hospital appointment or educational background, but to an official attachment to the
royal household. Twenty-nine licentiates and Fellows of the Royal
College of Physicians between 1701 and 1800 were knighted or raised
to a peerage. Amongst the backgrounds of this group (and one man
could of course appear in more than one category) were eight distinguished military careers, eleven hospital appointments, and nineteen appointments to the medical staff of the royal household. Of the
eight royal physicians in 1783, several had previously held hospital

35 These instances are taken from Munk, Roll of the Royal College; on the patronage
system, see N. Jewson, 'Medical Knowledge and the Patronage System in Eighteenth Century England', Sociology, VIII (1974), 369–85.
36 These figures have been compiled from the annual listings in the Royal Kalendar
(n. 2). On the general structure of the royal household for the earlier period, see J.
M. Beattie, The English Court in the Reign of George I (Cambridge, 1967). I am
currently investigating more systematically the medical arrangements of the royal
household. For the special case of George III's breakdown in 1788, see Ida
Macalpine and Richard Hunter, George III and the Mad-Business (London, 1969).

appointments, but none did in 1783. Typical was John Turton, of whom Munk said, '[His] progress as a physician was unusually rapid, and he accumulated a very ample fortune.' Another of the royal physicians, Richard Warren, had long since resigned his appointments at the Middlesex and St George's when the demands of private and royal practice grew too demanding.

IV

What, in conclusion, can we say about the relation of hospitals to medical careers, medical knowledge and the medical profession in eighteenth-century London? My own work to date can hardly assess Professor Holmes's thesis, particularly since in the end the 'coming of the doctor' above all meant for him the coming of the surgeon. But I do think that my own work has not seriously modified the more traditional accounts that date the corporate rise of the medical profession to the nineteenth century and that see this process as intimately linked to hospital medicine and the cluster of ideas, practices and educational patterns that accompanied it. None of this 'hospital medicine' was totally new, and in that sense the second half of the eighteenth century was markedly different from the first: For physicians, at least, a convincing account for social success could probably be drawn mid-way between Holmes's half century from 1680 to 1730, and the more familiar dates between the 1815 Apothecaries' Act and the 1858 Medical Act. For the London physicians, though, three brief conclusions may be suggested:

First, hospital appointments served as useful but not indispensable adjuncts to medical careers. An appointment was a means to success, not a way of rewarding success. Appointments were generally sought and made early in the career or not at all; there was little queuing of ambitious men who had spent years as resident physicians, or proved themselves with appointments to less prestigious institutions. In Victorian England (and after), a hospital post was a mark of recognition; in Enlightenment London it was the expectation of almost any physician who desired one.

Second, hospitals did not provide physicians with fields of experience from which publication was expected. Rather, for the more prestigious, more visible general voluntary and endowed hospitals, an appointment meant contacts with governors and a way of being seen by the public to be charitable.

Third, having stated the bold conclusions, some qualifications are inevitable. There are, of course, exceptions: individual medical men, but more particularly, institutional and chronological ones. Chrono-

logically, the second half of the century saw a marked increase of
hospital use for pedagogical purposes, both for bedside teaching and
for more formal lectures. Even in 1743–4 Richard Kay heard a variety
of hospital-based lectures, most, to be sure, delivered by the surgeons. Although the London surgeons never sought to open up hospitals more generally to the members of the Company of Surgeons
(e.g. along the lines of the rotational model employed at the Royal
Infirmary in Edinburgh),[37] they did make more systematic use of
hospitals than did their physic-professing colleagues. But even physicians were taking pupils at St Thomas's at least as early as 1750, and
by 1783 Simmons could list lectures on medicine and materia medica
by physicians at Guy's, the London, the Westminster and St Thomas's. Medical teaching became another avenue to the professional top
during the second half of the century, not only in the hospitals but
also through the private anatomy schools.[38] Many of the dispensaries
and some of the specialised hospitals became institutions used partially for clinical research, significantly enough, mostly staffed by
Edinburgh graduates denied Fellowship in the College and bent on
opening up the traditional hierarchies of the medical profession.
Symbolic of this new use of hospitals – for research – was a cancer
hospital, founded in 1802 (but short-lived), explicitly devoted to ex-
perimenting with new – and probably dangerous – remedies for dangerous diseases.

The changes, then, are gradual, and neither 1730, 1780, 1815 nor
1858 can be confidently placed as a date by which the doctor had
arrived. The changes are real and sometimes impressive, but then so
are the continuities, and British medicine never really underwent the
wholesale reorganisation and reorientation that French medicine did
from 1794. Thus, by 1850, the hospital *per se* was important for British
physicians, as a workplace as well as a symbol of medical power and
prestige. It was much less so in 1783. All the same, private practice
remained important, financially and professionally, for élite hospital
physicians throughout the nineteenth century, and the very *fact* that
the French model of full-time, hospital-based medical teachers who
were more or less expected to engage in research was never accepted
in Britain lends some credence to Holmes's proposal of a more piece-
meal, informal and individualistic development of the medical profession in this country. In that sense, my own research simply reinforces
Roy Porter's account of William Hunter, and in particular, suggests
that any description of the 'rise' of the medical profession in eigh-

37 See C. J. Lawrence, chap. 6, this volume.
38 See R. Porter and O. Keel, chaps. 1 and 8 respectively, this volume.

teenth-century Britain that cannot accommodate the case of Hunter, who created his own social space, has been blinkered by nineteenth-century corporatism, or twentieth-century sociology, and in this regard, is untrue to the complexities of William Hunter's world.

Acknowledgements

Earlier versions of this essay have been presented on several occasions and I have benefited from discussions. At the Wellcome Institute, Roy Porter has been particularly helpful. My research has been significantly aided by Ben Barkow, who amongst many other things, has been responsible for compiling the Appendix. Research expenses have been generously met by the Wellcome Trustees.

Appendix

Medical charities in eighteenth-century London

Institution	Foundation[1]	Medical staff in 1783[2]	Comments
St Bartholomew's Hospital	c. 1123	3P; 3S; 3AS; 1A	
St Thomas's Hospital	c. 1173	3P; 3S; 1A	
Bethlem Royal Hospital	c. 1247	1P; 1S; 1A	The medical staff of Bethlem & Bridewell are identical.
Christ's Hospital	1552	1P; 1S; 1A	
Bridewell Hospital	c. 1553	1P; 1S; 1A	
Charterhouse	1611	1P; 1S; 1A	
London Workhouse	c. 1649	1P; 1A (1778)	Opinions about the foundation date differ widely. No medical staff listed after 1778.
Royal Hospital, Chelsea	c. 1687	1P; 1S; 2AS; 1A	
Royal Hospital, Greenwich	c. 1705	1P; 1S; 2AS; 1D; 1AD	Date refers to entry of the first pensioners.
Hospital for Poor French Protestants	1718	1P; 1S/A	
Westminster Hospital	1719	3P; 3S; 1A	Also called Public Infirmary.
Guy's Hospital	1726	3P; 3S; 1A	
St George's Hospital	1734	4P; 4S; 1AS; 1HA; 5VA	
London Hospital	1740	3P; 3S; 1A	
Founding Hospital	1741	2P; 1S; 1A	Date refers to reception of patients.

124

Institution	Date	Staff	Notes
Middlesex Hospital	1745	2P; 2PMMW; 4S; 1HS; 1A	
Lock Hospital	1746	1P; 2S; 1HS; 2VA	
Small-pox Hospital	1746	1P; 2A	One apothecary at each of the two sites.
Corporation for Sick and Maimed Seamen	1747	1S	
British Lying-in Hospital	1749	2P; 2CP; 2S; 1A; 1MaMW	
City of London Lying-in Hospital	1750	1PO; 1MMWO; 1MMWE; 1PM-MWE; 1SO; 1SE; 1A; 1MaMW	Possibly 2 MMWE.
St Luke's Hospital for Lunatics	1751	1P; 1S; 1A	
Queen's Lying-in Hospital, Bayswater	1752	1CP; 1PO; 1SMMW; 1A	Medical staff are 1810.
Marine Society	c. 1756	1S; 1A	Medical staff are 1810.
Lying-in Charity for Delivering Poor Married Women	1757	3P	
Magdalen House	1758	1P; 2S; 1A	
Asylum for Orphan Girls (female orphans)	1758	1P; 2S; 1A	
Orphans Working School	1760	1P; 1S; 2A	Medical staff are 1810.
Westminster New Lying-in Hospital	1765	1PMMW; 1PMMWE; 1CP; 1S; 2SA	
General Dispensary for Relief of the Poor	1770	3P; 1CP; 2S; 1A	CP might be PE

(continued)

Medical charities in eighteenth-century London (continued)

Institution	Foundation[1]	Medical staff in 1783[2]	Comments
Dispensary for the Infant Poor[3]	c. 1772	2P; 1S	
Misericordia	1774	1P; 2S	
Westminster General Dispensary	1774	3P; 1CPMMW; 1PMMW; 1S; 1A	Possibly 2P
General Medical Asylum	1776	3P; 1PMMW; 2S; 1A	
London Dispensary	1777	1P; 1SAcc; 1A	
Surrey Dispensary	1777	3P; 1CP; 1SAcc	
Middlesex Dispensary	1778	2P; 1CP; 1S; 1A	
Benevolent Institution	1780	1P	
Finsbury Dispensary	1780	1P; 1PE; 1AP; 1S; 1A	
Eastern Dispensary	1782	1P; 1SAcc; 1A	
Public Dispensary	1782	1P; 1S; 1A	Medical staff are 1800.
St Marylebone General Dispensary	1785	1P; 1PMMW; 1S; 1A	Medical staff are 1810.
New Finsbury and Central Dispensary	1786	1PE; 1PO; 1S; 1A	Medical staff are 1810.
Freemasons Charity for Female Children	1788	2P; 2S; 1A	Medical staff are 1810.
Philanthropic Society	1788	1P; 1S; 1A	Medical staff are 1810.
Western Dispensary	1789	1CP; 2P; 1S; 1A	Medical staff are 1810.
Universal Medical Institution	1792	2P; 1S; 1A	Medical staff are 1810.
London Electrical Dispensary	1793	2P; 1S; 1E	Medical staff are 1800.
Sea-Bathing Infirmary	1796	3CP; 1PO; 2CS	Medical staff are 1800.
Masonic Charity	1798	1S	Medical staff is 1810.

126

Medical charities with unknown medical staff

Institution	Foundation[1]	Comments
Beth Holim (House for Infirm People)	1748	Mentioned in Highmore (1810)
Bayswater General Hospital	1752	Mentioned in F. K. Brown (1961)
Queen Charlotte's Lying-in Hospital	1752	Mentioned in F. K. Brown (1961)
Lying-in Hospital (Tottenham Court Rd.)	1767	Mentioned in F. K. Brown (1961)
Humane Society	1774	Mentioned in *Royal Kalendar* (1783)
General Lying-in Dispensary	1778	Mentioned in F. K. Brown (1961)
Metropolitan Dispensary	1779	Mentioned in Loudon (1981)
Society Known as the Sick Man's Friend	1784	Mentioned in F. K. Brown (1961)
National Truss Society for the Relief of the Ruptured Poor	1786	Mentioned in F. K. Brown (1961)
Benevolent Medical Society	1787	Mentioned in F. K. Brown (1961)
City Dispensary Society	1788	Mentioned in F. K. Brown (1961)
Lying-in Charity at Tottenham	1791	Mentioned in Highmore (1810)
Samaritan Society	1791	Mentioned in Highmore (1810)
Tower Hamlets Dispensary	1792	Mentioned in F. K. Brown (1961)
Bayswater General Lying-in Hospital	1792	Mentioned in F. K. Brown (1961)
Royal Infirmary for Sun Bathing	1796	Mentioned in F. K. Brown (1961)
Benevolent Medical Society (reorganised)	1799	Mentioned in F. K. Brown (1961)

Undated medical charities

Institution	Medical staff where known	Comments
Scots Hospital		Mentioned in *Royal Kalendar* (1783)
Welsh Charity	1P; 1S; 1AS; 1A	Mentioned in *Royal Kalendar* (1783)
St Clement's Dispensary	At least 1S	Mentioned in *Medical Register* (1783)

Key to medical staff

P   Physician
S   Surgeon
D   Dispenser
A   Apothecary
AD   Assistant Dispenser
AP   Assistant Physician
AS   Assistant Surgeon
HS   House Surgeon
HA   House Apothecary
VA   Visiting Apothecary
SA   Superintendent Apothecary
S/A Surgeon and Apothecary
CP   Consulting Physician
PE   Physician Extraordinary
PO   Physician in Ordinary
PMMW   Physician and Man-Midwife

PMMWE   Physician and Man-Midwife Extraordinary
CPMMW   Consulting Physician and Man-Midwife
MMWE   Man-Midwife Extraordinary
MMWO   Man-Midwife in Ordinary
SMMW   Surgeon and Man-Midwife
SE   Surgeon Extraordinary
SO   Surgeon-in-Ordinary
SAcc   Surgeon-*Accoucheur*
CS   Consulting Surgeon
MaMW   Matron and Midwife
E   Electrician

Notes to appendix

1. There are often ambiguities about the foundation dates of earlier institutions. Highmore generally gives a date in his short historical accounts, but his figures have been supplemented by other historical sources. Institutions whose date is given as *circa* retain an ambiguity between different historical sources.
2. The basic sources are the *Medical Register*, 1783 (see n. 1) and the *Royal Kalendar*, 1783 (see n. 2). Additional information about institutions has been taken from the *Royal Kalendar*, 1800; Highmore, 1810 (see n. 16), F. K. Brown, 1961 (see n. 16), and I. S. L. Loudon, 1981 (see n. 16).
3. Institution failed before 1800.

5

'Invite the philosopher, as well as the charitable': hospital teaching as private enterprise in Hunterian London

TOBY GELFAND

Hospital teaching in the eighteenth century is customarily distinguished from private medical instruction. In part this arises from their obviously different physical settings and also because the influential Hunterian tradition, which served as an exemplar for numerous private teaching ventures in late eighteenth- and early nineteenth-century London, was largely independent of hospitals. This essay will argue that any such distinction is superficial and ultimately misleading. From the perspective of eighteenth-century hospital medical men – most of whom were surgeons – hospital teaching was private teaching. Both hospital and extramural private instruction occurred within a common fee-for-educational-service nexus. Both were characterised by individual entrepreneurial initiatives. And both failed to survive beyond the heyday of unregulated capitalism, although hospital teaching evolved into a different type of enterprise.

After comparing private teaching with the traditional apprenticeship, I show that the private enterprise model of hospital teaching existed in Paris. The characterisation, however, is especially applicable to clinical instruction in London. Here, private enterprise in medical education emulated and benefited from broader cultural patterns. Understanding hospital teaching in this light helps explain why London emerged as the world centre for clinical learning during the second half of the eighteenth century. In the allied fields of surgery and midwifery, where Parisian superiority had been taken for granted until about 1750, the British developed an impressive reputation of their own, ultimately eclipsing their neighbours across the Channel.[1]

1 Several authors have noted in passing the essentially private nature of London hospital instruction during the eighteenth and early nineteenth centuries. See M. Jeanne Peterson, *The Medical Profession in Mid-Victorian London* (Berkeley, 1978), pp. 15, 157–8; Charles Newman, 'The Hospital as a Teaching Centre', in *The Evolution of Hospitals in Britain*, ed. F. N. L. Poynter (London, 1964), pp. 187–205, esp. 198–200; H. C. Cameron, *Mr. Guy's Hospital 1726–1948* (London, 1954), p. 88. On Paris teaching, see Toby Gelfand, 'The "Paris Manner" of Dissection: Student Anatomical

Private teaching

Private teaching in the eighteenth century resists clear-cut definition. The diverse manifestations of this kind of instruction shared in common only their *ex officio* status. Whether held in squalid cellars or garrets, private houses, spacious amphitheatres or in hospitals, private courses stood outside formal requirements for the aspiring surgeon or physician. By supplementing formal educational requirements, private courses sought to remedy perceived deficiencies in the apprenticeship experience and in public lecture courses on theoretical subjects. 'Private courses conducted by the great masters, such as the one I attend, were decidedly more profitable than those rigid and boring classes' (formal lectures at the Paris Medical Faculty), wrote an eighteenth-century Paris medical student expressing a generally held opinion.[2] What made private courses more profitable (as well as costly) for students was the privileged access they afforded to materials not generally available from masters or in the theatrical setting of free public lectures – to cadavers, experimental equipment, women in labour and hospital patients. For the instructor, profit lay in improving his knowledge and reputation, and literally, in the student fees.

Like the legal apprenticeship, private instruction represented a bargain between master and disciple sealed by a fee. There were, however, significant differences between the two arrangements. Private instruction remained an informal agreement in which neither notaries nor professional guild became involved. The duration of the contract was brief, seldom more than a few months or a year, compared with the multi-year apprenticeship. Private instruction at Paris or London thus held particular appeal to provincial and foreign students who had money but little time to spend in the capital. Most important, private instruction served a specific educational function. The student or *pensionnaire*, as he was known in France, paid to learn knowledge and skills from a master, not to work for him; he might live in the master's house, but he was not subjected to the menial tasks required of the young apprentice nor did he receive any formal credit towards qualification as a physician or surgeon. Finally, the master was not restricted as to the number of private students he could receive. Liberated from guild strictures, which generally limited masters to one apprentice at a time, private teaching readily evolved into a broad spectrum of courses that competed for students via advertisements in

Dissection in Early Eighteenth-Century Paris', *Bulletin of the History of Medicine* 46 (1972), 99–130.
2   Quoted in Gilbert Chinard, 'The Life of a Parisian Medical Student in the Eighteenth Century', *Bulletin of the History of Medicine* 7 (1939), 376; for similar views, see Gelfand, 'The "Paris Manner"', pp. 116–23.

the public press. Ambitious instructors, whether eminent practitioners or young men on the make, thus had an open market for their
services. They could take on virtually as many fee-paying students as
they could attract and accommodate. Conversely their mediocre or
indifferent confrères in the medical fraternity found themselves without students. Private teaching, in this respect, represented a penetration of Enlightenment liberal economic values of free competition into
medical education.[3]

By the early eighteenth century, private courses had found a niche in
the Paris hospitals. Surgeons who held posts in the major hospitals
brought their apprentices, journeymen, and *pensionnaires* along with
them to the wards and dissection rooms.[4] When Henri-François
Ledran, chief surgeon at the Paris Charité hospital, set up courses in
anatomy and surgical operations for young hospital surgeons in 1725,
his private students, such as the visiting Swiss physician, Albrecht
von Haller, also gained entry.[5] In the early 1740s, William Hunter
apparently attended Ledran's course of surgical operations, although
it is unclear whether Ledran still taught at the Charité.[6] Another Paris
surgeon, Sauveur-François Morand, used appointments at the Char-

3 This claim is admirably developed by Roy Porter, 'William Hunter: A Surgeon
and a Gentleman', chap. 1, this volume. The phenomenon of private courses in
medical, scientific and other disciplines deserves further exploration as a manifestation of entrepreneurial ideology and activity in education. Several essays in
Enseignement et diffusion des sciences en France au XVIIIᵉ siècle, ed. René Taton (Paris,
1964), provide data for such an enquiry. For a survey of the market in private
anatomical courses in London during the first half of the eighteenth century, see
George C. Peachey, *A Memoir of William and John Hunter* (Plymouth, 1924), pp. 8–52.
A medical register for 1783 listed twenty-eight lecture courses, eleven in hospitals
and seventeen extramural, mostly in private homes. All 'clinical lectures' took place
in hospitals. See Arnold Chaplin, *Medicine in England during the Reign of George III*
(London, 1919), pp. 137–8; Zachary Cope, 'The Private Medical Schools of London
(1746–1914)', in *The Evolution of Medical Education in Britain*, ed. F. N. L. Poynter
(London, 1966), pp. 89–109.
4 For examples, see Gabriel Mareschal de Bièvre, *Georges Mareschal* (Paris, 1906),
pp. 103–5; Antoine Louis, 'Eloge de Benomont', in *Eloges lus dans les séances publiques
de l'Académie royale de chirurgie de 1750 à 1792*, ed. E.-F. Dubois (Paris, 1859), pp. 191–
2 (hereafter cited as *Eloges ARC*).
5 Albrecht Haller, *Tagebuch der Studienreise nach London, Paris, Strassburg und Basel
1727 bis 1728*, ed. E. Hintzsche (Bern, 1942), pp. 25–34; 'Eloge de Ledran', *Eloges
ARC*, pp. 165–6.
6 Georges Arnaud, 'De Mr. Hunter', *Mémoires de chirurgie avec quelques remarques
historiques sur l'état de la médecine et de la chirurgie en France et en Angleterre*, 2 vols.
(London, 1768), xiii. Ledran stepped down as chief surgeon to the Charité in 1730,
but he may have continued to use the hospital for private courses. Arnaud's
statement that William Hunter attended Ledran's course 'in 1742', a connection not
mentioned by any other of Hunter's biographers, raises the intriguing possibility
that Hunter's own subsequent private course, where he introduced the 'Paris
manner' of dissection to London in 1746, may have been inspired by contact with
private *hospital* instruction at Paris. See Gelfand, 'The "Paris Manner"', p. 122.

ité and the Invalides hospitals to attract a large international retinue of private students to his 'school of anatomy and surgery'. Between 1726 and 1746 Morand had more than seventy foreign *pensionnaires*, many of whom were said to be English and Scottish.[7]

The Paris Charité had a reputation for opening its wards to students. A relatively small hospital (200 beds), the Charité proved responsive to the wishes of Paris surgeons, who during the Regency period (1715–23) in particular enjoyed support from the royal government against the monks entrusted with the hospital's administration.

At the immense Hôtel-Dieu, housing several thousand patients and administered by a secular board that stubbornly defended ancient traditions against infringement by either royal government or medical profession, the environment for private instruction appeared much less favourable. By the early eighteenth century, the Hôtel-Dieu admitted one hundred young surgeons to its wards. The primary job of this surgical hierarchy, which consisted of about twenty-five living in the hospital and the remainder coming to work as *externes* on a daily basis, was to care for patients. These hospital workers came under the close surveillance and supervision of the administrative board and the direct orders of the chief hospital surgeon and the senior resident surgeon or *gagnant-maîtrise*.[8] In return for their unpaid service, the house surgeons received occasional anatomical and clinical instruction. The administrators of the Hôtel-Dieu expected their chief surgeons to find time for such teaching, which was to be provided gratis to hospital surgeons and to be closed to outside students.[9] Thus, bureaucratic directive rather than private enterprise organised teaching at the Hôtel-Dieu.

Despite these regulations, the surgeons of the Hôtel-Dieu did not always resist the temptation to take in private fee-paying students. In the mid-seventeenth century, the administrators heard complaints that the chief surgeon, Jacques Petit, allowed his *pensionnaires* (*petits*

---

7 J.-F. Morand, *Lettre traduite du Latin sur feu M. Morand*, p. 12. 'Eloge de Morand', *Eloges ARC*, p. 209: 'Il avait établi dans chacune de ces maisons publique, et dans la sienne, une école d'anatomie et de chirurgie.'
8 See T. Gelfand, 'Gestation of the Clinic', *Medical History* 25 (1981), 169–80.
9 *Délibérations de l'ancien bureau de l'Hôtel Dieu*, in *Collection de documents pour servir à l'histoire des hôpitaux de Paris*, ed. Léon Briel, 2 vols. (Paris, 1881), I, p. 257 (31 December 1706) (hereafter cited as *Délibérations*). The regulation of 1706 establishing a regular winter series of anatomical dissection lessons forbade the attendance of 'les chirurgiens qui ne sont point de l'Hôtel Dieu' unless they had written permission from the administrators. The need to repeat this prohibition against outsiders suggests that it may not have been rigorously enforced. Major operations, such as lithotomies, often drew unruly crowds of students and medical men to the wards of the Hôtel-Dieu, despite protests from the religious nursing sisters. See *Délibérations*, I, pp. 306–7 (4 April 1730), 321–2 (3 May 1735).

garçons chirurgiens) to work on the wards while, at the same time, he tried to extort fees from the house *externes*.[10] Petit was not alone in seeking to use the Hôtel-Dieu for private profit. In 1687 a group of house resident surgeons, having obtained 'a few cadavers for dissection', let outsiders attend for a fee and denied *externes* free admission.[11]

A century later, in 1789, Pierre-Joseph Desault testified that his predecessor, Jean-Nicholas Moreau, chief surgeon of the Hôtel-Dieu from 1744 to 1786, 'permettait à qui bon lui semblait d'assister à ses leçons, qu'il y avait autant d'étrangers que d'élèves de la maison, qu'il y avait un cabinet d'anatomie où il faisait disséquer les chirurgiens du dehors, qu'il leur faisait pratiquer des opérations dans la salle des morts . . . il recevait de l'argent, même des élèves de la maison, pour les exercer à la pratique des opérations'.[12] Desault vigorously denied that he followed such venal practices in his own vastly expanded program of clinical teaching at the Hôtel-Dieu. But in November 1791, under attack from students who demanded open and gratis admission to the Hôtel-Dieu wards and teaching amphitheatre, Desault adamantly defended his policy of charging fees to outsiders. Although he continued to admit the one hundred house surgeons without charge to clinical lessons, he required several hundred outside students to pay one louis per course. Claiming that free public instruction was not characteristic of other Paris hospitals, Desault concluded, 'que l'éducation gratuite est la pire de toutes: qu'elle anéantit le zèle du professeur; qu'elle détruit l'activité de l'écolier'.[13]

A succinct and powerful formulation of medical education as private enterprise, Desault's plea to the Legislative Assembly probably fell upon deaf ears.[14] But the Hôtel-Dieu chief surgeon, despite his own unquestioned devotion to hospital service and teaching, clearly

---

10 *Délibérations*, I, pp. 112–13 (26 October 1655). Petit defended himself by claiming his predecessors had also taken money from young hospital surgeons. Ibid., p. 113 (3 December 1655). *Externes* were required to supply lancets to the resident surgeons when they first entered the Hôtel-Dieu. Ibid., p. 156 (7 July 1662).
11 *Délibérations*, I, p. 231 (17 January 1687).
12 Ibid., II, p. 241 (2 April 1789).
13 'Reclamation de M. Desault, chirurgien en chef de l'Hôtel-Dieu de Paris, contre une pétition présentée à l'assemblée nationale par des élèves en chirurgie', Archives Nationales, D XXXVIII, 3, 47. See T. Gelfand, 'A Confrontation over Clinical Instruction at the Hôtel-Dieu of Paris during the French Revolution', *Journal of the History of Medicine and Allied Sciences* 28 (1973), 268–82.
14 Gelfand, 'Confrontation over Clinical Practice', p. 282. Similar praise for private profit teaching came from another leading Paris surgeon of the period: 'Ce [private instructors] sont encore des maîtres d'autant meilleurs, que leur fortune dépend de leur enseignement et de la réputation bien meritée qu'ils se procurent.' Jacques Tenon, *Observation sur les obstacles qui s'opposent aux progrès de l'anatomie* (Paris, 1785), p. 30.

summarised the general attitude of eighteenth-century medical men towards clinical instruction. Education ought not to be a public service freely dispensed by the hospital. In a sense, even charity patients were expected to compensate hospital practitioners by serving as subjects for clinical teaching during life and for anatomical dissection after death.[15]

One further opportunity for instruction at the Hôtel-Dieu of Paris held special attraction for foreigners: admission to the pregnancy and delivery wards (*la salle des accouchées*). In the early eighteenth century, midwifery was a rapidly expanding field of much interest to male practitioners. At first surgeons, and then physicians, became aware of the lucrative profits available if attendance upon pregnant women and delivery of their babies could be wrested from female midwives. The Hôtel-Dieu had a reputation as one of the best places in Europe to gain experience in obstetrics.[16] Unfortunately for male professional aspirations, the nursing sisters of the Hôtel-Dieu vehemently opposed the admission of outside surgeons to their labour room, and, in a ruling in December 1720, the administrative board respected their views on the 'indecency' of permitting men to serve as *accoucheurs*.[17]

Although exceptions were made, the doors of the labour room of the Hôtel-Dieu had, by the 1730s, evidently been firmly closed to male visitors. It is worth noting that amongst the privileged few who gained admission during the Regency, the majority were English or Scottish. Hospital records indicate that five British medical men managed to be admitted to the labour room as a result of personal intervention by the regent on their behalf.[18] In October 1721, for example, 'docteur Campbel' was admitted for a three-month period to observe and 'même de travailler si les chirurgiens le jugent à propos'.[19]

15 Michel Foucault, *The Birth of the Clinic: An Archeology of Medical Perception*, trans. A. M. Sheridan Smith (New York, 1973), pp. 83–5, has described this quid pro quo as a tacit 'clinical contract' between indigent patient and hospital. In fact, eighteenth-century hospital authorities were more reticent than medical men to acknowledge such a bargain. One rare explicit statement came from the board of the Paris Hôpital Général in 1731, urging the poor 'à vaincre leur répugnance' towards serving as subjects for anatomical dissection. 'Délibération du Bureau de l'Hôpital Général . . . 12 mars 1731', Archives de la Préfecture de Police, Collection Lamoignon, vol. 30, fol. 281. See also T. Gelfand, 'A Clinical Ideal: Paris 1789', *Bulletin of the History of Medicine* 51 (1977), 397–411, esp. 406–9.
16 Marcel Fosseyeux, *L'Hôtel Dieu de Paris au XVIIe et au XVIIIe siécle* (Paris, 1912), pp. 286–95.
17 *Délibérations*, I, pp. 284–5 (31 December 1720).
18 Ibid., p. 274 (30 December 1716); pp. 276–7 (20 May 1718); p. 287 (24 October 1721); p. 288 (1 July 1722); p. 289 (28 July 1723).
19 Campbel obtained this favour by means of a letter from the king of England to the French regent, who in turn put pressure upon the hospital board via his chief minister, Cardinal Dubois, and the *procureur général*. As well, Campbel declared himself to be a Roman Catholic. Mention of an Irish surgeon working as an *externe* at the Hôtel-Dieu is in *Délibérations*, I, p. 292 (6 April 1925).

Although no fees were explicitly mentioned, this kind of opportunity clearly qualified as private hospital instruction.

Private teaching in the London hospitals during the second half of the eighteenth century can be understood as part of the British surgical élite's development of their own resources instead of depending, as earlier, on Parisian initiatives. Here, a comment by the exiled Paris surgeon, George Arnaud, provides a useful insight. Writing from London in 1768, Arnaud quoted an editorial remark that had appeared in the English translation of Ledran's *Traité des opérations* published twenty years earlier:

> It must be confessed, that both anatomy and surgery flourished much later in England than in France, where all possible encouragements were given to both: while, in London, the governors of the two hospitals, being mostly citizens, out of a false policy, entirely refused the education of pupils in one hospital, and allowed of but nine at a time in the other.[20]

To this passage, probably written by Cheselden, Arnaud added his own footnote: 'There were then only two hospitals in London; over the last twenty years, twelve or fifteen have been established and they all have extremely well-instructed students in abundance.'[21]

Arnaud referred, of course, to the remarkable proliferation of hospitals and infirmaries, usually known as the voluntary hospital movement, which began in London during the third decade of the eighteenth century.[22] Despite some chronological and numerical inaccuracies in his hospital count, the French surgeon had identified the crucial novelty in British medicine after mid-century.

London hospitals served the needs of late eighteenth-century clinical instruction better than their Paris counterparts, I suggest, because they fit better the then-dominant private enterprise style of medical education. As new foundations, most London hospitals were peculiarly sensitive to eighteenth-century conceptions of private enterprise. A voluntary hospital depended for its survival on an ability to compete effectively with a profusion of rival hospitals and other charitable institutions for limited funds from private philanthropists or subscribers.[23]

Cheselden's remark, quoted earlier, deplored the policies of 'mostly citizens' in neglecting medical education in London hospitals

20 *The Operations in Surgery of Monsieur LeDran*, trans. Thomas Gataker (London, 1749), p. 472, quoted in Arnaud, *Mémoires de chirurgie*, II, p. 824.
21 Arnaud, *Mémoires de chirurgie*, II, p. 824.
22 See John Woodward, *To Do the Sick No Harm: A Study of the British Voluntary Hospital System to 1875* (London, 1974).
23 See David Owen, *English Philanthropy 1660–1960* (Cambridge, Mass., 1965), pp. 36–61.

prior to 1750, and, clearly, hospital governors did not cede much power to their medical staffs until more than a century later.[24] Yet the hospital surgeons' very lack of administrative authority (and responsibility) may have encouraged them to take an entrepreneurial attitude towards the hospital, and to consider how the institution might best serve private professional interests, whether they be practical, didactic or research oriented. Receiving no salary at all (or a merely honorific £40 per year at St Thomas's and Guy's),[25] the voluntary hospital surgeons, themselves volunteers, did not share in kind or intensity the contractual obligations of their counterparts at the Hôtel-Dieu of Paris, who were paid a respectable, if modest, 2,000 livres. London hospital men could not be expected to provide the free instruction that constituted an official, if sometimes neglected, responsibility of the Hôtel-Dieu chief surgeon. Instead, they had every reason to view the hospital as an extension of their private practice and teaching.[26]

Private arrangements, in fact, defined the status of students in London hospitals: Apprentices and dressers purchased entrée and the right to work on the wards directly from surgeons to whom they paid substantial fees. Other pupils, who simply 'walked the wards' as observers, made similar financial settlements with medical professionals rather than with hospital authorities. In Paris, by contrast, reciprocal responsibilities and obligations linking worker-students and hospitals took precedence over private arrangements between surgeons and students. The Hôtel-Dieu compensated young surgeons for their work, not just with opportunities for practical experience and learning, but also with room, board, the status of a position in the hospital and, for the talented few, the prospect of a long-term post.[27] Whereas the London hospital pupil purchased instruction for a fee, the Paris hospital worker helped take care of patients and learned what he could by experience.

24 Peterson, *Medical Profession in Mid-Victorian London*, pp. 173–88; Brian Abel-Smith, *The Hospitals 1800–1948* (Cambridge, Mass., 1964), pp. 32–45.
25 Letter of Joseph Warner to John Gunning (29 December 1792), quoted in Cameron, *Mr. Guy's Hospital*, p. 92.
26 Hospital medical men, as a rule, could not sit on boards of governors. Although individual medical men were sometimes influential in the founding of hospitals and their subsequent administration, the profession as such remained marginal.
27 *Gagnants-maîtrise* at the major Paris hospitals served for six years in return for free entry into the Paris surgical company, a reward worth several thousand livres. At the Hôtel-Dieu, senior resident surgeons often served as long as fifteen years before becoming candidates for the *gagnat-maîtrise* post. See Gelfand, *Professionalizing Modern Medicine: Paris Surgeons and Medical Science and Institutions in the Eighteenth Century* (Westport, Conn., 1980), pp. 49–51, 101–2. The London hospital 'house-surgeon' enjoyed no such tenure or privileges during a relatively brief term of a year or two. See Peachey, *A Memoir of William and John Hunter*, pp. 106–8.

These contrasting educational experiences derived from basic differences between French and British hospitals. A product of state and church foundation and administration, the large French hospital marshalled human and material resources into an elaborate hierarchical chain of command. The Hôtel-Dieu functioned as an authoritarian and bureaucratic institution. British hospitals depended to a much greater extent upon private humanitarian and charitable initiatives for their foundation, administration and medical personnel. Students took advantage of opportunities available in the London hospitals in much the same spirit of voluntarist piety combined with self-improving investment in a career. Thus political realities and cultural values characteristic of the two nation-states manifested themselves in their respective ways of organising public assistance.[28]

From Paris to London

In 1750 an anonymous polemical essay appeared in London entitled *A Short Comparative View on the Practice of Surgery in the French Hospitals: with some remarks on the study of anatomy and midwifery. The whole endeavouring to prove that the advantages to students, in these professions, are greater at London than at Paris*. Probably written by the surgeon John Harrison, one of the founders of the London Hospital, *A Short Comparative View* denounced Paris surgery, impugned the skills and character of its practitioners and sought to persuade Britons to stay on their own side of the Channel:

> Let us rather embrace every opportunity our native country affords us, of excelling in our professions, and by observing and imitating those great examples which are at the head of our hospitals, show the French, that we need not copy anything from them but a self-sufficiency, and love for our own country.[29]

Harrison's chauvinistic harangue was somewhat undercut by the fact that he himself had evidently studied in the French capital. By his own admission, the trip was generally deemed essential to a complete training in surgery and midwifery, and he grudgingly conceded that Paris presented two advantages over London: free hospital attendance and an abundant supply of cadavers for dissection.[30]

28 See Owen, *English Philanthropy*; Olwen Hufton, *The Poor of Eighteenth-Century France, 1750–1789* (Oxford, 1974); Thomas M. Adams, 'Medicine and Bureaucracy: Jean Colombier's Regulation for the French *dépots de mendicité*', *Bulletin of the History of Medicine* 52 (1978), 529–41.
29 *A Short Comparative View*, p. 56. For further discussion of this work and its authorship, see Gelfand, 'The "Paris Manner"', pp. 124–5.
30 *A Short Comparative View*, pp. 4–8.

138   Toby Gelfand

Yet, even as Harrison wrote, the situation was shifting in favour of London, on its way to becoming, in the phrase of one American medical student visitor in the 1780s, 'the Metropolis of the whole world for practical medicine'.[31] Two other Americans, John Morgan (1735–89) and Benjamin Rush (1745–1813), who visited both London and Paris hospitals in the 1760s, judged the British learning experience superior; a third, William Shippen (1736–1808), did not bother to go to Paris, confining his studies in 1759 to London.[32] In 1787, Jacques Tenon, Paris surgeon and the leading European authority on hospitals, undertook a mission for the Académie des Sciences to report on British hospitals, prisons and workhouses. He found them, in general, much superior to their French counterparts. Although Tenon's primary concern on this visit went to matters of hospital construction, administration and sanitation, he also alluded to the advantages of British hospitals for medical education.[33]

These impressions of medical Anglophilia find support in an analysis of surgical and allied literature. Prior to mid-century, numerous English translations of French treatises were published but few English surgical authors beyond Samuel Sharp appeared in French translation (see Table 5.1). In all, French publications in anatomy, surgery and midwifery greatly exceeded English publications, perhaps by as much as fourfold.[34] British surgeons and translators openly praised French authors such as Dionis and Ledran as superior to their native products.[35] During the second half of the century, however, London surgical publications came to equal and perhaps surpass the number of Paris publications.[36] More significantly,

31 Quoted in Whitfield J. Bell, Jr., 'Philadelphia Medical Students in Europe, 1750–1800', in his The Colonial Physican and Other Essays (New York, 1975), p. 55.
32 Betsy Copping Corner, William Shippen, Jr.: Pioneer in American Medical Education (Philadelphia, 1951); Benjamin Rush, MS Journal of Trip to Paris (1769), in Historical Society of Pennsylvania, Philadelphia; Letter from John Morgan to Alexander Dick (20 February 1764) in Library of the College of Physicians, Philadelphia. Two other surgeons, the Italian Antonio Scarpa (1752–1832) and the Czech Johann Hunczovsky (1752–98), who visited Paris and London hospitals in the late eighteenth century, had a more favourable opinion of the latter.
33 Jacques Tenon, Mémoires sur les hôpitaux de Paris, pp. 229, 326. See Louis S. Greenbaum, 'The Commercial Treaty of Humanity. La tournée des hôpitaux anglais par Jacques Tenon en 1787', Revue d'Histoire des Sciences 24 (1971), 317–50.
34 During the period 1690–1746, seventy-one French surgical authors (fifty-five published at Paris) as compared with nineteen British (all London) are listed in a very extensive bibliography compiled in Robert James, Dictionnaire universel de Médecine, 6 vols. (Paris 1746–48), III, pp. 444–7 (original London edition published in 1745).
35 Gelfand, 'The "Paris Manner"', pp. 123–4.
36 I have found no bibliography comparable to James's for this period. The Index Catalogue of the Library of the Surgeon-General's Office, 1st ser., vol. 13 (Washington, D.C., 1892) contains under the rubric 'Surgery' nineteen authors who published at London and fourteen at Paris during the period 1750–99.

French translations of British surgical works became popular, in effect reversing the earlier pattern. The writings of Percivall Pott, in particular, were avidly translated into French (Table 5.1).

Paris did not, of course, abruptly cease after mid-century to be an important surgical center. Throughout the century, there were fruitful interchanges in both directions across the Channel.[37] The French capital maintained until well into the nineteenth century its reputation as the place of preference for anatomical dissection, a result, as John Harrison had noted, of a more accessible supply of cadavers.[38] As is well known, after the Revolution, Paris recovered European leadership, this time in medicine as well as surgery.[39] Nevertheless, for the period extending between approximately mid-century and the French Revolution, the centre of gravity for hospital instruction clearly shifted to London. On the eve of the Revolution, the most influential plan for reform of French medicine noted: 'cet usage [of hospitals for teaching] est à-peu-près suivi en Angleterre; on y trouve dans chaque hôpital une salle d'enseignement et des salles d'opérations et de dissection'.[40]

Why did Britain, and London in particular, gain, if only briefly, its position of leadership? This question has often been answered by singling out the private school of anatomy and surgery founded by William Hunter and carried on by his younger brother John, William Hewson, William Cruikshank, Matthew Baillie and others.[41] I have already suggested that the rise of private instruction in London hospitals probably overshadowed even the Great Windmill Street school; in any case, the latter's forte was anatomical and physiological, not clinical, teaching. Moreover, as we shall see in John Hunter's instance, the two teaching spheres overlapped, complementing as well

37   Pierre Huard, 'Les échanges médicaux franco-anglais au XVIIIe siècle', *Clio Medica* 3 (1968), 41–58.
38   See also Russell C. Maulitz, 'Channel Crossing: The Lure of French Pathology for English Medical Students, 1816–36', *Bulletin of the History of Medicine* 55 (1981), 475–96, esp. 482–3.
39   See Erwin H. Ackerknecht, *Medicine at the Paris Hospital 1794–1848* (Baltimore, 1967), esp. pp. 191–4.
40   *Nouveau plan de constitution pour la médecine en France*, in *Histoire de la Société Royale de Médecine, 1787 et 1788* (Paris, 1790), p. 64. The qualification of praise for British hospital teaching indicated by the 'à peu prés' suggests more subtlety than do recent revisionist historians who argue that the essential ingredients of the later Paris 'clinical-anatomical' school were anticipated at eighteenth-century London and Edinburgh. See Othmar Keel, *La généalogie de l'histopathologie: Une révision déchirante* (Paris, 1979), esp. pp. 51–7. A full-scale *étude d'ensemble* of late eighteenth-century London hospital medicine is still unavailable, but Susan Lawrence's doctoral dissertation, now in progress at the University of Toronto, should redress this gap.
41   Stewart Craig Thomson, 'The Great Windmill Street School', *Bulletin of the History of Medicine* 12 (1942), 377–91. The historiographical dominance of the Hunterian tradition is epitomised by the *Index Catalogue's* rubric 'Surgery (Ancient) [Prior to John Hunter's teachings – circa 1780]'.

Table 5.1. *Selected list of French-English and English-French translations of surgical and allied works in the eighteenth century*

Author	Short title	First edition	Translation
French to English			
Belloste	Chirurgien d'hôpital	Paris, 1695	London, 1701
Leclerc, G.	Chirurgie Complète	Paris, 1694	London, 1701
Dionis, P.	Anatomie de l'homme	Paris, 1690	London, 1703
	Cours d'Opérations	Paris, 1707	London, 1710
	Traité des accouchemens	Paris, 1718	London, 1719
Verduc, J. B.	Usage des parties	Paris, 1696	London, 1704
Portal, P.	Pratique des accouchemens	Paris, 1685	London, 1705
Verduc, L.	Manière de guérir les fractures	Paris, 1689	London, 1706
La Charrière	Traité des opérations	Paris, 1692	London, 1712
Garengeot	Traité des opérations	Paris, 1720	London, 1723
Petit, J. L.	Maladies des os	Paris, 1723	London, 1726
Winslow	Exposition anatomique	Paris, 1732	London, 1733–4
Astruc	De morbis venereis	Paris, 1736	London, 1737
Ledran	Parallèle . . . de tirer la pierre	Paris, 1730	London, 1738
	Obs. de Chirurgie	Paris, 1731	London, 1739
	Traité des opérations	Paris, 1742	London, 1749
Saviard	Obs. chirurgicales	Paris, 1702	London, 1740
La Motte	Accouchemens	Paris, 1721	London, 1746
Chirac	Obs. de Chirurgie	Paris, 1742	London, 1750
Astruc	Art d'accoucher	Paris, 1766	London, 1767
Goulard	Effets des preparations de plomb	Pezenas, 1760	London, 1769
	Maladies venériennes	Pezenas, 1760	London, 1772
Baudeloque	Art des accouchemens	Paris, 1781	London, 1790

English to French

Douglas, John	New Method of Cutting for the Stone	London, 1723	Paris, 1724
Taylor, J.	Mechanism of the Eye	Norwich, 1727	Paris, 1738
Sharp	Operations of Surgery	London, 1739	Paris, 1741
Turner	Critical Enquiry into the Present State of Surgery	London, 1750	Paris, 1751
	Diseases Incident to the Skin	London, 1714	Paris, 1743
	Syphilis	London, 1717	Paris, 1767
Ranby	Gunshot Wounds	London, 1744	Paris, 1745
Smellie	Theory and Practice of Midwifery	London, 1752	Paris, 1754–8
Warner	Cases in Surgery	London, 1754	Paris, 1757
Monro, A.	Anatomy of the Humane Bones	Edinburgh, 1726	Paris, 1759
Pott	Fractures and Dislocations	London, 1768	Paris, 1771
	Chirurgical Works	London, 1771	Paris, 1777–92
	Palsy of the Lower Limbs . . . Found to Accompany a Curvature of the Spine	London, 1779	Paris, 1783
Burton	New System of Midwifery	London, 1751	Paris, 1771–3
White	Pregnant and Lying-in Women	London, 1773	Paris, 1774
Underwood	Ulcers of the Leg	London, 1783	Paris, 1784
Clare	New and Easy Method of Curing the Lues	London, 1780 (3d ed.)	Paris, 1785
Hunter, John	Venereal Disease	London, 1786	Paris, 1787
	Blood, Inflammation, and Gunshot Wounds	London, 1797	Paris, 1798–9

A chronological order by date of translation is followed. Translations were not necessarily made from first edition of work as listed. See *A Short Title Catalogue of Eighteenth Century Printed Books in the National Library of Medicine*, compiled by John Blake (Washington: U.S. Government Printing Office, 1979). – – – – – = midcentury line of demarcation between Paris dominance during first half of eighteenth century and London dominance during second half.

as competing with one another. Before looking more closely at hospital teaching as private enterprise, I want first to consider several related factors in the ascendancy of London over Paris.

First, by mid-century, London medical men had effectively assimilated French clinical experience. One might date this process of cultural transmission back to the turn of the century when the surgeon Paul Buissière, a Huguenot refugee, apparently became one of the first to teach private courses of anatomy in London.[42] At mid-century, several leading London hospital surgeons, including Samuel Sharp at Guy's (1733–57), Caesar Hawkins at St George's (1735–74) and John Harrison at the London (1740–53) had availed themselves of opportunities for study in the French capital.[43] In 1746, the 'Paris manner' of providing cadavers to students in private anatomy courses became a London practice as well, first under William Hunter, and soon afterwards, generally. The Paris educational experience of Hunter and his British colleagues, imported and adapted for home consumption, made it less urgent for the next generation to cross the Channel. Hunter's fellow Scot, teacher and colleague, William Smellie, who studied at Paris in 1739 and then returned to London to establish the foremost private school of midwifery in Europe, epitomised the transfer process.[44]

Second, the rise and recognition of the Edinburgh medical school as a major centre for theoretical studies and, to a lesser extent, a clinical centre thanks to its Royal Infirmary, undoubtedly diverted English-speaking students from the Continent. In particular, the de-

42 Peachey, *A Memoir of William and John Hunter*, p. 9. Another Huguenot surgeon, Claudius Amyrand (1685–1740), served at Westminster Hospital and was involved in the establishment of St George's. Huard, 'Les échanges médicaux', p. 48. In this respect, it is worth noting that the French Protestant hospital, which opened in London in 1716, preceded the voluntary hospital foundations. See W. H. McMenemy, 'The Hospital Movement of the Eighteenth Century and Its Development', in Poynter, *Evolution of Hospitals*, pp. 43–71, esp. 46–7.
43 The dates given refer to each surgeon's tenure at the respective hospital. See Huard, 'Les échanges médicaux', pp. 45–6. In retrospect, John Hunter deprecated the outdated training of the older generation of surgeons who had been his colleagues at St George's when he arrived at the hospital in 1768: 'The late Mr. Hawkins and Bromfield the senior surgeons had got beyond the age of improvement; their education had been prior to the period of improvement in this country'; quoted in Peachey, *A Memoir of William and John Hunter*, p. 275.
44 John Glaister, *Dr. William Smellie and his Contemporaries* (Glasgow, 1894), esp. p. 29. Several of William Hunter's teachers and colleagues studied at Paris. See Gelfand, 'The "Paris Manner"', pp. 102–3. John Hunter boasted that his brother's achievement had single-handedly turned British medical students away from Contental studies: 'He [William Hunter] was the only one that stem'd the course of our young Gentlemen going to Holland and France for their medical education, he even inverted the stream.' Samuel Foart Simmons and John Hunter, *William Hunter 1718–1783, A Memoir*, ed. C. H. Brock (Glasgow, 1983), p. 6.

gree-granting privileges of Edinburgh and other Scottish medical schools proved attractive to young British and American medical men who, prior to mid-century, had ventured across to Rheims for the easy degrees dispensed by that French university.[45]

Third, the dissolution of the Barbers-Surgeons' Company in 1745 gave a stimulus to private instruction. The Company of Surgeons, now dominated by hospital surgeons, repealed a by-law that until then had effectively prohibited dissection courses from competing with the anatomy lessons held at Barber-Surgeons' Hall. The new hands-off policy gave free rein to the entrepreneurial teaching inclinations of leading surgeons, many of whom readily paid fines rather than fulfil routine obligations to serve as officers and lecturers for the surgical company.[46]

Finally, there was evidence of an absolute decline in educational opportunities in Paris during the decades after mid-century. Practical training in surgery and midwifery suffered a series of reverses, such as the closure of the labour wards at the Hôtel-Dieu and, in 1761, a loss of direct professional control over the surgical wards of the Charité Hospital.[47] At a time when the reputation of the Hunter brothers was becoming international, the Paris Academy of Surgery appeared on the wane, the publication of its *Mémoires* ceasing after 1774. Never a prestigious centre for the study of medicine, Paris anatomy, surgery and midwifery now also seemed diminished in stature especially when compared with British counterparts. Given British ascendancy over its traditional rival in the military, political and economic spheres during the second half of the century, it is not surprising to find the same in medicine and, specifically, in the use of hospitals for private teaching.

The London hospital as private school

I conceived that to give the hospital a reputation for improvement it was to invite the philosopher, as well as the charitable to contribute to its support. Other hospitals were beginning to participate in the improving spirit of the times, more especial-

45   Huard, 'Les échanges médicaux', pp. 45–6; Bell, 'Philadelphia Medical Students in Europe'; Joseph F. Kett, 'Provincial medical practice in England, 1730–1815', *Journal of the History of Medicine* 19 (1964), 17–29. Kett notes (pp. 26–7) that by 1791, 60 percent of all medical degrees held by practitioners outside of London had been conferred by the four Scottish universities: Edinburgh, Glasgow, Aberdeen and St Andrews.
46   Cecil Wall, *The History of the Surgeons' Company, 1745–1800* (London, 1937), p. 60.
47   Gelfand, *Professionalizing Modern Medicine*, p. 106.

ly those into which the younger surgeons had been elected.
They united their powers and had lectures given to their
pupils not only in surgery but in every branch of the healing
art.[48]
So wrote John Hunter in 1793 about his unsuccessful effort over the
preceding quarter-century to establish a 'regular school of medicine'
at St George's Hospital where he had been a surgeon since 1768.
Embroiled in what was to be the final confrontation with his surgical
colleagues, Hunter took the stance of an aggressive champion of private instruction. His letters to the governors of St George's and his
adversaries' replies exposed tensions in the hospital as private
enterprise.

The 1792–3 conflict also reflected how the organisation of hospital
teaching had matured since William Cheselden's comment that 'the
governors of the two hospitals . . . entirely refused the education of
pupils in one hospital, and allowed of but nine at a time in the other'.
Cheselden most likely referred to practices at St Bartholomew's and
St Thomas's hospitals during the early decades of the century when
the two medieval foundations remained the only general hospitals in
London. According to an historian of St Thomas's, the governors of
the hospital actively discouraged medical instruction and in fact limited the admission of pupils to the hospital to three per surgeon for a
total of nine.[49] At St Bartholomew's, students apparently were admitted to the wards as early as the mid-seventeenth century, but the
evidence of teaching remains thin until more than a century later.[50]

By the second half of the century, potential resources for clinical
teaching had increased dramatically. The two royal hospitals had
been rebuilt and expanded; in rapid succession, between 1720 and
1745 five new general hospitals – Westminster, Guy's, St George's,
London and Middlesex – were established by private philanthropy.
Numerous maternity hospitals, perhaps as many as seven in London,
also the result of voluntary subscription campaigns, opened their
doors between 1740 and 1760. Lastly, other speciality hospitals like
the Lock for venereal diseases (1746), St Luke's for lunacy (1751) and

48 'John Hunter to the Governors of St. George's Hospital' (28 February 1793),
quoted in Peachey, *A Memoir of William and John Hunter*, pp. 275–6.
49 F. G. Parsons, *The History of St. Thomas's Hospital*, 2 vols. (London, 1934), II pp.
182–3.
50 *The Royal Hospital of Saint Bartholomew 1123–1973*, ed. Victor C. Medvei and John
L. Thornton (London, 1974), pp. 44–9. Hospital instruction began in earnest with
Percivall Pott's courses in the late 1760s. Pott evidently did not charge fees for the
courses *per se*, but pupils' fees for entry into the wards at St Bartholomew's, as
elsewhere, were divided amongst the surgical and medical staff.

various dispensaries offered opportunities for clinical learning.[51] Before the century's end, four hospitals – St Thomas's and Guy's (the United), St Bartholomew's and the London – housed recognised schools of medicine, defined at the time as 'the whole course of lectures for the improvement of pupils in chirurgical and medical knowledge . . . concentrated within the verge of the respective hospitals'.[52] In addition, as Arnaud had noted, numerous other hospitals provided instruction to students.

Hospital schools were private inasmuch as the pupils paid fees to their instructors and not to the hospitals. The essential part of the hospital learning experience lay in access to the wards where the pupil could accompany physicians and surgeons during rounds, visit patients on his own, observe operations and perform an occasional autopsy. Pupils' fees purchased learning experiences sold by the medical staff.[53] Having no clinical responsibilities to the hospital, pupils remained free to organise their own program of studies: 'The pupil's business is only to look on and to make such enquiry as he shall choose of the surgeon who is attending . . . They [pupils] may quit the hospital whenever they please and return when they chuse.'[54]

A few selections from William Shippen's diary vividly illustrate the opportunities available to and the freedom enjoyed by a London hospital pupil in 1759:

> (30 July) went thro the hospital by myself to examine the patients . . . spent 2 hours in examining a dead body at

---

51 See Owen, *English Philanthropy*, pp. 36–61; Donna Andrew, 'Obstetrics and Maternity Charities in 18th-Century London' (Paper read at University of Ottawa, 12 February 1981).

52 Surgeons' letter to governors of St George's Hospital (27 May 1793), quoted in Peachey, *A Memoir of William and John Hunter*, p. 300. Monographs on the various hospitals provide only a sketchy account of medical education. In 1768–9, St Thomas's and Guy's formally agreed to unite teaching so that pupils at either hospital could attend anatomy and surgery lectures at St Thomas's and medical lectures at Guy's. See Cameron, *Mr. Guy's Hospital*, pp. 88–90; Pott's lectures, begun at St Bartholomew's in 1767, formed the centerpiece of the hospital school. At the London Hospital, a medical school opened in 1785 largely through the efforts of the surgeon William Blizard. See A. E. Clark-Kennedy, *The London*, 2 vols. (London, 1962), I, pp. 164–8. At mid-century, John Harrison, who had been lecturing at the London for several years, argued that the hospital should be thought of as a 'university'. *A Short Comparative View*, p. 54.

53 For pupils' "walking" fees at the major hospitals, see Peachey, *A Memoir of William and John Hunter*, pp. 300–1. The price rose in relative terms as the term shortened from one year to three months. The Edinburgh Royal Infirmary, where students paid their fees directly to the managers, appears to be an exception to this system. Personal communication from Dr Stephanie Blackden.

54 Joseph Warner, quoted in Cameron, *Mr. Guy's Hospital*, pp. 92–3.

hospital who died suddenly . . . (4 August) saw Mr. Way
surgeon to Guy's hospital amputate a leg above the knee very
dexterously 3 ligatures . . . (23 August) attended Dr. Akenside
in taking in patients and prescribing for them, 56 taken in . . .
(5 September) examined particulars in hospital several smallpox 3 out of 4 die, saw Mr. Baker perform 3 operations, a leg,
breast and tumor from girl's lower jaw inside, very well
operated. Mr. Warner extracted a large stone from urethra
of a man and pinn'd the incision up as in harelip . . . (2
November) went to Georges Hospital and saw Hawkins and
Bromfield operate, stone and amputation . . . (7 November)
went to Bartholomews Hospital and saw the neatest operation
of bubonocele that I ever saw by Mr. Pott a very clever neat
surgeon.[55]

All in all, Shippen, who seems to have been a 'pupil at large'
primarily affiliated with St Thomas's, witnessed more than a dozen
major surgical operations performed by London's leading hospital
surgeons at four different institutions. At the same time, he saw
medical patients both in the hospital and privately, enrolled in dissection courses with the Hunter brothers and took extramural private
courses in midwivery.

Private medical education conferred mobility and flexibility upon
pupils who could afford its benefits. In hospitals and large private
schools, the one-on-one character of the traditional master–apprentice relationship broke down for both parties: Masters took on numerous private students, students in turn followed multiple masters.
Even in the case of apprentices and dressers, who contracted with
individual surgeons, multiple rather than exclusive allegiances were
common. James Hutchinson, who paid a fifty-guinea yearly fee to be
Percivall Pott's dresser in 1775–6, noted:

Tho' I am a pupil of Bartholomew's Hospital only, yet there
are few curious cases, that are worthy of particular observation, in the other hospitals but what I have an opportunity of
seeing, and there are but few capital operations performed,
that I am not invited to . . . I am a perpetual pupil to both
Pott and John Hunter; and I shall be to Fordyce.[56]

By the latter eighteenth century, private instruction within and outside the London hospitals served the educational needs of the medi-

55 Corner, *William Shippen*, pp. 13, 14, 18, 21, 28.
56 Quoted in Whitfield Bell, Jr., 'James Hutchinson (1752–1793): Letters from an
American Student in London', *Transactions and Studies of the College of Physicians of
Philadelphia*, 4th ser., 34 (1966), 23.

cal élite. Derived from the traditional apprenticeship, which continued to train ordinary practitioners, private instruction permitted young medical men to negotiate a flexible post-apprenticeship experience.[57] Private enterprise education conserved the cash bond between teacher and pupil but did away with corporative requirements of service, residence, lengthy tenure and exclusivity. 'Formerly they brought certificates of their apprenticeship, but now they bring only their money', wrote Joseph Warner, retired surgeon at Guy's, about hospital surgical pupils in 1792. 'There are customs understood but no rules . . . The pupils are considered as belonging to the hospitals, not to one particular surgeon'.[58]

Warner's final remark about the pupils 'belonging to the hospitals' was somewhat misleading. He meant that pupils' fees at the united hospitals became the common property of *all* the hospital surgeons, each of whom received an equal portion, rather going to the individual surgeons under whom they had been admitted as was the practice with apprentices' and dressers' fees. As always, the hospital itself received no share of the profits from the educational transaction.

John Hunter at St George's

In 1792 John Hunter challenged the custom of equal division of pupils' fees.[59] Declaring his intention to keep all fees from pupils henceforth admitted under him to St George's Hospital, Hunter sought in effect to push to its logical extreme the notion of the hospital as a private school. In the ensuing debate, Hunter's colleagues won their case with the hospital governors, but they also defined (although they may not have wished to) a concept of a hospital-school that transcended the special private interests of its medical staff.

Hunter, not surprisingly, denied that considerations of financial gain motivated his decision to keep pupils' fees. Amongst 'many reasons' for his resolution, he first noted his wish to provide 'an incitement to the surgeons of the hospital . . . to instruct the pu-

---

57 On the persistence of apprenticeship, see Joan Lane, chap. 3, this volume. Kett, 'Provincial Medical Practice', p. 19, suggests that by the end of the century hospital experience was not uncommon; in 1791, 40 per cent of surgeon-apothecaries in Lincolnshire and Essex had attended one of the three London hospitals for which pupil registers are available.
58 Quoted in Cameron, *Mr. Guy's Hospital*, p. 92.
59 This discussion is based on six letters exchanged between Hunter, his surgical colleagues and the governors of St George's Hospital from 9 July 1792 to 27 May 1793. The letters are published in Peachey, *A Memoir of William and John Hunter*, pp. 272–303.

pils'.[60] On several occasions since his arrival at St George's in 1768, Hunter had tried to set up lecture courses at the hospital only to be thwarted by his fellow surgeons' lack of co-operation. He claimed sole credit for a steep rise in numbers of hospital pupils during the period 1769–79 and attributed their subsequent decline to his withdrawal of 'attention' from the hospital. Hunter underlined the disinterestedness of his action by pledging not to compete for future hospital pupils as he was already too busy, presumably with his private research and teaching. He simply wanted St George's to take its place with other London hospitals as a teaching centre and thereby provide 'not only immediate relief to the poor and distressed . . . but diffuse its influence to mankind in general'.[61]

Hunter was nevertheless keenly aware of the financial dimension of hospital teaching. When, sometime after mid-century, St George's and the other London hospitals removed limitations on the numbers of fee-paying pupils, substantial sums began to be generated. Hunter himself drew attention to this fact by measuring numbers of pupils at St George's in terms of revenue produced: He pointed to an increase from a low of £107 per annum in 1769 to £266 in 1779 for each surgeon. Even the lower figure represented an extremely lucrative perquisite at a time when the total annual income of most London practitioners rarely amounted to £1,000.[62] Hunter attacked a system that limited the most industrious surgical teacher at St George's to 'one fourth of the whole profit' while others 'by doing nothing . . . still got a fourth'.[63] And, in his own case, Hunter claimed his share to have been more than 50 per cent of the 834 pupils who had entered St George's since 1770.

I do not think financial profit was the primary motive of Hunter's manoeuvre of 1792. He clearly wanted to improve the voluntary hospital's role in the diffusion of knowledge, to make the hospital an institution patronised by 'the philosopher, as well as the charitable'. In addition, Hunter nursed complicated long-standing personal and political grudges against his surgical colleagues at St George's, as they did against him.[64] These mutual hostilities burst loose in 1792. Hunter's argument, however, did confirm the extent to which the ideology of private enterprise pervaded teaching at St George's, structur-

---

60 Ibid., p. 272 (9 July 1792).
61 Ibid., p. 275 (20 February 1793).
62 Letter from Richard Huck to Benjamin Rush (31 August 1774) in Historical Society of Pennsylvania, Philadelphia.
63 Quoted in Peachey, *A Memoir of William and John Hunter*, p. 280 (28 February 1793).
64 Ibid., pp. 196–205.

ing the conditions of admission, tenure, cost and career connections for hospital pupils. Beyond the narrow technical issue of how fees were to be divided, the hospital school remained the private enterprise of its medical staff.

Hunter's surgical colleagues fundamentally accepted the entrepreneurial nature of the ties between medical men and students in the hospital setting. But provoked by Hunter's attack on their own teaching performance and his self-serving claim to have brought in a majority of the pupils, the other surgeons at St George's had to counter-attack. Seeking to preserve the status quo, namely collective surgical control over fees and teaching, Gunning, Williams and Keate expressed their 'entire disapprobation' of Hunter's proposal.[65] In the process, they came precariously close to inviting the hospital governors to assume direction of the teaching enterprise.

Hunter's adversaries urged the governors of St George's to enforce existing regulations that vested formal control over pupils in the administrator's hands. They expressed particular displeasure with the increasing numbers of 'quarterly' pupils who entered the hospital for periods of only three months. Such pupils purchased hospital instruction 'in the retail' while their main interests and loyalities lay outside the charitable institution, at Hunter's private lessons for example.[66] Hunter's colleagues pointedly accused him of harming 'the chirurgical credit of this hospital' by attracting pupils to his private lectures and demonstrations and of neglecting for more than ten years his own attendance at St George's.[67] During William Hunter's lifetime, the hospital surgeons had recommended the anatomical lessons at nearby Great Windmill Street to their pupils, and Dr Hunter returned the favour to the mutual financial advantage of both parties: 'We had supported them and they supported us.'[68] William Hunter naturally sent students to his brother. This, rather than any exceptional merit as a teacher, was one reason why John Hunter had the greatest number of hospital pupils. Now, with William Hunter dead, John withdrawn from active involvement at St George's and, in any case, threatening to keep all pupils' fees, the cosy system of fee-splitting between Great Windmill Street and St George's had collapsed.

The surgeons' concluding proposal called for a centralised hospital

---

65 Ibid., p. 274 (4 October 1792).
66 Ibid., pp. 289, 291–2.
67 Ibid., pp. 291–2; Peachey notes that prior to 1793, John Hunter's name 'scarcely appears in the minutes of St George's hospital despite his 24 years as a surgeon to the hospital'. Ibid., p. 196.
68 Ibid., p. 288.

school at St George's. Their recommendations were clearly directed against John Hunter's spotty hospital attendance, his casual use of the institution for private teaching and his extramural courses:

> It will be indispensably necessary for the four surgeons belonging to this hospital to visit all their patients twice a week, and to be present themselves at the dressing of them once, and to visit them on the remaining days of the week as often as may be necessary . . . close attendance of the surgeons is indispensably necessary for the instruction of the pupils . . . no pupils shall be entered for a less period than one year, or half a year, excepting during the time of war . . . every pupil shall be considered as receiving his instructions from the hospital at large and consequently under the care of all the surgeons alike . . . give us leave to bring home the different professors [of outside private courses] to the hospital.[69]

Conclusion

Private enterprise continued to supplement public medical instruction well into the nineteenth century. And, typically, private fees purchased a superior educational experience. This remained true even at Paris during the apotheosis of public clinical instruction in the first half of the nineteenth century.[70]

More important than the continuing distinction between public and private instruction, however, was the extent to which hospitals began to endorse the clinical enterprise and to cede administrative authority to their physicians and surgeons. Once this took place (and more than a century would pass before the process that began at the end of the eighteenth century at Paris and London reached maturity), private instruction was doomed. The medical élite captured control over teaching hospitals, and the hospitals in turn captured a professional élite increasingly dependent upon large institutions for research and teaching, referrals, technology and prestige, if not yet for full-time employment and income.

This essay has shown how hospitals served medical education during a period before the profession acquired much authority within the charitable institutions. Individual medical men and students struck private arrangements making use of the hospital as the site for a modified form of apprenticeship-style training. Medical individual-

69   Ibid., pp. 297–303 (27 May 1793).
70   See Russell M. Jones, ed., *The Parisian Education of an American Surgeon: Letters of Jonathan Mason Warner (1832–1835)* (Philadelphia, 1978), pp. 48–53.

ism and free enterprise sustained an educational pattern that drew strength from values conspicuous in eighteenth-century British society.

I have argued that voluntarism in this broad sense of giving free rein to private initiative and competition contributed to the shift of clinical leadership from Paris to London after 1750. But free enterprise hospital instruction had definite limitations. By the turn of the century, a more intensive immersion in the clinic along with a more authoritarian supervision of students had made Paris once again the model for medical education, this time powerfully supported by the Napoleonic state.[71] Tighter reciprocal responsibilities linking medical students and professionals more intimately with hospitals eliminated the space within which private teaching had flourished.

John Hunter's vision of a hospital for 'the philosopher', a centre for the production and diffusion of clinical knowledge, was realised during the nineteenth century, first in Paris and then throughout Europe. But the private enterprise pattern, epitomised by the Hunter brothers' school and warmly defended by John Hunter and Pierre-Joseph Desault in the 1790s, would not be the vehicle for the new clinical medicine. When the Great Windmill Street school finally closed its doors in 1831, it signified not only the end of the Hunterian enterprise dating back to William Hunter's first course eighty-five years earlier, but also the end of an era in which private enterprise dominated advanced medical training. Henceforth large corporate and, ultimately, public bureaucracies, namely the hospital medical schools and university hospitals, would take control of medical education.[72]

Acknowledgment

I thank Professor Deborah Gorham, Department of History, Carleton University, Ottawa, for her helpful criticism.

71 See Foucault, *The Birth of the Clinic*.
72 A different chronology applied to medical education in the United States. Here private enterprises, in the form of proprietary medical schools, persisted until the end of the nineteenth century. But, unlike earlier European private teaching, the proprietary schools tended to be mediocre in quality.

6

Ornate physicians and learned artisans: Edinburgh medical men, 1726–1776

CHRISTOPHER LAWRENCE

The medical department of the University of Edinburgh was always remark-able for the order of its scholastic arrangements, so that a student, who might be in difficulty respecting his proper course of study, could here acquire the system best adapted to the fulfilment of his object.

Bransby Blake Cooper, *The Life of Sir Astley Cooper, Bart.*, 2 vols. (London, 1843), II, p. 174.

The Edinburgh Medical School

Within fifty years of its foundation in 1726, the Edinburgh Medical School became the pre-eminent centre of medical education in the English-speaking world. By the 1770s students flocked there from all over Britain as well as the colonies, a few to attend the whole medical programme and graduate as MDs, others to enrol for only one or two courses and so complete or commence their education as surgeons or apothecaries. In this essay I will examine the medical courses available at Edinburgh in order to elucidate what it was in the lectures that gave them such appeal to an extremely diverse student audience. In doing so I will point to some of the important consequences for the intellectual and social relations between medicine and surgery that arose from the professorial exploitation of the unique institutional organisation existing at Edinburgh University.

The history of the Edinburgh Medical School in its first fifty years can be conveniently divided into three periods. During the first twenty years the teaching was characterised by the use of a foreign medical system, although within the anatomy classes elements of a unique Scottish programme began to emerge. During the second twenty years, from 1746 to 1766, the foreign model was partially abandoned and distinctive local elements appeared in the lectures. Within the

154 Christopher Lawrence

last decade, 1766–76, it is possible to speak of an authentic Scottish medical school, characterised both by its institutional structure and its intellectual coherence. Throughout the period under consideration certain elements in the arrangement of the medical courses and the clinical teaching remained constant. These features highlight the tight control the professoriate had over teaching in Edinburgh, in contrast to which medical education in London seems a free-for-all. It is this very exclusivity that helps explain why an ambitious young man like William Hunter, who attended Edinburgh for a brief period between 1739–40, would eventually choose the high road to London and not return.

Early years, 1726–46

The Edinburgh Medical School began its formal life in 1726. Its complex origin has been related to the attempt, by a small number of men, to create an attractive educational focus in a city that was both economically depressed and divided by religious and political issues that had arisen, in part, from the union of Scotland with England in 1707.[1] The school was located in the reformed university, where a unique Scottish pedagogical model was eventually utilised by the medical teachers to serve the demands of a new student clientele.[2] The medicine that was first taught at the new school was virtually a copy of that expounded by Hermann Boerhaave at Leiden.[3] There are several reasons for this. Leiden was a flourishing school, attracting many students, including Scots, and thus the Edinburgh curriculum was deliberately intended to compete for these paying customers. The fact that the university welcomed Dissenters, unlike Oxford and Cambridge, also made it a step on the educational ladder for many English students. Besides being adopted for its structural virtues, however, the establishment of Boerhaave's course in Edinburgh was used to signify the increasing power in the city of pro-Union, improvement-minded Scots committed to the values of the Enlighten-

1 J. R. R. Christie, 'The Origins and Development of the Scottish Scientific Community', History of Science, XII (1974), 122–41.
2 J. B. Morrell, 'The University of Edinburgh in the Late Eighteenth Century: Its Scientific Eminence and Academic Structure', Isis, LXII (1970), 152–71. See also his excellent review, 'Medicine and Science in the Eighteenth Century' in Gordon Donaldson (ed.), Four Centuries of Edinburgh University Life 1583–1983 (Edinburgh, 1983), pp. 38–52. I cannot agree, however, with his assertion that 'The rational medicine taught at Edinburgh, so different from London, encouraged the separation of medicine from surgery' (p. 50).
3 C. J. Lawrence, 'Early Edinburgh Medicine: Theory and Practice', in R. G. W. Anderson and A. D. C. Simpson (eds.), The Early Years of the Edinburgh Medical School (Edinburgh, 1976), pp. 81–94.

ment.[4] Boerhaave's medicine was based on the same teleological and experimental Newtonian philosophy enlisted into the Whig cause in England.[5]

The Edinburgh medical course changed little in the first two decades of the school's existence, and the medical students attending it could expect to receive a very specific education. Lectures at Edinburgh, however, were not obligatory, students attending whichever professor they wished.[6] An educated young man with a knowledge of Latin, able to pay three guineas for a course and find the cost of lodgings, could expect the following: All his professors would teach him that the practice of medicine was an art and that this practice required the prior learning of a system. Systematic medicine had several related meanings. At the most general level it meant that learning began with particular facts and progressed to general principles. More specifically it meant ascending through natural philosophy, anatomy, chemistry, physiology, botany, general pathology and materia medica to the theory of the practice of physic. Thus in understanding the general causes of health and disease the student was equipped for practice itself. More specifically still, learning by system in Edinburgh meant learning the system of Boerhaave. This embodied Newtonian natural philosophy, an experimental approach to chemistry, a physiology based on the mechanical philosophy and a medical theory drawn from a vast range of ancient and modern authors. Systematic medicine, also called by contemporaries rational or dogmatic medicine, was by no means the approach to practice approved of by all medical men. Although naked empiricism of the type advocated by John Wesley had, as far as I know, few medical defenders in the eighteenth century, a less systematic medicine certainly did. Scepticism that general medical principles were attainable had as one of its ablest defenders the most cited medical man of the age, Thomas Sydenham.[7] In effect, of course, the polar opposites of rationalism and empiricism as theoretical positions were defended by few. The point is, however. that the student attending the *full*

---

4   This question has not been the subject of any one paper, but see J. R. R. Christie, 'The Rise and Fall of Scottish Science', in M. Crosland (ed.), *The Emergence of Science in Western Europe* (London, 1975), pp. 116–26.
5   Margaret C. Jacob, *The Newtonians and the English Revolution* (Hassocks, 1976). Although the details of Jacob's account are the subject of dispute the broad claim seems incontrovertible.
6   Morrell, 'The University of Edinburgh'.
7   The whole question of learning medicine by system, and the objections to it, is dealt with by Andrew Robert Cunningham in 'Aspects of the History of Medical Education in Britain in the Seventeenth and Eighteenth Centuries' (PhD thesis, University of London, 1974).

medical course at Edinburgh was endorsing a particular ideological
position. This was that medicine was a *learned* occupation, practised
properly only by a relatively small, Latin-speaking élite. Edinburgh
medicine was thoroughly modern in that it was based on the new
sciences, but it was also linked to humanism and the arts through its
ancient constituents. For the student aspiring to this end of the medical market the content of the Edinburgh course properly equipped
him for practice as a genteel physician. The aetiological theory taught
by the medical professors Andrew St Clair and John Rutherford was
based on the non-naturals and stressed the importance of personal
moral responsibility in the maintenance of health and cited moral
failure as the cause of disease. Loose living, over-indulgence, ex-
posure to cold or a badly managed diet all brought sickness in their
train. This sickness was unique to the sufferer. It was conceptualised
by the physicians within what has been termed a physiological
model.[8] Disease was essentially a disturbance of fluid equilibrium to
be managed by a personal attendant.[9] Ontological theories of disease,
though implicit in the teachings on special pathology, played little
part in the physician's training. The medical model I have described
here fits well with the sociological explanation of eighteenth-century
medicine given by Jewson.[10] In Jewson's account a medicine of symptoms is seen as the appropriate response to a client-dominated medical world. The medical student getting the full course of treatment at
Edinburgh would be well turned out to practise amongst an élite and
cultured clientele. It is not surprising that this was the educational
commodity the Edinburgh medical professors offered. They were,
after all, men of substance in a very hierarchical society. That is they
were all successful, sought-after practitioners themselves. They had
learned an élite medicine at Leiden and, impressed by its success as a
marketable product, offered it on their home ground. Weight is added to this interpretation by a factor usually held to demonstrate the
reverse: clinical teaching. Edinburgh is usually hailed for its pro-
gressiveness in its early establishment of clinical teaching. Yet it was
not until *twenty-two years* after the founding of the school that Rutherford gave his first clinical lecture, and even then probably only be-

8   I employ the distinction between physiological and ontological theories of disease
as explained by Owsei Temkin in his important paper, 'The Scientific Approach to
Disease: Specific Entity and Individual Sickness', in A. C. Crombie (ed.), *Scientific
Change* (London, 1963), pp. 629–47.
9   Charles E. Rosenberg, 'The Therapeutic Revolution: Medicine, Meaning and
Social Change in Nineteenth Century America', in Morris J. Vogel and Charles E.
Rosenberg (eds.), *The Therapeutic Revolution* (Philadelphia, 1979), pp. 3–26.
10 N. D. Jewson, 'Medical Knowledge and the Patronage System in Eighteenth-
Century England', *Sociology*, VIII (1974), 369–85.

cause of his own dwindling class size (professors were paid per cap-
ita). The establishment of clinical lectures in Edinburgh probably
owed far more to the farsightedness of Provost George Drummond,
who saw in them a way to entice a different breed of students to the
capital.[11] Clinical teaching, in other words, was not a commodity
demanded by aspirants to élite practice.

Yet Edinburgh was not Leiden and from the earliest days this pure
medical model was adulterated with elements that promised the extinction of the élite physician. From the first there were teachers at
Edinburgh who used the institutional structure to capture a different
audience. By far the most important of these was Alexander Monro
primus. Monro was a member of the Incorporation of Surgeons in
Edinburgh and the first incumbent of the Anatomy Chair in the new
medical school. Monro, with his father and Provost Drummond, had
participated in the attempt to bring Boerhaavian medicine to Edinburgh. Monro was an important figure for several reasons. First,
although he was a surgeon it is quite clear that he effectively excluded
his surgical brethren from the university and the infirmary, but at the
same time systematically taught anatomy, physiology, pathology and
surgery to large numbers of surgical apprentices in the medical
school.[12] Monro taught in English and attracted to his lectures medical students besides formally indentured surgical apprentices.
Corpses for dissection were not common in Edinburgh yet Monro's
anatomy course flourished. At this time, however, London was by no
means the centre of choice for anatomical instruction it was to become
in the days of William Hunter. Besides, Monro more than offset the
deficit of cadavers by the use of anatomical models, an attractive
oratorical style, and the production of a very comprehensive lecture
course. It is highly likely that more students attended Monro's English presentation of Boerhaave's physiology than attended the Latin
version given by St Clair.[13] As a Boerhaavian, Monro, like his col-

11 On Drummond see J. B. Morrell, 'The Edinburgh Town Council and its
University 1717–1766', in Anderson and Simpson, *Early Years*, pp. 46–65.
12 The role of the Edinburgh surgeons throughout the eighteenth century would
repay study. Rosalie Stott has already shown what an important educational
institution the Incorporation was in the early years of the century. In a way Monro
simply took into the university context a curriculum that would have been as well
received in Surgeons' Hall. See Rosalie Mary Stott, 'The Origins of the Edinburgh
Medical School 1696–1755' (PhD thesis, University of Edinburgh, 1984).
13 A fundamental feature of all the teaching at Edinburgh was the use of the
method of commentary. The medical professors commented solely on the works of
Boerhaave. I know of only one copy of St Clair's commentaries (in the Royal College
of Physicians, Edinburgh). As a grateful student, John Fothergill remembered St
Clair's lectures thus: 'With what grace and elegance and with what minuteness and
precision would the humane, the inimitable Sinclair explain the Institutes of the

leagues, taught the importance of learning medicine by system. But he also taught that surgery should be learned that way as well. The operations of surgery were the conclusion of his own theoretical course. Monro's lectures then were unusual. By attending them surgical apprentices would be exposed to the medical theory of Boerhaave and medical students to accounts of surgical operations and surgical concepts of disease. Thus there was taking shape in Edinburgh a medical curriculum that could eventually break down traditional medical and surgical boundaries.

Monro's teaching, where it used a particular theory of disease, drew mainly on the Boerhaavian system. But as a surgeon his main concerns were topographical anatomy and the differentiation of local conditions. Not surprisingly, therefore, he stressed the need for straightforward clinical description. This emphasis clearly relates to his concern with surgical therapy. These points are well illustrated by the text of his lectures on tumours.[14] It is noteworthy first that Monro chose to lecture on tumours as a single clinical topic for in Boerhaave's works different tumours are described at widely dispersed intervals.[15] Monro, on the other hand, was concerned with visible, localisable and potentially excisable disorders. Tumours, Monro

master, whose nervous simplicity he studied to exemplify though not with servile imitation.' John Fothergill, 'An Essay on the Character of the late Alexander Russell M.D. F.R.S.', in *The Works of John Fothergill M.D.* (London, 1784), 431. St Clair's lectures may well have been poorly attended. Alexander Monro also taught by commentary, both on Boerhaave's texts and on his own. See Douglass Taylor, *The Monro Collection in the Medical Library of the University of Otago* (Dunedin, 1979), p. 85. Monro also had published a fundamental anatomical text, *The Anatomy of the Humane Bones* (Edinburgh 1726), which could be used for teaching osteology by commentary.
14   Monro had included a lecture on tumours in a surgical course he gave in 1722. Many student copies of this course existed and Monro was not particularly proud of them. See H. D. Erlam, 'Alexander Monro *primus*', *University of Edinburgh Journal*, XVII (1954), 84. Taylor, *Monro Collection*, seems to conclude that Monro did not give the lectures again. However, Wellcome Institute for the History of Medicine, MS. 934, 'A treatise of tumours', notes of lectures by Robert Hamilton, finishes with Hamilton's saying he took the lectures down in 1734 (Wellcome Institute MS. catalogue dates them as 1736). There was a Robert Hamilton in Edinburgh in 1734. See Monro's student list, Edinburgh University Library, MS. DC. 5. 95. Medical Society of London, MS. 33, 'Lectures on tumours', states that they were taken down from Monro in 1735 and Medical Society of London MS. 74, between 1731 and 1733.
15   Cancer and aneurysm for instance are separated, one as a species of inflammation and the other as a species of wound, though van Swieten discusses how aneurysms may be 'distinguished from other tumours'. Ascites, however, is treated independently as a species of dropsy. Gerard van Swieten, *The Commentaries upon the Aphorisms of Dr. Hermann Boerhaave*, 18 vols. (London, 1744–73), II, p. 142. There were medical precedents for teaching on all tumours as a single group, notably in Galen for example; see *Ueber die krankhaften Geschwülste*, trans. Paul Richter (Leipzig, 1913). Galen was comprehensive and included among tumours, cancer, ascites and varicose veins.

taught, fall into three broad groups; those of the vessels, such as varices and aneurysms; dropsical disorders, for example hydrocoele; and finally inflammation and its consequences – suppuration, gangrene, scirrhus and cancer.

Inflammation was universally regarded as the origin of the best known of all tumours, the phlegmon, a 'red hard and painful tumour accompanied with fever'. Monro's theoretical account of inflammation did not differ from Boerhaave's. A phlegmon is 'occasioned by obstruction in the small vessels in which the red globules of blood circulate . . . the liquids are constantly driven on towards the obstructed parts'.[16] Like physicians, Monro taught that the causes of phlegmon were individual moral lapses and that these gave rise to its characteristic pathological qualities. The causes included 'violent motions, furious passions, drinking hard spiritous liquors'. But, he said, it was important for the surgeon to view phlegmon with respect to its site, whether superficial or 'near those parts . . . necessary for life'.[17] In dealing with cases of phlegmon he taught that the first therapeutic aim of the surgeon was to prevent suppuration. Such a resolution could be affected by diminishing the impetus of the blood by evacuation and a strict regimen of the non-naturals.[18] If, however, the phlegmon is the precursor of a critical discharge the surgeon should encourage suppuration. But if the suppurating phlegmon is deep and bursts before it reaches the skin,

> The heat of the body turns it acrid and it insinuates itself into the neighbouring parts all about it, it produces sinuses, ulcers, fistulae, caries in bones, opens into some of the cavities, is perhaps absorbed into the mass of the blood, brings on an hectic fever, phthisis pulmonalis, ulcers of the liver.[19]

What is significant here is Monro's stress on local anatomical spread of disease and the consequent structural abnormalities. His account of such local spread used a theory of 'acridity' yet the clinical observations were virtually independent of the theory. Monro's students were thus being exposed to the most up-to-date medical theory, capped by a surgical, natural historical account of disease.

---

16   Medical Society of London, MS. 74, 'A Treatise of Tumours and Ulcers by Mr. Alexander Monro', part 5, p. 21.
17   Wellcome Institute for the History of Medicine, MS. 934, pp. 37, 34.
18   Ibid., p. 37. Monro at first seems quite happy here to deal in the sort of therapeutic recommendations usually thought of as pertaining to physicians. However, he adds (p. 38) that in the treatment of phlegmon the appropriate internal medicines are diluents and attentuents, but he would go no further, being 'afraid he would be thought encroaching on a subject that does not properly belong to us'.
19   Ibid., p. 46.

A similar concern with surgical therapy is seen in his account of caries, the terminal stage of necrotic bone disease. Monro proposed a new classification of the disease. He began by reviewing the most important authors on the subject from Hippocrates onward. Monro considered that the two most significant contemporary authors on caries were, from a surgical point of view, Jean-Louis Petit (1674–1750) and, from a medical one, Boerhaave. Both of these authors regarded bone disease as identical to those of the softer parts, but different in manifestation because of the density of bone. But here the similarity of their views ended. Boerhaave's account of bone disease was consistent with his logical deductive approach to disease. He divided it into five anatomical components, each with its own distinct disorder depending on the proximate causes, for example inflammation, acrimony and so forth. The outcome of any of these could be caries.[20]

As Toby Gelfand has suggested, Petit on the other hand epitomised a particular French surgical approach to disease, that of 'therapeutically orientated pathology'. Within such an approach,

> The surgeons of the Academy did not perform autopsies simply to satisfy curiosity as to the causes of death. Rather they studied morbid anatomy in order to visualize and thus understand and, ultimately, treat diseases inside the body in terms of the familiar categories of external diseases: inflammations, abscesses, ulcers, gangrene, and tumours.[21]

Petit, says Monro, divided caries into four 'species'. These were clinical descriptions subservient to the demands of therapy. Monro's classification was an extension of this *method*. His primary concern was to describe different clinical appearances requiring different therapies, though he was aware that such appearances might result from a variety of causes:

> It would be very improper to pretend to give here directions for the cure of the lues venerea, scrophula, scurvy, gangrenes, abscesses, wounds, contusions and all the other diseases which occasion caries. I must confine myself to the topical management of the caries without any regard to the habit of the patient or to any other disease.[22]

Monro's classification is very little theory dependent. He divides caries into seven types depending on its similarity to gangrene, ab-

20 Van Swieten, *Commentaries upon . . . Boerhaave*, IV, 353–456.
21 Toby Gelfand, *Professionalizing Modern Medicine: Paris Surgeons and Medical Science and Institutions in the Eighteenth Century* (Westport, Conn., 1980), p. 181.
22 Alexander Monro, *The Works of Alexander Monro* (Edinburgh, 1781), p. 296.

scesses, ulcers, white swelling, scrofula and cancer. In other words the descriptions were simple, clinical, natural histories dictated by the demands of surgical intervention.

Monro's preoccupation with clinical phenomena led him to value post-mortems, accounts of which are frequent in his works. Most of his necropsies show a decided emphasis on local pathology intended to explain the patient's symptoms and lay the basis for future diagnoses. The pathological terminology was intended to be descriptive rather than theoretical. A tumour of the knee dissected after amputation revealed 'glairy matter' in the joint.[23] Beneath another leg swelling was a 'pappy substance', which had appeared as 'fungus' on the skin.[24] In this instance Monro's concern was to use the necropsy information to help him differentiate in future between such a tumour and a similar swelling caused by the presence of pus. The indications to interfere surgically in each instance were quite different. In a woman who had died after a chronic abdominal complaint, post mortem revealed a 'large body . . . distended . . . with a firm steatomatous substance' and identified by Monro as an ovarian tumour.[25] Later on the basis of this experience he was able to make this diagnosis in a patient who displayed similar symptoms. He could then suggest, in the absence of a post-mortem, that the symptoms were explainable in the following manner: 'The ovarian being supposed monstrously swelled, adhering to the colon, at last inflamed and suppurated, with the pus eroding a hole through the coats of the ovarium and the continguous adhering colon.'[26] Such an account shows a remarkable concern for local anatomical spread. It can be seen then that Monro accepted, in general, the Boerhaavian synthesis, but he modified it in several ways because of his surgical orientation. Notably, he was much more concerned to identify the natural history of a clinical entity, with a view to treatment, than he was to postulate proximate causes. Not unexpectedly he showed a strong anatomical bias in his description of the location and progress of disease. Within Monro's course, therefore, Edinburgh surgical students learned something of the science of medicine. Medical students, though, also encountered a local anatomical, surgical approach to disease.

In 1756 Monro consummated this marriage of medicine and surgery when he was awarded the MD degree. In 1757 he became a

23 Ibid., p. 461.
24 Ibid., p. 464.
25 Ibid., p. 510.
26 Ibid., p. 283.

Fellow of the College of Physicians. Within the span of thirty years then Monro effectively policed the public teaching of surgery in Edinburgh and in doing so changed it from a practice learned by apprenticeship at an incorporation to an academic discipline. In a way, though, the fact that the subject was learned at the university was purely fortuitous. The students who came to hear Monro probably did not come to hear him *because he was in a university*. Rather, the extremely favourable institutional arrangements at the university had made it a suitable setting for him to develop a systematic or learned anatomical and surgical course. Students would presumably have come in equal numbers to a private school if it had offered the appropriate curricular blend. That was no doubt the case in London. The lessons of Edinburgh were almost certainly not lost on the young William Hunter. Whatever specific anatomy he had learned from Monro, he certainly gathered the importance of methodically planning a course with a wide appeal and delivering it with clarity and conviction. He also saw a working model for policing intellectual work and for excluding competitors. It was this latter factor perhaps that directed Hunter's vision southwards. There was no chance of his becoming Monro's protégé, for Monro had three sons, any one of whom might assume his father's mantle. Indeed, so effective was the Monro grip on Edinburgh life that there was no one else of equivalent stature with whom Hunter could rise to fame. London offered quite different possibilities.

Development, 1746–66

The principal feature of this period is continuity rather than radical change. John Rutherford remained in the Chair of the Practice of Physic throughout the twenty years and continued to deliver lectures on Boerhaavian medicine in Latin. His class sizes, however, may have been small.[27] The Chair of the Institutes of Medicine, however, was filled in 1747 by a new incumbent, Robert Whytt, who remained there until his death in 1766. Whytt probably lectured in Latin at first and commented on the works of Boerhaave and, later, Gaubius. At some point he switched to lecturing in English. He had no great flair

27 Rutherford's lectures after all were only commentaries on Boerhaave's aphorisms, which by this time were being published by van Swieten. Many copies of commentaries from the Leiden period also existed in manuscript. I know of only one MS copy of Rutherford's commentaries (at the Royal College of Physicians, Edinburgh).

for lecturing.[28] Whytt, like his colleague, offered a course in dogmatic physic, primarily for those aspiring to elevated status within the profession. His theory of a sentient principle and his novel account of the nervous system may have enticed to Edinburgh a few students interested in the new physiological developments of the mid-century, but in the main his course was much like that of his predecessor. His decision to lecture in English seems to suggest a sensitivity to the success of his anatomical colleagues.

The Monro succession at Edinburgh on the other hand, ever the source of anecdote, was actually a very shrewd consolidation of an important interest. Alexander Monro *secundus* began teaching anatomy, physiology and surgery in 1754. Like his father he taught in English and he also emphasised the importance of learning by system. Unlike his father, though, Monro was never a surgeon. He became an MD in 1755, and a Fellow of the Edinburgh College in 1759. Twenty years later he was its president. With all the adroitness of his parent, *Secundus* cornered the market in the university teaching of surgery, successfully excluding the brethren of the Incorporation. The Monros also kept a tight grip on the surgical attendance at the Royal Infirmary. Comparison with London is instructive here. Surgeons in Edinburgh attended the infirmary by rotation, a system that was to some extent the result of the friction between the Monros and the Incorporation. This coupled with official status of clinical lectures, plus the professorial position of the Monros, meant that no surgeon was able to use the infirmary to build up a vast private course as was the case in London.[29] *Secundus*, like his father, was in great demand as a teacher. This extraordinarily truculent man was very alive to medical change and brought to his courses all the new concerns of the mid-century. He rejected much of the Boerhaavian corpus and proposed a vitalist physiological model based on the nervous system. He dissected, experimented and used the microscope. Although corpses for anatomical purposes remained less plentiful in Edinburgh than

28 I know of only one copy of Whytt's physiology lectures and these are very truncated and consist of rather random commentaries on Boerhaave. The randomness presumably was of student origin. Wellcome Institute for the History of Medicine, MS. 3781. 'Dr. Roberti Whytt, in institutiones Medicinae', Edinburgh, 20 Nov. 1756. There is a copy of Whytt's general pathology lectures, in English, at Edinburgh University Library, MS. 745D. Whytt had the same problem as Rutherford; just when he began teaching, English commentaries on Boerhaave's Institutes began to appear.
29 For an account of the relations between physicians and surgeons in Edinburgh see W. S. Craig, *History of the Royal College of Physicians of Edinburgh* (Oxford, 1976), chaps. 18, 19. On teaching in London see Gelfand, chap 5, this volume. No London hospital had a rotational system; see Bynum, chap. 4, this volume.

London, there were wax models in abundance, and before there is evidence to prove the point, the historian should not assume that students looked for the same degree of practical dissecting experience as later became the case. In addition to its necessary surgical orientation, Monro's teaching outstripped that of his father in its endorsement of an ontological model of disease, in its praise of pathological anatomy and its stress on the importance of physical examination at the bedside. In his later lectures Monro openly esteemed the value of nosology. His physiology course was full of suggestions that questioned traditional medical theory. For example, although physicians were, in one sense, clearly aware of the specificity of glandular function, urine being secreted only from the kidney or perspirable matter solely from the skin, in clinical practice they regarded glands as interchangeable. A poor urine output might be aided by catharsis or sweating, obstructed perspiration might be treated with a diuretic and so forth. Monro, however, argued on theoretical grounds for the uniqueness of glandular function and then pointed to the real therapeutic consequence that 'we can't supply a want of secretion from the kidneys by increase of secretion from the skin'.[30]

The most obvious feature of Monro's teaching is his strongly developed concept of local disease, and the associated idea of invasion along the planes defined by topographical anatomy. In general, as with his contemporaries, he seemed to show little regard for time-scale but there is a distinct sense of Monro's imposing, as Foucault has said, 'the configuration of the disease' on the sick man.[31] At the empirical level Monro clearly seems to have performed far more post-mortem examinations than did his predecessors. A common-place book in the Otago collection describes thirty-six performed in the 1750s and 1760s.[32]

More significant than the number of necropsies he performed is that Monro, like his father, apparently used them for a rather different purpose than did his physician colleagues. He opened the body not just to identify a specific cause but also to collect a series of cases

30 Royal College of Surgeons, England, MS. 42d 43. Alexander Monro *secundus*, 'Lectures on physiology 1772', II, p. 141. Some of my evidence for Monro *secundus*'s teaching is drawn from the period outside that under discussion. There is no doubt though that he was an iconoclastic presence in the medical school from the time of his appointment. See for instance his radical questioning of Boerhaave's theory of the lymphatics; Nellie B. Eales, 'The History of the Lymphatic System with Special Reference to the Hunter-Monro controversy', *Journal of the History of Medicine*, XXIX (1974), 280–94.
31 Michel Foucault, *The Birth of the Clinic*, trans. A. M. Sheridan Smith (London, 1973), p. 1.
32 Taylor, *Monro Collection*, Otago MS. M 174.

in order to define the pathological nature of a particular disease. He notes for instance that hydrocephalous is commonly considered to occur in two forms: internal (intraventricular) and external (on the brain surface). He then points out that in '20 or more post-mortems in such cases, I believe the latter [external hydrocephalous] has hardly, if ever, occured'.[33] He repeatedly referred to post-mortems to elucidate perplexing cases, often making special references to local pathology. In a lecture describing the nature of dropsy he added 'and on dissection of a case of ascites I have found the interstices of the vessels of the kidneys filled with sebaceous matter, the pressure of which on the vessels must have prevented the free secretion of urine'.[34] It is notable how in such instances Monro still resorts to a mechanical explanation of the clinical event.

He went into great detail when describing diseases of the arterial system, notably 'ossification'. He pointed out that such a process might obstruct the arterial cavity, and he referred to a post-mortem on a man who died after 'mortification' of the leg, dissection of which showed severe arterial ossification. He made no reference to the possible origins of such pathology. He further noted that such ossification might 'contract the Passage between the Ventricles and Arteries and, by preventing the blood from getting into the Arteries, occasion a dilation of the Heart'.[35] He illustrated this by reference to a case in which ossification of the aortic valve had gone so far as not to allow the passage of a goose quill. Such an increase in size of the heart, he pointed out, was accompanied by thickening of the muscle fibres. Monro was by no means the first to discuss such matters, and all his observations can be found in Giovanni Lancisi's classic *On the Motion of the Heart and on Aneurysms*, which appeared in 1728. However, what is significant is that such an approach dominated his course even more than it had done his father's.

The idea of local anatomical spread in breast cancer received particular prominence in Monro's writing. This was a consequence of two factors: first, his own putative discovery of the anatomy of the origin of the lymphatics, and second, the work of Jean-Louis Petit, who had drawn attention to the enlarged lymph glands in breast cancer and the necessity to remove them in order to effect a complete cure. Monro, in fact, had engaged in a vigorous priority dispute with

33 Royal College of Surgeons, England, MS 42a 62, Alexander Monro *secundus*, 'Lectures on Surgery', 1776, II, pp. 217–18.
34 Ibid., pp. 220–1, stated anachronistically, Monro was describing what was later known as Bright's disease.
35 Wellcome Institute for the History of Medicine, MS. 4216, 'Lectures anatomical and physiological', by A. Monro, taken by Joshua Rigg, *c*.1775, pp. 78–9.

William Hunter over the discovery of the origin of the lymphatics. In a way the dispute was a microcosm of the competing claims of Edinburgh and London, priority being seen as enhancing the prestige of the lecturer to delivering the anatomy course. In his lectures Monro stressed the general role of the lymphatics in spreading disease and paid particular attention to their place in cancer of the breast. This disease, he taught, arose from an ulcerated scirrhus and begins without previous inflammation. When presented with a case the surgeon should 'examine' the lymphatic glands at the edge of the pectoral muscle and in the axillae. These glands 'are felt by relaxing the arm and pressing the points of the fingers deep into the axilla'. Untreated, the disease progresses through the stage of adhesion to the skin (which is accompanied by itching), to local erosion and finally to death within twelve months. For any hope of a cure the lymph glands must be removed: 'My father has mentioned that of 60 cases where he had the operation performed not above five remained free of the disorder five years after the operation.' Monro himself gave a breakdown of eighteen cases and their relative survivals, but the time periods are not clear.[36] One of the Otago manuscripts contains an analysis of 106 cases of the same operation.[37] Monro drew attention to the importance of the lymphatic diseases other than breast cancer. He described a patient with a liver abscess who had died and had had a post-mortem, and he noted that 'two lymphatic glands were swelled and hard which points out the way Nature takes to relieve herself'.[38]

Some of Monro's most remarkable pathological investigations occurred in his lectures on oedema. He classified it by anatomical site, as was usual even among physicians, and attempted to distinguish between hydrothorax and a pericardial effusion. Both, he said, may produce scanty urine, oppression of the breast, dyspnoea, a dry cough and nocturnal ankle oedema. However, he went on to say that it may be possible to distinguish between them 'by feeling the strokes of the heart'[39] – in other words, by precordial palpation. In a similar set of lectures, Monro described one further method of distinguishing the two: 'It is Percussio Thoracis, it does not sound like a drum containing air.'[40] Monro had seemingly been percussing the chest of

---

36 Monro, 'Lectures on Surgery', pp. 280–6.
37 Taylor, *Monro Collection*, Otago MS. M 183. On the use of the statistical method by Edinburgh-trained physicians see Ulrich Tröhler, 'Quantification in British Medicine and Surgery 1750–1830, with Special Reference to Its Introduction into Therapeutics' (PhD thesis, University of London, 1978).
38 Monro, 'Lectures anatomical and physiological', pp. 155–7.
39 Monro, 'Lectures on Surgery', p. 257.
40 Royal College of Surgeons, England, MS. 42a 54, 'Lectures on surgery' by Alexander Monro M.D., n.d., probably about 1772. I, p. 230.

his patients, though apparently with relatively little success. An un-dated set of notes, apparently from about 1772, has the following difficult paragraph:

> I have not enough trial, whether the stroke on the abdomen in ascites will give a different sound from that in health or filled with air – we might try this easily in the dead body, by filling one pleura with water and striking the hand against it I think the sound of the one side would be higher than the other but the trial requires great accuracy and would also suffer from the quantity of fat under the skin.[41]

Leopold Auenbrugger's account of percussion had been published in 1761 with further editions in 1763 and 1775. Almost nothing is known about the fate of the work in Britain. It is acknowledged in Cullen's *First Lines of the Practice of Physic* in editions after 1778. Cullen stated: 'How far the method proposed by Auenbrugger will apply to ascer-tain the presence of water and the quantity of it in the chest I have not had occasion or opportunity to observe.' Auenbrugger's book, how-ever, was reviewed in a London newspaper in 1761, and the reviewer was probably Oliver Goldsmith, a former Edinburgh student.[42] It would seem almost certain that Monro knew of Auenbrugger's work, and he had probably read it. His account of percussion gives the impression of an unsuccessful attempt, because of inexperience, to apply a new technique. The significance of the event, however, lies in Monro's interest in establishing clinical correlations with local inter-nal pathology.

Monro's course was a big attraction. Class sizes increased and with it, his income. The Town Council were sufficiently impressed to build him a new lecture theatre. Monro, however, was not simply educat-ing an élite group that once would have gone to Leiden. He was teaching apothecaries, dilettantes, surgeons and others who were taking an anatomy course at Edinburgh before moving on to the London schools and hospitals. Furthermore Monro was a physician who, in his surgical teaching, was using the most recent medical theory. At the same time he was dealing sceptically with some of the most hallowed axioms of élite medical practice. Monro was educating students who would move in different circles than those who had once attended Boerhaave.

As well as the arrival of a second Monro other things changed during this period. Most famous perhaps was the establishment of clinical teaching at the Royal Infirmary, a hospital that began as a

41 Royal College of Surgeons, England, MS. 42d 42, 'Lectures on the operations of surgery by Alexander Monro Junior', n.d., p. 172.
42 See Saul Jarcho, 'A Review of Auenbrugger's *Inventum Novum*, attributed to Oliver Goldsmith', *Bulletin of the History of Medicine*, XXIII (1959), 47.

small house in 1729 and that later achieved the grandeur of a purpose-built institution. It is important to note, however, the comparatively small size of the Infirmary. From the beginning complaints
were heard of overcrowding with students and apprentices, the patients being 'frightened with so great numbers of persons'.[43] An issue
of tickets solved this problem by boosting revenues and controlling
the chaos. These attendances were not at clinical lectures but rather
the daily round of physicians and surgeons where the students and
apprentices trailed behind the surgeons and physicians listening, and
possibly writing. Some thought was given to students who could gain
clinical experience by eavesdropping.

> In acute cases [the physician] will find it necessary to examine
> the symptoms accurately every day; and he ought to dictate
> them to the clerk so audibly and deliberately, that the stu-
> dents may have time to take them down in writing.[44]

In 1748 John Rutherford was given permission to use the 'operation
room' for clinical lectures, and in 1750 a special ward was opened
comprising ten beds specially intended for clinical teaching. In 1756
this was increased to twenty-nine.[45] Extolled as the paternal institution of clinical teaching in Britain it is probable that comparatively few
students received clinical instruction at the Royal Infirmary during
this period. Most students went off to the London hospitals during
the summer to receive instruction and gain experience on the wards.
Joseph Black for instance, after his unusually prolonged medical education, 'proposed to go immediately to London to spend some time in
the Hospitals there'.[46] David Skene complained of the paucity of
instruction on a number of occasions. In 1752 he wrote, 'We have no
great variety of patients for our clinical lectures.'[47] Eight years later he
remarked, 'What I am most surprised at is the scarcity of surgical
cases here.'[48] He had seen only one operation, an amputation, in two
months. The trip to London became a must for many Edinburgh
students.[49] One problem was the shortage of beds. In 1728 there were

43 Royal Infirmary of Edinburgh Minutes, 2 Nov. 1730.
44 *History and Statutes of the Royal Infirmary of Edinburgh* (Edinburgh, 1778), p. 83.
45 A. Logan Turner, *Story of a Great Hospital. The Royal Infirmary of Edinburgh*
(Edinburgh, 1937), p. 135; cf. the essay by Othmar Keel, chap. 8, this volume.
46 Joseph Black to his father, 1 June 1754. Cited in William Ramsay, *The Life and
Letters of Joseph Black* (London, 1918), p. 18. Black did not in fact go immediately, but
the letter makes it quite clear that it was necessary to go to London to 'acquire this
part of medicine'.
47 King's College, Aberdeen, MS. 38/17. David Skene to Andrew Skene, Feb. 25
1752.
48 King's College, Aberdeen, MS. 38/64, 6 Jan. 1760.
49 See the evidence in C. Helen Brock, 'Scotland and American Medicine', in
William R. Brock (ed.), *Scotus Americanus* (Edinburgh, 1982), pp. 114–26.

a mere six and in 1741, in the first section of the new infirmary, only thirty-four. By 1748 the 228-bed edifice was complete. However, because of shortage of funds, only forty beds were in use in 1749. In 1763, the first year for which matriculation figures are available, 223 students registered of whom 93 enrolled for formal clinical lectures.[50] But even by this time opportunities to see new patients were rare, and clinical lectures were given only twice a week and only for five months of the year. The opportunity to acquire clinical experience then was by no means the major attraction of the Edinburgh Medical School in the 1750s. Its appeal to students must have had much more to do with the lectures available, and other extramural possibilities.

By the late 1750s there were indeed other attractions. In 1755 the audacious and iconoclastic William Cullen arrived to teach chemistry. Cullen also gave private medical lectures as well as offering official clinical ones. Cullen's reputation went before him as the chemistry classrooms at Glasgow emptied and those at Edinburgh filled. For the student who aspired to master a medicine based on the new natural sciences Cullen was the *only* teacher from whom to learn chemistry. Cullen of course lectured in English, but there were other reasons for being in Edinburgh. For instance, students could attend other courses, such as botany, materia medica or natural philosophy. Moreover, the Royal Infirmary offered the students the chance to learn some midwifery, and the surgeons in the town seemed only too glad to have students attend their 'shops'.[51] By this period the Medical Society, a lively student organisation, had been established, but the claim made by the Society's own historians in the 1770s that this institution was the source of intellectual change in Edinburgh has to be treated with care. Student dissertations at this time were relatively orthodox, that is they cited Boerhaave and Gaubius. Only later did the students come to have more intellectual and social 'muscle'. Then they rewrote the history of the Society accordingly.[52]

The curious feature of Edinburgh medicine at this period then is the slight incongruity between the medical teaching and the other courses offered. Students could attend regular medical courses, given

50 Turner, *Royal Infirmary*, p. 151.
51 B. Cozens-Hardy (ed.), *The Diary of Silas Neville* (London, 1950), p. 137. Joseph Black decided to remain in Edinburgh on account of 'the shop'. John Thomson, *An Account of the Life, Lectures and Writings of William Cullen M.D.*, 2 vols. (Edinburgh, 1859), II, p. 574. It should be noted that the Edinburgh College of Surgeons exchanged class tickets for the College diploma. See Clarendon Hyde Creswell, *The Royal College of Surgeons of Edinburgh* (Edinburgh, 1926), pp. 169–90.
52 For an outline analysis of the Society later in the century see J. R. R. Christie, 'Edinburgh Medicine in the Eighteenth Century, the View from the Students', *Bulletin of the Society for the Social History of Medicine*, XIX (1976), 13–15.

in Latin, aimed at producing ornate and learned physicians. But they could also attend vernacular courses, which stressed surgery, ontology and local pathology. The next ten years partially resolved this dichotomy.

Maturity, 1766–76

This ten-year period is conveniently marked at the one end by the appointments of John Gregory and William Cullen as professors of the Practice and Institutes respectively, and at the other by Cullen's decision to give up clinical lecturing and the appointment of James Gregory in succession to his father in 1776. In fact, during these years Cullen and Gregory shared the lectures on the Institutes and the Practice. Within this period the lectures of the younger Monro continued to flourish, and the appointment of Joseph Black to the Chair of Chemistry gave extra dash to the school. From the numbers of student notes extant and the testimony of former pupils the evidence is that the medical classes filled out during these years.[53] Both Cullen and Gregory were cultured men and aimed to impress on their students that medicine was a learned and genteel occupation.[54] Like their predecessors both were dogmatic physicians and stressed the importance of practising medicine within a system. In Cullen's case the defence of a systematic medicine was underwritten by a new and sophisticated philosophy of science derived from David Hume.[55] Traditionalists though they were, the teachings of both these men also showed a sharp awareness of the medical changes that had taken place since the school's foundation. Both lectured in English and both presented medicine in such a way that an audience with heterogeneous demands could be satisfied. Cullen's lectures in particular embody the sort of synthesis that has been held by Ludmilla Jordanova to identify the 'increasingly self confident medical profession' of the late Enlightenment.[56] The medical systems of Cullen's French contemporaries have been analysed by Jordanova, but many of the

---

53 Thomson, *Cullen*.
54 See [John Gregory], *Observations on the Duties and Offices of a Physician* (London, 1770). Gregory gave these lectures as an introduction to his course. The first edition was anonymous, being taken from a student's notes. An authorised edition appeared in 1772.
55 See J. R. R. Christie, 'Ether and the Science of Chemistry 1740–1790', in G. N. Cantor and M. J. S. Hodge (eds.), *Conceptions of Ether* (Cambridge, 1981), pp. 85–110.
56 L. J. Jordanova, 'Earth Science and Environmental Medicine: The Synthesis of the Late Enlightenment', in L. J. Jordanova and Roy Porter (eds.), *Images of the Earth* (Chalfont St Giles, 1979), pp. 119–46.

elements she describes can be found in Cullen's work. Cullen's system presented a totally naturalistic account of health and disease based on the laws of the environment–organism relationship. For Cullen these laws were essentially those of sensibility and irritability. Developing Whytt's account of the sentient principle, Cullen used these concepts to create a model of the reactive organism, drawing attention on the one hand to the determining power of the environment and on the other to the original human constitution. These laws were used by him to construct a physiology, a psychology and then, in turn, an anthropology. They were also used as the foundation of pathology and, with natural history, to explain the geography of disease and the laws of hygiene.

Cullen's success lay in his ability to incorporate the new medical concerns of the time within a single system that clearly delineated a possible role for medical men either as traditional physicians or as new social architects. The most important new features of mid-eighteenth-century medicine to which his system paid reference were the increasing concern with slow and nervous fevers, the interest in the diseases of the military, the worry about the healthiness of institutions and the question of dirt, overcrowding and contagion. These epidemiological issues that took shape at this time have been related by several writers to more general factors. The most important of these are cameralism and the origins of medical police. It has been suggested that during the eighteenth century British physicians increasingly turned to meteorology, pneumatics and the powers of the atmosphere to demonstrate the whole system of nature and in turn explain health and disease. This medical understanding of the circulation in the atmospheric economy created a role for physicians in the policing of health and the managing of sickness in society at large. Hygiene and health were coupled with descriptions of how the whole system operated naturally and harmoniously. Diseases on the other hand were associated with sources of putrefaction, corruption and decay, where pathology resulted from the stagnation of the vital circulation. The practical result was in the management of those institutions where these conditions prevailed, the camp, the garrison, the ship, the prison and the hospital.[57] Cullen's system embraced all these issues by including a wide-ranging account of the diseases of foreign climes and directions for the management of civilian populations explained by the fundamental laws of physiology. Gregory's medical teaching lay in Cullen's shadow and was, moreover, much

57 Simon Schaffer, 'Natural Philosophy and Public Spectacle', *History of Science,* XXI (1983), 1–43.

more sceptical and tentative in its conclusions. However, the same sorts of questions were brought to the fore in his lectures making the emphasis in his work far closer to Cullen's than to that of his predecessors.

Cullen's system also included one area that has proved puzzling to historians, his nosology, often thought of as a fruitless labour. Properly regarded, however, the nosology can be seen to have served several ends. First, it was an unequivocal statement of an ontological theory of diseases discernible by natural historical methods. Second, it was a simple didactic device in that the order of Cullen's lectures followed the order of his nosology. Third, the subordinating principles on which the nosology was based were the function of the nervous system, and thus the nosology was a way of imparting the whole of Cullen's system and showing its points of contact with the tangible reality of disease. In other words, to learn the nosology properly was to learn the whole of Cullen's system. Finally it was intended not as a finished product, but as structure within which to study pathological anatomy and pursue nosography. Cullen wanted disease species to be defined ultimately by the results of many postmortems. Here was the dovetailing of Cullen's course with that of his anatomical colleague. Likewise Cullen held that in most instances the clinical description of diseases was in its infancy and that there was still a great deal of cautious nosographical work to be done, both at the bedside and at the epidemiological level in, for example, the military camp.[58] It was, it should be recalled, Cullen's astuteness as a clinician that many students remembered most fondly about him.[59] Not surprisingly, then, the evidence, in terms of numbers of clinical notes, suggests the increasing importance of infirmary attendance in this decade. This systematically informed clinical medicine was later called, with much praise, 'rational empiricism'.[60]

Thus in the 1770s the student attending Edinburgh could find in Cullen's system the description of a role for the educated doctor as personal physician, natural historian or nosographer, but also an account of how, through his knowledge of the natural economy, the medical man was best fitted to be the manager of civil and military

58   See, e.g., Medical Society of London, MS. 63a, p. 56.
59   Astley Cooper, who was in Edinburgh in 1787, wrote, 'Never shall I forget the veneration with which I viewed Cullen; he was then an old man; physic may have much improved since this time, but if Hippocrates was its father, Cullen was its favoured son'; Bransby Blake Cooper, *The Life of Sir Astley Cooper Bart.*, 2 vols. (London, 1843), I, p. 172.
60   J. Bostock, 'History of Medicine', in John Forbes, Alexander Tweedie and John Conolly (eds.), *The Cyclopedia of Medical Practice*, 4 vols. (London, 1833), I, p. 69.

institutions. This in fact is what many of Cullen's pupils went on to become.[61]

It was then the range and topicality of the medicine taught at Edinburgh at this time that made it the Mecca of medical education. The spectrum of courses on offer produced some interesting consequences for surgery and medicine. Considered passively, the Monros provide a perfect example of the rising status of surgeons and the consequent transfer of surgical ideas into medical thought.[62] Considered more actively, however, not in terms of 'surgery rising' but in terms of real individuals, it can be seen that the Monros successfully cornered anatomical and surgical teaching in Edinburgh and provided courses that were both learned, in that they were based on medical theory, and practical. For the ambitious young practitioner anxious to break into the expanding Enlightenment medical market the Monros' course provided the necessary cultural equipment in terms of training in the most up-to-date science.[63] This entrepreneurial success was, as it happened, pursued in an institutional framework within which they were considered equals by medical colleagues. Indeed, Monro *secundus* was a titular as well as a social equal. These were perfect conditions for the potential interchange of medical and surgical ideas and were exploited to that end by Cullen. Cullen's lectures have a far greater intellectual continuity with those of Monro *secundus* than did Rutherford's with those of Monro *primus*. At the one extreme Cullen's lectures were part of a tradition that offered an education to genteel physicians. At the other it provided a cultural and practical training for the new artisans of the medical world. Most students probably clustered around the middle of the spectrum, intent on becoming learned, but not élite practitioners, elegant but not afraid to use their hands. Cullen, it might be said, was the first mass medical educator in the vernacular. Testimony to Cullen's pulling power came from William Hunter, who had always remained on good terms with his former teacher. In 1765 he wrote to Cullen urging him to join him in establishing a medical school in Glasgow: 'We should at once draw all the English, and, I presume

61 The careers of former Edinburgh students clearly deserve study. Some idea of their multifarious destinies can be gained from Bostock, 'History of Medicine', in Forbes et al., and Tröhler, 'Quantification in British Medicine'.
62 The importance of this event was first pointed out by Owsei Temkin in 'The Role of Surgery in the Rise of Modern Medical Thought', *Bulletin of the History of Medicine*, XXV (1951), 248–59. Temkin, of course, does not reify 'surgery' in the way I have suggested.
63 I am thinking here less of medicine as a technical procedure than as a cultural passport. Cf. Arnold Thackray, 'Natural Knowledge in Cultural Context: The Manchester Model', *American Historical Review*, LXXIX (1974), 672–709.

most of the Scotch students. Among other reasons, I should not dislike teaching anatomy near my two friends, the Monroes, [*sic*] to whom I owe so much.'[64] This remark is revealing in several ways. To begin with it finishes on an obvious note of sarcasm; Hunter had so little love for the Monros that he was prepared to take their students away. The irony of the remark is that he did owe Monro *primus* a great deal, as pointed out earlier. Indirectly too, the letter is also more than simple testimony to Cullen's skill for what it really pays tribute to is the *combined* pulling power of an eminent anatomist (Monro *secundus*) and a physician. Hunter clearly saw that geography was no bar to large audiences, as the student market for the teaching in a Scottish medical school was clearly not just the Edinburgh hinterland.

The dialectics of medical education

At least two important questions arise in regard to the educational skills of these northern pedagogues. First, what was it about Scotland that made them so peculiarly able to provide courses that were crowded out with students most of whom would leave Scotland? Second, to what extent did they simply respond to a new medical demand, and how far did they actually shape the medical consciousness of the late eighteenth century? Both questions admit of extended discussion. In regard to the first question, however, the answer lies in part in the peculiarly Scottish post-Union context, where an ideology of cultural 'improvement' had been shaped that placed a particularly high value on practical knowledge and that esteemed natural science in this regard.[65] This ideology was forged within a culture that had always valued the training of young men to be of service to the state and had educational institutions well structured to serve a large market.[66] Scottish professors then were intent on educating students in a practical discipline but by way of a sound philosophical or theoretical training. Thus these teachers whilst teaching systematically were prepared to organise their courses so that their practical applications were apparent. Cullen's nosology is

64   Thomson, *Cullen*, William Hunter to William Cullen, 1 April 1765, I, p. 151.
65   Nicholas Phillipson, 'The Scottish Enlightenment', in Roy Porter and Mikuláš Teich (eds.), *The Enlightenment in National Context* (Cambridge, 1981), pp. 19–40. See also Phillipson's earlier articles cited in his notes.
66   It was a long-standing Scottish conviction that 'the primary function of the universities was to train young men of appropriate talents for the service of society in Church and state'. Ronald G. Cant, 'Origins of the Enlightenment in Scotland: The Universities', in R. H. Campbell and Andrew S. Skinner (eds.), *The Origins and Nature of the Scottish Enlightenment* (Edinburgh, 1982), p. 44.

the most obvious example of this. The answer to the second question – Who shaped whose consciousness? – shades into this. There was an expanding medical educational market in the eighteenth century, where, in an increasingly fluid and pleasure-orientated society, upward mobility could be achieved through medical practice.[67] The professors catered to this demand for a learned medical education.[68] Factors such as these shaped the form of medical lectures and no doubt their content to some extent. But this is not to suggest that the whole of the intellectual substance of Edinburgh medicine was a response to the student audience. International and local concerns, material interests and intellectual problems all played their part. Besides, the relations between professors and students were not unidirectional. Students did not demand and professors merely perform. There was a much more subtle dialectical involvement. Just as students came to be taught how to practise medicine so the professors in turn taught them to evaluate highly practical knowledge. They also taught them respect or distaste for theory, and a love or repugnance for scepticism. Students turned up at lectures for what their professors had told them to value. To take one example, the overwhelming emphasis on the nervous system in the lectures of all the teachers arose almost entirely from preoccupations relating to the Scottish cultural context.[69] Yet this did not inhibit students such as Benjamin Rush from adopting the model, modifying it and using it elsewhere. There was no anomaly in Scottish medicine being a home-grown product appropriate for mass international consumption.

Acknowledgements

Many of the points raised in this essay are dealt with in much greater detail in my doctoral thesis, 'Medicine as Culture: Edinburgh and the Scottish Enlightenment' (University of London, 1984). The importance of the 'ornate' in Scottish medical education was pointed out to me by J. B. Morrell, to whom I am very grateful. For permission to

67 For the significance of health and its relation to pleasure in the Enlightenment see Roy Porter, 'Was There a Medical Enlightenment in Eighteenth Century England?' *British Journal for Eighteenth Century Studies*, V (1982), 49–63.
68 See the attempt by Vern Bullough and Bonnie Bullough to explain the flowering of Edinburgh medicine by simple statistical appeal to changes in the Scottish population structure in 'The Causes of the Scottish Medical Renaissance of the Eighteenth Century', *Bulletin of the History of Medicine*, XLV (1971), 13–28. John Christie, in an unpublished paper, first exposed the deficiencies of this approach.
69 Christopher Lawrence. 'The Nervous System and Society in the Scottish Enlightenment', in Barry Barnes and Steven Shapin (eds.), *Natural Order* (Beverly Hills, Calif., 1979), pp. 19–40.

quote from manuscripts I should like to thank the libraries of Edinburgh University; King's College, Aberdeen; the Medical Society of London; the Royal College of Physicians, Edinburgh; the Royal College of Surgeons, England; the Royal Infirmary of Edinburgh; the Royal Medical Society; and the Wellcome Institute for the History of Medicine.

7

German medical education in the eighteenth century: the Prussian context and its influence

JOHANNA GEYER-KORDESCH

No claim for a proper assessment of medical education in the eighteenth century is possible if it rests solely on an analysis of internal organisation. In considering medical education at the Universities of Halle and Berlin (founded in 1694 and 1810, respectively) one is already *in media res* in regard to both the history of universities in Germany and their political and cultural significance. The universities of the German-speaking world were more subject to the vicissitudes of religious, cultural and political pressures than, say, the insular, élite and strangely traditional medieval foundations of Oxford and Cambridge. Whereas the traditions of monasticism in these two towns still strike the eye today, much of what was formerly the extensive, amoebalike contour of the Holy Roman Empire *Deutscher Nation* has disappeared or changed beyond recognition.

A brief historical survey shows how diverse and turbulent was the background against which the fortunes of the universities waxed and waned. North of the Alps the renaissance of higher learning began later than at Oxford and Cambridge: at Prague in 1348; Cracow, 1364; and Vienna, 1365. It then spread northward and eastward to Heidelberg, Cologne, Erfurt, Leipzig, Rostock, Greifswald, Freiburg/ Breisgau, Ingolstadt, Trier, Mainz, Wittenberg, Tübingen and Frankfurt-an-der-Oder. With the great disruption of the Reformation the mould of scholasticism and humanism was broken and a new intellectual map was drawn, repositioning faculties according to sovereign and creed. The Reformation also triggered the founding of the first Protestant universities, financed and protected by the local *Landesfürst*, the reigning duke, these being Marburg (1527), Königsberg (1544), Jena (1558), Helmstedt (1576), Giessen (1607) and Rinteln (1621). In the seventeenth century the universities, both old and new, were battered by various religious and political controversies, particularly that between Calvinism and Lutheranism, which caused disruption in reigning houses and amongst their subjects, as well as the larger tensions created by the Catholic Counter-Reformation.

Within the House of Habsburg's sphere of influence the magnificent opulence of Austrian baroque emerged, built on the shadowy and questionable foundation of reconversion to the old faith.[1] The Jesuit university in Vienna became more powerful than the older, traditional one. The Austrian lands, which had been largely Protestant, saw, in the course of the seventeenth century, punitive measures enforced whose effect was expulsion or, alternatively, the nominal adoption of Roman Catholicism. The highly literate and book-oriented culture of Protestantism moved elsewhere with those whose consciences clung to their religion. The same was true of the French Huguenots coming to Protestant lands (England, the Netherlands, Prussia) after the revocation of the Edict of Nantes (1685).

These religious issues and the political interests that prodded and used them had their effect.[2] Again, universities rose and declined with emigrant talent or they bled in the fractious financial or succession disputes that loomed large in the sovereign tapestry of the German lands (often there was no rule of primogeniture in the smaller reigning houses). Another ruinous influence during this period was the duration of the Thirty Years War. In times of war, with its concomitant plundering and hunger, its general effect of impoverishment, institutionalised learning does not blossom. Most universities survived but their intellectual impact was restricted to a few outstanding personalities and publications that shine through the tempestuous climate of the period.

In Prussia, once peace had been restored, a new era began. The *Grosse Kurfürst*, Frederick William (1620–88), laid the foundation for the growth of wealth and power. His successor, Frederick I (1657–1713), and his court were preoccupied with the outward trappings of power. From Habsburg (the Holy Roman Emperor) he bought (literally) the right to be called king *in* Prussia, and was duly crowned in Königsberg in 1701. In 1680 the territory of Magdeburg came under Prussian dominion. On its outskirts lay the city of Halle with its nascent academy.[3] Across the border, in the dukedom of Saxony, the

1 For a fine exposition of these problems, and literature, see Friedrich Heer, *Der Kampf um die österreichische Identität* (Vienna, 1981), pp. 40–92.

2 For a detailed analysis of a German university that did not survive religious, political and financial pressures, see Gerhard Schormann, *Academia Ernestina, Die schaumburgische Universität zu Rinteln an der Weser (1610/21–1810)* (Marburg, 1982). For the most recent survey of literature on universities, see the excellent review by N. Hammerstein, 'Jubiläumsschrift und Alltagsarbeit. Tendenzen bildungsgeschichtlicher Literatur', *Historische Zeitschrift*, No. 3 (1983), pp. 601–33.

3 E. Neuß, 'Die vorakademischen Akademien in Halle', *Hallische Universitätsreden*, Neue Folge 44, 1961; F. Paulsen, *Geschichte des gelehrten Unterrichts*, 2 vols., 3rd ed. (Berlin, 1919), I, pp. 514ff.

University of Leipzig was an old institution (founded 1409) and continued to be a stronghold of orthodox Lutheran power.[4] To the south
and west of Halle, in the duchies of Sachsen-Gotha-Weimar, the University of Jena (a post-Reformation university, founded 1548–58)[5] catered for a different sort of clientele: By the end of the seventeenth
century its faculties of mathematics, medicine and theology were notable. The teachers here included Erhard Weigel (1625–99), an eccen-
tric, unorthodox man who was the foremost teacher of mathematics
and astronomy at the time, and Kaspar Sagittarius (1643–94), one of
the very few professors of history and a supporter of enthusiastic
religion. Such men overstepped the boundaries of tradition. Weigel
went so far as to teach in the vernacular, an affront that Christian
Thomasius (1655–1728) copied conscientiously, both at Leipzig and
when he came to Halle. It is also to be noted that these small territories were strongholds of a new religious and cultural force, Lutheran
Pietism. This was a mainstream revivalist movement whose network
of support had been steadily expanding since the 1670s and that was
not subjected to the same persecution by either the resident theological faculty at Jena or the local secular authorities as were the
more radical religious sects.

The *founding* of the University of Halle,[6] though not its crucial
importance for the eighteenth century, is to be explained in terms of
the dynastic interests of the rulers of Prussia (the reigning house was
nominally Calvinist). Their concern was to provide their Lutheran
subjects with another prominent university (Frankfurt-an-der-Oder
and Königsberg, both to the east, were the others of immediate relevance). Of the universities established in the period between the
foundation of Halle and that of Berlin – and there were six in Germany proper – only one other, Göttingen (1737), rose to decisive
cultural prominence, although many made intellectual contributions.

In assessing medical teaching at Halle and its later establishment in
Berlin more than the structural organisation is at stake. The impor-

---

4 'Die Leipziger Theologen im Kampf gegen Synkretismus und Pietismus 1592–
1699', in *Festschrift zur Feier des 500jährigen Bestehens der Universität Leipzig*, 2 vols.
(Leipzig, 1909), I, pp. 108–33.
5 For the history of Jena see *Geschichte der Universität Jena 1548/58–1958* (Jena,
1962). For E. Weigel, Kaspar Sagittarius, Johann Franz Buddeus and early Pietism,
see in particular chap. 4, pp. 486ff; the volume contains an excellent bibliography.
6 Much has been written on Halle. The official history is still Wilhelm Schrader,
Geschichte der Friedrichs-Universität Halle, 2 vols. (Berlin, 1894). The most recent
bibliography (including eighteenth-century works) can be found in Notker Hammerstein, *Jus und Historie* (Göttingen, 1972), although he treats mainly the faculty of
law. See also N. Hammerstein, 'Zur Geschichte der Deutschen Universität im
Zeitalter der Aufklärung', in H. Rössler and G. Franz (eds.), *Universität und
Gelehrtenstand 1400–1800* (Limburg/Lahn, 1970); *450-Jahre Martin-Luther-Universität
Halle-Wittenberg*, 2 vols. (Halle, 1952), vol. 2.

tance of medicine at Halle and then in Berlin depended on more than what we would now call the curriculum or programme offered. The taste of the new, the flavour of being at centre stage, was not technocratic, but rather that of intellectual tension and discussion. At Halle, as we shall see in greater detail, Enlightenment and enthusiastic religion, two trends formed and articulated by the turn of the century, vied for allegiance. In mid-century the Hanoverian university of Göttingen,[7] financed and protected by George I, the English king, and structurally modelled after Halle, advocated the natural-scientific approach to medicine[8] early championed by Hermann Boerhaave in Leiden. In this it achieved a counterpoint to the concerns prevalent at Halle. At the Prussian university medicine had not yet disengaged itself from the broader spectrum of debate concerning the nature of man or the theological discussion of his ultimate purpose. In Berlin, the third centre of influence, another pattern of medical education emerged. Its inception, as will be shown, rested upon a curious liaison. The Pietist university exported talent to the centre of administrative power, Berlin. Practical matters, three in particular, were at issue: (1) bureaucratic control of medical qualifications; (2) better surgical and medical care for the expansion of the Prussian army; and (3) expanded hospital facilities for the sick poor.

In Berlin these three areas of medical expansion and institutionalisation progressed on the basis of personal influence and recruitment managed along a Berlin–Halle axis. When Wilhelm von Humboldt master-minded the founding of the University of Berlin in 1810,[9] medical courses *and* clinical instruction were already a going concern. One could even state that the Berlin university grew up around a medical nucleus that had fostered the educational and professional standards in that discipline for nearly a century. Besides Berlin, the scientific allure of Göttingen, with its small 'academic' clinics, including the early teaching clinic (hospital is too grand a word) for male and female midwives (1751), pales just a bit.[10]

Before discussing medicine at Halle and Berlin, a structural comparison with other universities of relevence should be made. In the

---

7 Literature on Göttingen is contained in Wilhelm Ebel (ed.), *Die Privilegien und ältesten Statuten der Georg-August-Universität zu Göttingen* (Göttingen, 1961); W. Ebel, *Catalogus Professorum Göttingensium 1734–1962* (Göttingen, 1962); Hammerstein, *Jus und Historie*, chap. 7 'Die Universität Göttingen', pp. 309ff; G. von Selle, *Die Georg-August-Universität zu Göttingen 1737–1937* (Göttingen, 1937).

8 Medical history has tended to emphasise this above all else. See Brita Thode, 'Die Göttinger Anatomie 1733–1828' (Ph.D. Diss., Göttingen, 1979); W. Brednow, *Jena und Göttingen, Medizinische Beziehungen im 18. und 19. Jahrhundert* (Jena, 1949).

9 The standard work on the University of Berlin is Max Lenz, *Geschichte der Universität Berlin*, 2 vols. (Halle, 1910).

10 H. Martius, *Die Universitäts-Frauenklinik in Göttingen. Von ihrer Gründung im Jahre 1751 als Accouchirhospital . . . bis . . . 1951* (Stuttgart, 1951).

North those that serve best as a guide to medical teaching would be Jena, Leiden and Göttingen. Leiden is included here as one of the leading medical faculties of the time and one of the centres to which students travelled from various countries. It is well to note at this juncture that at best small numbers were involved in the education of learned doctors.[11] The faculties with the most numbers of students were still those of law and theology. Juridical training, which served the bureaucratic concerns of the small German states, drew students from aristocratic families and those of middle-class urban backgrounds with a stake in the civil service.[12] The training for clergymen was socially less dependent on élites, although many came from church-connected families. However, the churches required full theological studies and held fast to their own methods of doctrinal surveillance. Only practical medicine in the eighteenth century was suffused with empirics of various persuasions and with practitioners in fields outside university training (surgeons, midwives, apothecaries).[13] A medical doctorate was not essential for practice. However, the higher administrative posts (such as court physicians, city physicians, university teaching) were the province of the learned doctor. It was here that the pattern of medical influence and effectiveness made its presence felt. It instituted change in medical organisation and administration. In this regard the university, with its professors and graduates, the qualifications it insisted upon, and in terms of recommendations, was a broker of talent. That is why the intellectual and personal constellations at Halle and Berlin were so significant for Prussia. A lonely faculty of medicine without its networks was a ship without moorings.

11 The literature on student numbers is complex. The main references in respect to medicine, exclusive of published matriculation lists are F. Eulenburg, *Die Frequenz der deutschen Universitäten von ihrer Gründung bis zur Gegenwart* (Leipzig, 1904); E. Th. Nauck, 'Die Zahl der Medizinstudenten der deutschen Hochschulen im 14.–18. Jahrhundert', in *Sudhoffs Archiv*, 38 (1954), pp. 175–86; F. Zimmermann, 'Materialien zur Herkunft der Studenten der Universität Halle in der Zeit von 1696–1730', in *450 Jahre Martin-Luther-Universität Halle-Wittenberg*, II, pp. 95–100; H. Mitgau, 'Soziale Herkunft der deutschen Studenten bis 1900', in Rössler and Franz, *Universität und Gelehrtenstand 1400–1800*, pp. 232–68 (mainly mid-eighteenth century onward). The problem of numbers is further complicated by the fact that matriculation is not graduation and also by the habit of studying at different universities.
12 Typical of the attitude of the aristocracy with regard to juridical training are the pressures exerted by the family of N. L. Count Zinzendorf (all high-placed civil servants) when he wanted to study theology. He studied law. A. G. Spangenberg, *Leben des Herrn Nikolaus Ludwig Grafen Zinzendorf . . .* , 8 vols., n.d. (preface signed 1755), n.p.; F. W. Euler, 'Entstehung und Entwicklung Deutscher Gelehrtengeschlechter', in Rössler and Franz, *Universität und Gelehrtenstand 1400–1800*, pp. 183–232; Hans Rosenberg, *Bureaucracy, Aristocracy and Autocracy: The Prussian Experience 1660–1815* (Boston, 1958).
13 For an attempt to illustrate medical care in Berlin, see M. Sturzbecher, *Beiträge zur Berliner Medizingeschichte* (Berlin, 1966), pp. 67ff.

The medical faculty at Jena was a substantial one at a university strong in one of the important developments of the period, the chemiatric interpretation of physiology and therapeutics.[14] In the seventeenth century Werner Rolfinck (1599–1673) was one of the most enthusiastic adherents and defenders of Harvey's discovery of circulation. Towards the end of the seventeenth century the faculty had three full professors of medicine, Rudolph Wilhelm Krause (1642–1718), Georg Wolfgang Wedel (1645–1721) and August Heinrich Fasch (1639–1690). After 1690 the faculty had four or five full-time members. There are no readily available figures for the medical students or for the graduates or near graduates who held lectures on their own (*extraordinarien; doctores legentes*). All in all, Jena was influential in medicine because of the number and high quality of its full faculty. Most of the professors mentioned had travelled widely (England, Holland, Italy). Krause and Wedel especially had absorbed the theories of Sylvius in Leiden and were experts in chemistry. Both Georg Ernst Stahl (1660–1734) and Friedrich Hoffmann (1660–1742), the two professors of medicine at Halle, and fine chemists in their own right, studied under Wedel and received their doctorates at Jena. Judging from the courses offered and the high number of dissertations completed in medicine towards the end of the seventeenth century, medical education at Jena was broadly effective. It did not so much decline as recede before the changes in approach wrought by Stahl and his opponents of the 'mechanist' school with its Boerhaavian-trained adherents. An interesting comparison is provided by a survey of medical faculties of 1828, at which time Jena had ten professors of medicine out of a faculty of fifty to fifty-seven, with between 450 and 500 students at the university. In 1828, then, the total number of students at Jena was equal to the number of students of medicine at Halle in the eighteenth century at its peak.[15]

The University of Leiden in the seventeenth and eighteenth centuries was a pole-star of medical learning, attracting students and medical visitors from many nations. Its attraction lay in the teaching of anatomy (the *theatrum anatomicum* was not only well equipped, but

---

14 Information taken from E. Giese and B. von Hagen, *Geschichte der Medizinischen Fakultät der Friedrich-Schiller-Universität Jena* (Jena, 1958). This book is too sporadic and eclectic to be entirely useful. An excellent description of the eighteenth-century history of the University of Jena (including economic and social history) in chaps. 3–4 of *Geschichte der Universität Jena 1548/58–1958*; medical faculty, pp. 156–160; student matriculation, pp. 174–6.
15 Figures for 1828 are given in H. F. Kilian, *Die Universitäten Deutschlands in medicin-naturwissenschaftlicher Hinsicht* (1828; reprint, Amsterdam, 1966), p. 282. No published material is available on medical students at Jena in the eighteenth century. The highpoint of student matriculation was the period in Jena 1711–20, with 720 new matriculations per year. See *Geschichte*, p. 175.

also had frequent public dissections) and in Hermann Boerhaave's lectures. The influence of medicine at Leiden is well documented, accessible and need not be duplicated here.[16] What should be pointed out is that in the eighteenth century (Boerhaave died in 1738) in the Protestant north (Holland and Germany proper) only three university medical faculties had peak student numbers: Leiden with over 300 after 1709; Halle with 529 in 1730; Göttingen (founded 1737) with 491 in 1800. The number of matriculated students in medical faculties in the German-speaking lands (excluding Vienna and Jena and including Salzburg and Basel) rose steadily, from 308 in 1660 to 3,234 in 1800. Halle from 1710 onward consistently ranged over 300, making that university's medical faculty with its two to three full professors one of the largest next to Leiden.[17]

Expansion in medical education in the latter half of the eighteenth century is quite clear. Not only did full professorships rise with the student numbers, but Göttingen and Berlin established themselves almost immediately as centres of the natural sciences. Subjects subsumed under medical teaching, such as botany and chemistry, in the latter half of the eighteenth century received their own chairs. Anatomy, surgery and gynaecology became teaching subjects no longer linked to an apprenticeship, guild-oriented or empiric (midwives) structure of learning. In a book on the medical faculties at universities in Germany proper of 1828 the expanded teaching subjects were as follows: Berlin, with 29 faculty members in medicine out of 104 professorships; Göttingen with 18 out of 85 to 87 professorships; Halle with 9 out of 60 to 65 professorships. Total student matriculation at these universities ran between 1,500 (Göttingen), 1,400 (Berlin) and 1,300 (Halle) in 1828. Law and theology, however, still carried the day.[18]

Although numbers and structural changes indicate university dominance of the qualifications expected in medicine, they do not explain entirely why or how this came about. In the following discussion one aspect of this change will be pursued. This is the link between Halle and Berlin, a link clasping disparate purposes at a time *before*

16 See G. A. Lindeboom, *A Classified Bibliography of the History of Dutch Medicine 1900–1974* (The Hague, 1975), 'Leyden', pp. 418ff. There has been much work on foreign students, on the seventeenth century, on Boerhaave and the anatomical theatre, but none on the total student numbers in medicine in the eighteenth century or on the medical faculty and its composition.

17 These figures are from Nauck, 'Die Zahl', p. 182. See also Heinz Schneppen, *Niederländische Universitäten und deutsches Geistesleben. Von der Gründung der Universität Leiden bis ins späte 18. Jahrhundert* (Münster, 1960), p. 109.

18 H. F. Kilian, *Die Universitäten Deutschlands*, p. 54 (Berlin); p. 79 (Göttingen); p. 126 (Halle); medical faculty members are listed under each university.

university medical faculties were integrated primarily with the natural sciences and developed their familiar nineteenth-century pattern. We return therefore to the beginning of the eighteenth century and the social and intellectual movements of that time, in a word, to its cultural context. The focus is on Prussia in the first years of its monarchy until the time of its dynastic consolidation under Frederick the Great. Halle had a role to play immediately after its founding in 1694 as the leading Prussian university comprising a faculty of luminaries in the juridical, theological and medical fields. These were university teachers recently appointed who were much more than specialists in their subjects. They had been immersed in the great ideological currents of the time, and emerged in spanking shape: Stahl and Hoffmann from training at Jena, atop the field in chemistry and the often eclectic medicine of the age, with Stahl willing and able to integrate theoretically questions of theology and philosophy with medicine; Christian Thomasius and the juridical faculty aiming for a new secularised conception of law, undoing religious influences (problem of witchcraft; problem of interfaith marriages) and hoisting the banner of enlightenment, another word for secular morals; August Hermann Francke and his staffing of the theological faculty with the type of committed clergyman who does not think religion is solely an academic subject. Common to these wonderfully inharmonious aims were the dissatisfaction with tradition and a solid intellectual ability to argue new and useful (however they were later judged) directions.

In Berlin before 1810 there was no intellectual centre other than the Prussian Academy founded by Gottfried Wilhelm Leibniz in 1700.[19] In the medical section of the academy nothing much was happening, the physicians who were members in Berlin being of minor stature and held in check by Andreas von Gundelsheimer, first court physician to Frederick I, who opposed the academy. Friedrich Hoffmann, who brought scientific light and organisational abilities to the academy when he went to Berlin in 1708, was forced out in 1712. The *Medizinal Ordnung* of 1685 had instituted professional criteria for physicians, but they were hardly enforceable. A *collegium medicum* of the normal type, (i.e., a body of learned physicians of the town that met regularly) existed. In 1713 all this changed as Frederick William I (1688–1740) ascended the throne. A practical king, he admired pragmatic instaurations. As with finances and the army, so with medicine: It would have to carry its practical weight.

---

19 The standard work is Adolf Harnack, *Geschichte der Königlich Preussischen Akademie der Wissenschaften zu Berlin*, 4 vols. (Berlin, 1900).

I

The University of Halle was officially inaugurated in 1694 with all the pomp and circumstance of the baroque.[20] The preliminary skirmishes leading to its foundation had been fought in Berlin. This was wholly natural considering that the seat of power resided in the administrative apparatus responsible to the monarch. However, the intentions of bureaucracy were almost immediately superseded by the counsel and motivation of personalities outside the circle of responsible ministers. This was due to social and intellectual pressures on the new university. These were not narrowly political, in the sense of accomplishing what today might be called a 'party' or ideological programme, but were determined by groups and interests that had to be recognised within Brandenburg-Prussia.[21] These interests were part of larger socio-cultural changes in Germany, and if they found elbow-room in Prussia, it was due to the very porous nature of eighteenth-century German frontiers and to Prussia's still relatively weak economic and political condition.

The inaugural ceremony of 1694 was – although historians have not called it such – an acknowledgement of the value of dissidents. The new members of the three major faculties were distinguished in their respective fields, but the leading personalities had come to Halle following various processes of disruption. The great upheavals within German Lutheranism, provoked by the broadly based revivalist movement within its own ranks (Pietism), had caused bitter splits across North Germany, especially in the more established universities such as Jena, Leipzig and Erfurt. All of these universities were outside Brandenburg-Prussia's borders. Near these borders, in the neighbouring territories of Sachsen-Weimar and its smaller splinter-

20 Schrader, *Geschichte der Friedrichs-Universität Halle,* vol. I; Hammerstein, *Jus und Historie,* pp. 148ff; Paulsen, *Geschichte des gelehrten Unterrichts,* I, pp. 524ff; J. C. Hoffbauer, *Geschichte der Universität Halle bis zum Jahre 1805* (Halle, 1805); J. C. Förster, *Übersicht der Geschichte der Universität Halle in ihrem ersten Jahrhundert* (Halle, 1794). Because Halle was *the* exemplary university of the German Enlightenment, there has always been a great debate as to which elements were 'more progressive'. My interpretation differs from current interpretations and stems from readings into Pietist biographies and scholarship: Paul Grünberg, *Philipp Jacob Spener,* 3 vols. (Göttingen, 1893–1906); Gustav Kramer, *A. H. Francke, Ein Lebensbild,* 2 vols. (Halle, 1880–2).
21 Carl Hinrichs, *Preußentum und Pietismus. Der Pietismus in Brandenburg-Preußen als religiös-soziale Reformbewegung* (Göttingen, 1971); K. Deppermann, *Der hallesche Pietismus und der preußische Staat unter Friedrich III. (I.)* (Göttingen, 1961); 'Die Anfänge des Pietismus', in *Pietismus und Neuzeit, Ein Jahrbuch zur Geschichte des Neueren Pietismus,* vol. 4 (Göttingen, 1979); H. Lehmann, *Das Zeitalter des Absolutismus* (Stuttgart, 1980); W. Hubatsch, *Absolutismus* (Darmstadt, 1973). This is, of course, selective. Economic and diplomatic scholarship on Prussia is legion.

ings – although somewhat less in Saxony, the stronghold of orthodoxy (Leipzig) – Lutheran Pietism had recruited its most determined
following. The men who came to the University of Halle had all been
involved.

Two main groups wished to perpetuate their cultural ascendancy in
Halle. As ideas are not separate from men, these moved with their
proponents to the newly founded institution of learning. They represented powers of a different sort: On the one hand there was Christian Thomasius,[22] a brilliant and showy master of jurisprudence, who
increasingly represented (after his own spiritual turmoil) secularised
critical thinking. In the new faculty of law, a powerful assembly as far
as money-earning and the arbitration of civil life were concerned,
Thomasius became the symbol of self-conscious success. Those
qualities of the German Enlightenment, which later found their voice
in the sceptical, emancipated and yet morally didactic writings of G.
E. Lessing, Moses Mendelssohn or Friedrich Nicolai, had their intellectual predecessor here. Thomasius represented an individualistic
flair, in the ironic wit of his writings, in his disdain for the Latin of his
caste, in his fashionable dress. He was not aloof from political power,
however, and when he used his connections in the Berlin court, he
wilfully caused trouble for the administrative alignments within the
new university.[23] His juridical colleagues, Samuel Stryck and Justus
Henning Böhmer, later Johann Peter Ludewig amongst others, were
progressive. Their ability to earn outside fees made them relatively
independent of the university, and they were well aware of the an-
choring weight (high student numbers, knowledge of legalistic matters, law faculty opinions) their professorships constituted. Only
Thomasius, perfectly aware of these more sober qualities of power,
drew out other characteristics: those of a cultural rebelliousness that
indicated that thinking and habits were on the verge of change.

On the other hand there were the theologians. They also possessed
a network of patronage that struck root in Halle.[24] In contrast to the
law faculty, or for that matter the theological faculties elsewhere, they

22 Hammerstein, *Jus und Historie*, chap. 2: Christian Thomasius; G. Schubart-
Fikentscher, *Unbekannter Thomasius* (Weimar, 1954); Max Fleischmann, *Christian
Thomasius* (Halle, 1931); *Christian Thomasius in Schrift, Buch und Bild* (Catalogue of an
exhibition, containing bibliography) (Halle, 1928).
23 The most famous case is his criticism of the university on a visit to Berlin in
1713. It resulted in a commission. A university *consilium*, signed among others by
Stahl, opposed Thomasius. See Universitätsarchiv Halle, Rep. 3, Nr. 70; Schrader,
Geschichte der Friedrichs-Universität Halle, I, pp. 242ff.
24 See the discussion of posts, personalities and commitment in any of the
published or unpublished Pietist correspondences; e.g., Peter Schicketanz (ed.), *Der
Briefwechsel Carl Hildebrand von Cansteins mit August Hermann Francke* (Berlin, 1972).

were not committed solely to the advancement of academic learning. The turbulent beginnings of the rise of Lutheran Pietism had already produced some highly public academic dismissals. August Hermann Francke, whose influence was to be singularly dominant in Halle, had been 'routed' – that would be the correct term for the outcome of the sharp conflicts between his followers and the orthodox Lutheran theologians – from his teaching post in Leipzig and his revival efforts in Erfurt, events that caused these universities considerable discomfort. He had held Bible meetings from which he barred no one. He had drawn many listeners, including, perhaps most alarmingly, those training for clerical office. He was teaching Christian action based on a more literal understanding of the Bible than that current in orthodox circles, did not apply learning only to academicians, and did not heed the bounds of the conventional.[25] His followers were devoted to him.

When he was thrown out he saw it as being thrown onto the providence of God – and God acknowledged His own. His protector in Berlin was Philipp Jacob Spener,[26] who had left his position at the court of Dresden, unpopular with the ruler of Saxony because he did not condone his life-style, and had gone to Berlin, the second major centre of power for Lutherans. Spener had early on stood fast for religious renewal and reform and had been rewarded with biting attacks for what was meant to be a slur: 'Pietism'. His defender in the 1680s was Veit Ludwig von Seckendorff, one of the ablest administrators of the time, whose acclaimed talents had been well used by the smaller courts of the territories east and south of Prussia (those small lands from which Francke himself came). Veit Ludwig von Seckendorff's abilities were tapped by Bradenburg-Prussia when he was made first pro-rector (the rector or chancellor was always the king himself) of Halle University. It was not surprising that Francke received one of the first posts (initially in oriental languages) open at Halle. Other theologians, such as Joachim Justus Breithaupt and Johann Franz Buddeus, were drawn from the University of Jena. These men too were inclined towards the activism of Pietist Lutheran revival.

25   Francke's dismissals and the *collegium philobiblicum* are treated in G. Kramer, *A. H. Francke. Ein Lebensbild*. By Francke himself in 'Lebensnachrichten', in G. Kramer, *Beiträge zur Geschichte A. H. Franckes* (Halle, 1861). For Francke's distrust of 'reasoned religion', see F. de Boor, 'Erfahrung gegen Vernunft. Das Bekehrungserlebnis A. H. Franckes als Grundlage für den Kampf des Hallischen Pietismus gegen die Aufklärung', in H. Bornkamm (ed.), *Der Pietismus in Gestalten und Wirkungen* (Bielefeld, 1975).
26   J. Wallmann, *Philipp Jacob Spener und die Anfänge des Pietismus* (Tübingen, 1970); Veit Ludwig von Seckendorff, *Imago Pietatis* (n.p., 1692), countered the attacks against Spener and Pietism. On V. L. v. Seckendorff see *Allgemeine Deutsche Biographie*. Spener was instrumental in Francke's installation in Halle.

Francke arrived in Halle in 1691, three years before the official inauguration. He was certainly one of the most formative influences on the new university. His manner was quiet, but he rarely backed down on an issue he considered important. He also had the talent of inspiring confidence, remarkable because not only students and those dependent on him responded but also those who were his equals in learning, age and talent. Heinrich Julius Elers, for example, gave up a promising theological career and all prospects of personal wealth to make common cause with Francke. Elers, who died owning one suit of clothes and a bible, built up the *Waisenhaus Verlag* (publishing house). This included presses and an extensive distribution system for books by eminent authors, largely Pietist, but also prominent juridical and medical authorities. The publishing house was located in and administered by the *Waisenhaus* institutions and its directorship. The *Waisenhaus* took its name from its inception as an orphanage, but homeless children were only a small part of its work. When Francke died (1727) it was engaged in such varied activities as Old Testament translation (*Oriental Seminar*), schools for boys from different social backgrounds, the education of girls, better training for teachers, a laboratory for medical remedies and the distribution of the most famous of these, the *Essentia dulcis*, to patients far afield, and the production of a German bible everybody could afford, the *Canstein Bibel*. Elers's launching of a publishing house was a great success amongst eighteenth-century endeavours of this kind.[27] In 1691, however, Francke had only a nominal appointment at an as yet unchartered university and an additional post in one of the poorest parishes outside the gates of Halle. Some ten years later he had guided the extensive pedagogical institutions collectively known as the *Waisenhaus*[28] to prominence and working order – including a building programme praised by the king himself. The Prussian monarch had thought only the official purse capable of creating such impressive institutions.

The institutional results of Francke's influence made for a curious situation. On the one hand he dominated what had traditionally been the 'first' faculty at any university, that of theology; on the other he was the independent director of educational facilities that provided pre-university training and gave the best students tutorial posts

27 J. Böhme, *Heinrich Julius Elers, ein Freund und Mitarbeiter A. H. Franckes* (PhD Diss., Freie Universität Berlin, 1956).
28 An English version of Francke's first laudatory description of 'his' institutions exists: *An abstract of the Marvellous Footsteps of Divine Providence, In the building of a very large Hospital, or rather, a Spacious College, for Charitable and Excellent Uses; and the maintaining of many Orphans and other Poor People therein; at Glaucha near Hall, in the Dominions of the King of Prussia,* . . . (London, 1706).

whilst offering them and other students food and lodging. For many eminent individuals it was the *Waisenhaus*, with its opportunities for their children, that attracted them to Halle.[29] Physically, too, it could sometimes overshadow the less institutionalised quarters of university teaching. *Privatissimae* were held in the homes of professors and only the public disputations had a ceremonial room, but it was the centre of town, in the *Waage*, and was also used for other functions.

Lutheran Pietism,[30] the movement with which Francke, as one of its central figures, was identified, should be briefly characterised: It was not sectarian; that is it never separated from the Lutheran church, as did more 'enthusiastic' groups. There was no dissension on central matters of belief. And yet there was a clear-cut antagonism, for the orthodox did not care for the revivalist activism. Pietism differed from Lutheran orthodoxy in that a fervent Christianity came first and other details of life – money, clothes, careers – came second. These beliefs made for an 'equality before God', and aristocrats could be reminded of the fact. Pietism also represented a revival of Lutheran thought on the nature of man, a non-materialist emphasis (counter to solely empiricist mechanics), and it therefore influenced medical teaching at Halle.

In Halle then, in 1694, the founding of the university drew men who were not imbued with traditional, conservative values, but who were the upstarts of eighteenth-century thought: the proponents of an 'enlightened' mode of expression as well as those who were causing rifts in religious self-definition. The faculties of law and theology formed exciting counterpoints. For this very reason Halle attracted students from the Protestant enclaves of the Holy Roman Empire, and for a time it eclipsed all the older universities.

Without knowledge of this background neither the medical faculty nor its influence can be understood. Nor can the later developments towards the end of the century in Berlin be fully appreciated. The medical faculty at Halle was, at first, a grey zone. At the inception an attempt was made to recruit from local medical men. No one particularly wanted the appointments.[31] Official histories of the university mention only the sudden appearance of Friedrich Hoffmann,[32] who is then made responsible for enticing Georg Ernst Stahl to come,

29 Francke reserved the 'paedagogium' largely for the sons of aristocratic families. The correspondence in the Archiv der Francke'schen Stiftungen attests to innumerable requests for admission to the educational facilities of the *Waisenhaus*.
30 Literature on all these aspects of Pietism can be found in the extensive bibliography published in the journal *Pietismus und Neuzeit* 1, 1974.
31 Zentrales Staatsarchiv, Dienststelle Merseburg, Ministerium des Innern, Rep. 52, Nr. 159 N3c Fasz. 22.
32 Schrader, *Geschichte der Friedrichs-Universität Halle* I, pp. 56ff.

resigning his post as court physician to Johann Ernst von Sachsen-Weimar. Archival sources point to a different connection. August Hermann Francke had always maintained close relationships with the various Pietist circles, especially those in Gotha and Quedlinburg. Both cities were outside Brandenburg-Prussia proper. Stahl was sometimes in Gotha, one of the residences of the Sachsen-Gotha-Weimar line. Hoffmann was city physician in Halberstadt, not terribly far from the Thuringian territories. In 1691, when Francke already knew that he would probably go to Halle he was travelling from Gotha via Quedlinburg to Berlin (to see Spener).

In Quedlinburg, amongst convinced Pietists such as Johann Heinrich Sprögel,[33] Christian Scriver had officiated as chaplain to the *Damenstift* (a Protestant convent for aristocratic ladies). Scriver was known for his emotionally expressive religious writings; he was a friend of Spener and Francke and had strong Pietist leanings. When he was seriously ill in 1693 (the year of his death), one of the physicians consulted was Georg Ernst Stahl.[34] This is not the only proof of pre-Halle contacts. On the journey of 1691, after the fateful eviction for his religious activities in Erfurt, Francke himself wrote that after his sermon at the Augustinerkirche in Gotha, Dr Stahl approached him with a commission from Johann Ernst von Sachsen-Weimar.[35] The duke wished to ask him to take the position of court chaplain and that of educational supervisor to his son. Francke declined, having other intentions, and in 1692 the position went to Kaspar Johann Weydenhain, an adamant Pietist and one of Francke's long-time correspondents.

Pre-Halle contacts are also in evidence in regard to Friedrich Hoffmann. In a letter from Halberstadt dated 21 January 1692, Hoffmann congratulates Francke on his appointment as professor at the nascent university.[36] Furthermore, Hoffmann mentions, in tones not at all adverse to Francke's thinking, the manifestation of 'God's Glory' through the 'speaking in tongues' of servant girls who were part of the Pietist circle around Sprögel in Quedlinburg. Hoffmann had been called upon to judge these matters from a medical standpoint and his opinion (later published) did nothing to undermine Pietist claims.[37]

33 Martin Schulz, 'Johann Heinrich Sprögel und die pietistische Bewegung Quedlinburgs' (PhD Diss., Halle, 1974).
34 *Leichenpredigt* (funeral oration) Christian Scriver (d. 1693).
35 Diary of A. H. Francke, 1691/92, in Kramer, *Beiträge zur Geschichte A. H. Franckes*, p. 155.
36 Archiv der Francke'schen Stiftungen, C 65a 1: letter from Hoffmann to Francke, 21 Jan. 1692; C 65a 2, dated 17 Oct. 1697.
37 F. Hoffmann, *Unlängst gestelltes Teutsches Judicium von der Quedlinburgischen Magd Magdalenen an Hn. Sprögeln* (Quedlinburg, 1692).

The evidence suggests then, that the positions on the medical faculty at Halle were within the long reach of those Francke considered favourable to his cause. Persuasion must have mattered, as did conviction, because the records show that financial gain (in terms of salary) was not guaranteed in Halle. Berlin was notoriously stingy.[38] Stahl's salary, as court physician to Johann Ernst von Sachsen-Weimar, was not less than he was offered in Halle.[39]

What difference, then, did the medical faculty make, with its two appointed professors, Friedrich Hoffmann and Georg Ernst Stahl?

In the general politics of the university both Hoffmann and Stahl were quite decisive figures. Not because of an intrinsic desire for political management, but rather in the eighteenth-century sense of being 'politick' with its implication of prudence. The University of Halle, all suppositions of Absolutism to the contrary, was highly autonomous. It could block appointments for example. But much depended on an inner cohesion. In cases of internal conflict committees were set up, and these were recruited from the faculties. Other decisions as well required representations from faculty professors.[40] Considering the even balance between the juridical and the theological faculties, the two professors of medicine were able to exercise a great deal of influence.

Almost everything at Halle in the first decades was fraught with controversy. Several incidents illustrate the way in which the medical professors supported certain positions. Much of the following material is new and has not been mentioned in writings about Hoffmann or Stahl.

Christian Thomasius had already acquired a reputation as a liberal agent of Enlightenment with publications in periodical form, horrifying to the learned community because they were in the vernacular and (his book reviews in particular) were sharp-tongued.[41] Another controversial publication appeared in 1700, this time in Latin: the *Observationes selectae ad rem litterariam* . . . , ten volumes with supplements appearing until 1705. Thomasius's two collaborators from the Halle faculties were Johann Franz Buddeus (professor of moral

---

38 Alberti and Juncker, after years of service on the medical faculty in Halle, were still applying for their salaries; Zentrales Staatsarchiv, Dienststelle Merseburg, Ministerium des Innern, Rep. 52, Nr. 159 N3c Fasz. 53; Rep. 52, Nr. 159 Nbc Fasz. 61.

39 Two hundred thaler increased in 1708 by one hundred thaler because of diligence. Universitäts archiv Halle, Rep. 3, Nr. 243, Bl. 18–18v. and Nr. 62, Bl. 125 (12 Nov. 1694).

40 Stahl and Hoffmann were both *Prorektor*, the administrative head of the university. Stahl was involved in the controversy over Thomasius's criticism of the university (1713).

41 *Freymüthige . . . Monatsgespräche*, appearing 1688–9. Collectively published in three parts (1690).

philosophy) and Georg Ernst Stahl. The *Observationes selectae* were erudite and polemical. They argued an antischolastic, anti-Aristotelian and antimechanistic line. If one separates 'Enlightenment' from its French determinant of anticlerical secularism, then one of the German cultural meanings here becomes clear: 'Enlightened' meant breaking the orthodox mode; with respect to Lutheranism it could mean accepting the value of sectarian enthusiasm; with respect to medicine, distrusting atomism and mechanics as an explanation of the living body; in cultural values (Thomasius's strong point) it involved calling into question the canon of scholastic logic in favour of scepticism and individualist opinion.

The very fact that specialists from different disciplines moved away from the *acta eruditorum* and joined forces to produce a polemical periodical shows a willingness to provoke thought and to make opinion, and not received knowledge, a touchstone of education. It was an acknowledged contribution, as evidenced by the German encyclopaedia, Zedler's *Universal-lexikon*, which mentions the *Observationes selectae* as one of the accomplishments of Stahl's career.[42]

The medical faculty were also prominent in another innovative area. As we have seen, one of Lutheran Pietism's outstanding social traits was its lack of discrimination or snobbery. University education was expensive. Law students generally came from wealthier backgrounds, but for theological students (many of whom went into teaching), medical students and those studying philosophy, food, lodging and fees were not simple matters. Francke was very sensitive with regard to both talented and needy scholars. With the founding of his institutions he evolved supportive measures for poor students. His practical bent of mind led him to the organisation of *Freytische*,[43] an arrangement whereby poor students received meals at no cost. Other universities may have had numerically insignificant arrangements of the same sort, but as a report of 1704 put it, more students received aid at Halle than the entire student population at some other institutions. Francke was the driving force, although Samuel Stryck, professor of jurisprudence, helped with the draft put before the king.

42　*Großes vollständiges Universal-Lexicon* . . . , (Leipzig and Halle, 1744), (published by J. H. Zedler), vol. 39, p. 888.
43　Francke began the *Freytische* in 1696 (1697: forty-two students; fifty-two orphans). Information given in the text comes from the following sources: *Hallesche Correspondenz*: June, 1704; Sept. 1705; Oct. 1705; Hoffbauer, *Geschichte der Universität Halle*, pp. 118–19; Schrader, *Geschichte der Friedrichs-Universität Halle*, I, p. 92; Franz Zimmermann, *Matrikel der Martin-Luther Universität Halle-Wittenberg 1690–1730*(Halle, 1960). Universitätsarchiv Halle, Rep. 3, Nr. 504; Nr. 529; Zentrales Staatsarchiv, Dienststelle Merseburg, Ministerium des Innern, Rep. 52, Nr. 159 N8; Much work still has to be done on the significance of the *Freytische*.

On 16 May 1704, the initiative of Francke and Stryck stimulated a royal order that, in the lands ruled by the crown, collections were to be taken after the main sermon in all churches every three months for this purpose. With twelve needy students to a *Freytisch* and between ten and thirteen 'tables' of this sort the number was indeed large (120–160 students). These tables were open to students of all faculties.

Both Hoffmann and Stahl were active in support of the *Freytische*. Hoffmann persuaded the provincial councils of Magdeburg and Halberstadt to finance three 'tables'.[44] They were among the first, founded in 1696, the year of Hoffmann's first chancellorship. Georg Ernst Stahl was involved in another and more permanent way: He was a member of the council (Ephoria) of four professors (Stryck, Stahl, Anton, Michaelis) who supervised the finances, admissions, complaints and other matters relating to the *Freytische*.[45] Stahl never sought to avoid this duty, which was highly important on two counts: First, it involved large sums of money from sources outside the university, for which the Ephoria was accountable to the state; and second, it was a selection process for talented students. Judging from the archival records, it cost much time and energy. Stahl was very careful, when he left his professorship for Berlin, to ensure that his successor, Michael Alberti, became a member of the Ephoria. The number of medical students who completed their studies by this method has yet to be calculated. But at least two professors of medicine, Alberti and Johann Juncker, could not have studied had they not had the support of meals and lodging at the *Waisenhaus*.[46]

The *Freytische* were, socially speaking, revolutionary. A more conservative chronicler of the university in 1805 complained that too many students at Halle were poor and could not buy the *compendia* for the lectures.[47] The poor could come only because of the *Freytische*. 'Poor', it must be said, at the time applied also to much of the middle classes. These, however, were the backbone of the Prussian state, as

44 Schrader, *Geschichte der Friedrichs-Universität Halle*, I, p. 92.
45 *Hallesche Correspondenz*, June 1704. Archival records. Alberti succeeded Stahl in 1716.
46 For the careers of Alberti and Juncker and the composition of the medical faculty at Halle, see W. Kaiser and A. Völker, 'Michael Alberti (1682–1757)', *Wissenschaftliche Beiträge der Martin-Luther-Universität Halle-Wittenberg* (Halle, 1982/4); W. Kaiser, 'In Memoriam Johann Juncker (1679–1759)', in *Johann Juncker (1679–1759) und seine Zeit (I)*, *Wissenschaftliche Beiträge der Martin-Luther-Universität Halle-Wittenberg* (Halle, 1979/29); *250 Jahre Collegium Clinicum Halense 1717–1967* (Halle, 1967); W. Kaiser and Karl-Heinz Krosch, 'Zur Geschichte der Medizinischen Fakultät der Universität Halle im 18. Jht', Beiträge XIII–XX, *Wissenschaftliche Zeitschrift der Martin-Luther Universität Halle-Wittenberg* (1967), Nos. 3 and 4.
47 Hoffbauer, *Geschichte der Universität Halle*, pp. 118–19.

it became a well-organised and bureaucratically administered nation. This applied also to the medical practitioners, once the regulation of the profession took root.

Just as revolutionary was an intellectually creative symbiosis developed from the unorthodoxies collectively present at Halle. If it were possible to imagine an Oxford whose medical thinking had assimilated conceptual problems such as those written about and expounded by John Henry Newman, then one would have, in a conservative mirror image, an idea of what was happening in Halle. The man whose mind was capable of such breadth of purpose was Stahl. Friedrich Hoffmann's character was too pliable to resist the pressure of medical fashion, whose outlines were clear by then: The body was solely of a material order and its dysfunctions were to be explained in material terms. No matter if the explanation were atomist, or iatromechanist, or sought for in the behaviour of chemical substances and processes, the underlying determinant was clear: to have done with supposed 'forces', innate powers, spiritual ephemera. This was the solid ground, prepared by English empiricists and Cartesian philosophy in the seventeenth century on which the Enlightenment aligned itself firmly with science. The relationship was dynastic; it conquered much new territory in its rapid advance. It was exemplified in Halle by Christian Thomasius's insistence that crimes of witchcraft were insupportable superstitions, bound up with belief in a devil who could not be identified juridically.[48] Law should be culturally sanitised, especially against beliefs in the material manifestations of the powers of darkness.

Although this was laudable, it had its price: the complete denial of the spiritual side of mankind, in particular of the soul as an integral element of human nature. Medicine wished to ignore the question. The only medical 'school' that still wrote consistently about themes such as the influence of the emotions and the imagination on the body was that of Stahl.[49] Stahl objected, from a professorial position and on principle, to medical explanations that denied mental influence and that approached the body as a substance capable only of reactive behaviour.[50] He saw most clearly that neither illness, which is related to person and personal habit, nor the reinstitution of health

48 C. Thomasius, *De Crimine Magiae* (Halle, 1701); *Kurtze Lehrsätze von dem Laster der Zauberey* (Halle, 1703); *Gelehrte Streitschrift von dem Verbrechen der Zauber- und Hexerey* (n.p., 1775).
49 For example M. Alberti, *De Therapia imaginaria* (Halle, 1721); *De Valetudinariis imaginariis* (Halle, 1723).
50 G. E. Stahl, *De mechanismi et organismi diversitate* (Halle, 1706); *De mixti et vivi corporis vera diversitate* (Halle, 1707).

(cure through the stimuli of medication), was in essence material. Even pigeons, he wrote, are not automatons that react to the sensual stimuli of grain kernels strewn on the ground. They can circle uselessly and can err.[51]

Stahl's refusal to give way before a scientific advance that also threatened established views on human nature, disassociating what in terms of biblical revelation can be called the 'indwelling of the Holy Spirit' from man's material being, marked him as a possible ally of Lutheran Pietists. Their belief systems, or the nature of their fundamental assumptions, were compatible. Elsewhere I have given details of their intellectual co-operation.[52] Here we must be satisfied with the more general assertion of a symbiosis that remains historically relevant even into the era of nineteenth-century German romanticism.[53] Lutheran Pietism, in contrast to orthodoxy, emphasised spiritual change. This was introspective and attuned to feelings; emotive cognizance was not pushed away as irrational.[54] It was very close to Stahl's medical sensitivity. To Lutheran Pietism the cure of illness without concern for man's spiritual condition was akin to atheism. For Stahl, too, the dynamics of illness and health were inseparable from mental and emotional states, although his area was medical, and he did not, as did William James, link the religious with the psychological.

A symbiosis, by definition, leaves the interacting entities their own separate lives. Stahl's medical theory and Lutheran Pietism had this quality. They passed on stimuli to writers and thinkers in Germany whose themes went beyond the narrow confines of the scientific, including the dramatic arts, the theory of knowledge as it relates to sensual perception and aesthetics (A. Baumgarten, I. Kant), and popular medicine. Each took strands from these mutually supportive and articulate movements (Stahl's medicine was acknowledged as a 'school'). Halle had given them room to develop their identities and the legacy was a fruitful one. This constellation of individual determination and intellectual depth determined the efficacy and attrac-

51 G. E. Stahl, *Theoria medica vera* (Halle, 1708), p. 39.
52 J. Geyer-Kordesch, 'Illness and Cultural Values: The Dilemma of Science and Medicine in Eighteenth Century Germany', *The Social History of the Bio-Medical Sciences* (in press); 'Die Medizin im Spannungsfeld zwischen Aufklärung und Pietismus. Das unbequeme Werk Georg Ernst Stahls und dessen kulturelle Bedeutung', *Wolfenbüttler Beiträge* (in press).
53 For romanticism and medicine see N. Tsouyopoulos, *A. Röschlaub und die Romantische Medizin* (Stuttgart, 1982).
54 For two views on the subject see H.-J. Schings, *Melancholie und Aufklärung* (Stuttgart, 1977), and Gerhard Sauder, *Empfindsamkeit* (Stuttgart, 1976).

tion of medicine in Halle. It is well to remember that for its first decades Halle had no *theatrum anatomicum* or even a *hortus medicus*. Alberti and Juncker, the Stahlian succession, were not even paid properly. Compared to Leiden, 'science' was at a minimum. The medical faculty was held at two professorships, extended to three in 1718, reaching five by 1780 and eight by 1788. Structurally this was slow progress. Yet the students came in greater numbers than elsewhere and the graduates held important posts. We must conclude that the working order established through the Pietist institutions and their claim upon those who were not privileged, that is dependent on ability and learning, influenced medical recruitment. Stahl's teaching especially was more than medical fact. It was theory. It sought an enlightenment contrary to its usual link with secularised science. It was not Helmontian or Paracelsian, but anthropocentrically comprehensive, akin to the contemporary philosophical strategies of Leibniz or Christian Wolff (1679–1754), who were not in agreement with Stahl, but whose approaches addressed the question of man's nature in similar ways. This drew attention to, and seemed to solve, the Enlightenment's pressing needs, seemed even 'to enlighten' in a manner that Calvinist pragmatism (Leiden's science) or 'reductive' science (Göttingen's) could not. Regular medical teaching was, of course, offered consistently – Hoffmann, Stahl and the rest – but it was the other dimension that shaped Halle.

Berlin had a different quality: It was an administrative and court centre. It is remarkable that it became a centre of medical teaching, but that was due to the men who found scope for their work there. Stahl was the only medical professor who did not die an incumbent of his chair in Halle. He went to Berlin.

II

Georg Ernst Stahl succeeded Andreas von Gundelsheimer as first court physician (*Hof- und Leibmedicus*) on 15 July 1715. On 2 Novembr 1715 he was appointed president of the *collegium medicum*.[55] In Prussia the Berlin *collegium medicum* had a different function than these medical bodies had in other places. Since the Edict of 1685 (*Medizinal Ordnung*),[56] inaugurating the *collegium medicum* in Berlin, it had an administrative role to play. Whereas usually such a 'college' merely

55 M. Pistor, *Grundzüge einer Geschichte der Preussischen Medizinalverwaltung bis Ende 1907* (Braunschweig, 1909), pp. 8–9.
56 Reprinted in M. Stürzbecher, *Beiträge zur Berliner Medizingeschichte* (Berlin, 1966), pp. 27ff.

represented the professional interests of the physicians of a city, the edict defined the function of the *collegium medicum* in Berlin to be that of a central organ for the regulation of medical concerns in all its branches.[57] The *collegium medicum* of Berlin therefore became an administrative arm of the government although its effectiveness cannot be proven until after the reign of Frederick William I.[58] Structurally it was composed of the *Hof- und Leibmedici* and other physicians, whose services could also be co-opted. Originally its president came from the king's advisory cabinet, the *Geheime Rath*. Stahl was *ex officio* a powerful member as first court physician. In 1715 when he assumed his duties his position was considerably strengthened because Frederick William I made him president as well.[59] He was therefore personally responsible to the king and to the cabinet for medical matters throughout Prussia. Since the basic structure of the 'college' was never changed (although its duties and powers were altered in successive proclamations), and Stahl was never relieved from his posts until his death in 1734, he remained the key man, the *éminence grise*, behind medical developments. It is worthy of note that the changes from 1717 onward could never have been instituted without reference to the *collegium medicum* and its president.[60]

The second strand whose interweaving with medical reorganisation altered the fabric of medical training available in Berlin was the establishment of the *theatrum anatomicum*.[61] None of the Prussian universities had such an institution, but this does *not* mean there were no dissections.[62] Leiden was closest and it can be observed that the

57 Ibid., p. 34. Stürzbecher, however, sees the various court proclamations as decisive and misses two vital points: The administrative set-up gave particular physicians power, and second, the *interplay* of the structures was more important than the history of one institution.
58 Ibid., p. 65. See also M. Stürzbecher, 'Aus der Geschichte des Collegium medico-chirurgicum in Berlin', in *Medizinische Mitteilungen der Schering AG* (21. Jahrgang, 1960), pp. 110–14.
59 Pistor, *Grundzüge*, p. 9.
60 Stahl, in the protocol-conscious eighteenth century, still signs first on letters of approbation (this time for an apothecary) of the *collegium medico-chirurgicum* in 1732: Zentrales Staatsarchiv, Dienststelle Merseburg, Ministerium des Innern, Kurmark Tit. CXV, Stadt Berlin, Sect-O, 1, Apoth. Nr. 3 and Nr. 5.
61 Much information on the *theatrum anatomicum* and its finances is presented in A. Harnack, *Geschichte der Königlichen Preussischen Akademie der Wissenschaften zu Berlin*, vol. I/1 (Berlin, 1900).
62 For Halle, see W. Kaiser, K.-H. Krosch, W. Piechocki, 'Collegium clinicum Halense', in W. Kaiser et al., *250 Jahre Collegium Clinicum Halense 1717–1967* (Halle, 1967), p. 23; W. Kaiser, 'In Memoriam Johann Juncker', in *Johann Juncker . . . und seine Zeit* (I), pp. 10ff. The term *collegium clinicum* is *not* here equivalent to a teaching group or an administrative body. The dissections on cadavers were occasional; those on animals were more frequent.

important teachers of anatomy in Berlin had visited Leiden, more for this than for Boerhaave's teaching.[63] The establishment of an anatomical theatre was of prime significance because it became the focal point for expanded medical teaching. The teaching went beyond anatomical demonstration into traditional medical teaching (therapeutics, pathology, fevers and other subjects related to 'internal' medicine) and related subjects (pharmaceutical chemistry, chemistry, botany). This expansion began in 1724. After the first years the lecture catalogue was printed and became publically accessible.[64]

The history of the *theatrum anatomicum* is not a simple one, nor does it do credit to the old-guard court physicians who dominated the medical side of the Academy of Science in Berlin.[65] The teaching expansion was the result of a considerable struggle with the Academy. No matter how one evaluates the initial impetus for anatomical instruction – and some credit Ernst Konrad Holtzendorff (1688–1751), Frederick William's chief army surgeon and *Leibmedicus* (1716), with this suggestion[66] – it was a long-drawn-out financial struggle whose resolution depended on the king and the president of the *collegium medicum*. Archival evidence shows that Stahl was centrally involved in wresting funds for medicine from the Academy.[67] When they offered him membership – not without political motivation – he declined.[68]

One has to understand the personality and objectives of Frederick William I in order to give due credit to his role in advancing professional medical expertise in Berlin. Frederick William I[69] had suc-

63 The most prominent were Theodor Eller, who was the assistant of J. J. Rau in Leiden. August Buddeus also studied anatomy in Leiden. No publication exists giving the full members and their medical education for the *collegium medico-chirurgicum*.
64 Archiv der Akademie der Wissenschaften (AAW), Berlin, German Democratic Republic, Akte I, XIV, Nr. 24, contains the programme of lectures.
65 A. Harnack, *Geschichte der Akademie*, shows how prominent members even diverted the salary of Leibniz, pp. 197ff. The archives show an even more drastic refusal to give money for medical purposes: AAW, Sitzungsprotokolle (minutes of meetings of the society) of 7 Oct. 1716 showed that they planned to oppose Stahl, and how the battle continued: 19 Nov. 1716, 7 Jan. 1717, 9 June 1717, 23 Sept. 1717.
66 See H. Lehmann, 'Das Collegium medico-chirurgicum in Berlin als Lehrstätte der Botanik und der Pharmazie' (PhD Diss., Berlin, 1936) p. 10. This would bear some reassessment; Holtzendorff enters the academy only through von Gundling's suggestion 12 Feb. 1724 (AAW I, IV, Nr. 36, p. 54). Lehmann's dissertation is often cited because he was able to study the archival material before World War II. However, I find his general history of the *collegium medico-chirurgicum* erroneous.
67 AAW I, XIV, Nr. 1, Stahl's letter of 23 Nov. 1717. Frederick William comments on this request for funds *gutt* (good). See also minutes cited in note 65.
68 AAW I, IV, Nr. 6, minutes of 9 June 1717 shows the Academy asking Stahl to join – at a politically opportune moment. Stahl never became a member.
69 Carl Hinrichs, *Friedrich Wilhelm I, König in Preussen. Eine Biographie*. Revised edition including 'Der Regierungsantritt Friedrich Wilhelms I' and 'Die Preussische

ceeded his father, Frederick I, on 25 February 1713. It was more than a mere succession. The changes were drastic: From a largely ceremonial court with chaotic finances, Frederick William created an ordered, solvent, bureaucratically directed system. Naturally he encountered resistance, and one point of opposition was the Academy of Sciences where, after Leibniz's death (1716), the entrenched old-guard court physicians wished, first of all, to keep the money allotted to the Academy and, second, to continue a programme of scientific enquiry that consisted mainly of internal reports and specialised discussions.

But precisely this conception of what the medical section of the Academy should do went against the king's plans of reform. Frederick William I was not interested in pomp and circumstance, nor in idle speculation. Even more troubling, he had a talent for economics and finances. In other words, he was not a puppet of ministerial advice. The result was the appropriation of the Academy's money for the establishment and upkeep of the *theatrum anatomicum*. After Stahl had taken office (1716) the financial onslaught on the Academy of Sciences had taken a systematic turn. Only after the Academy agreed to take over the maintenance and teaching connected with the *theatrum anatomicum* did the king ratify its charter (1717).[70] One can name the king and Stahl in the same breath because a certain temper united them: It was the heritage of Pietist Halle, for which both had deep affinities, and it is describable in terms of personal commitment. I refer here not to 'Prussian' duty – that would be much too bland and self-satisfied a term – but to a commitment to spiritual life that sought to use a man's short time on earth to create as much of value as possible. This was the quality that characterised the men around Francke (Elers, Neumann, Freylinghausen, Canstein) or the immediate successors of Stahl in Halle (Michael Alberti, Johann Juncker). All of these men laboured to accomplish something they believed was useful. None of them found money a worthwhile object in life. Their common trait was a painstaking conscientiousness and religious commitment.

We should not idealise them, but visualising these traits helps us understand a decisive change. It makes Stahl's key position in Berlin clear: He had no qualms about extracting money for practical medical purposes from men like Krug von Nidda and Jaegewitz, the two physicians to the court from the reign of Frederick I, who headed the medical division of the Academy and who produced a great deal of

Zentralverwaltung in den Anfängen Friedrich Wilhelms I' (reprint, Darmstadt, 1968); *Preußentum und Pietismus* (Göttingen, 1971); Jochen Klepper, *Der Vater, Roman eines Königs* (1st ed., 1937; paperback reprint, Stuttgart, 1977).
70   Harnack, *Geschichte der Akademie*, p. 228 (14 Aug. 1717). A new president for the Academy was appointed very late, in March 1718 (p. 220).

obfuscation and delay, as well as money for themselves. It also explains why Stahl insisted on new medical talent, selected on the basis of productive work and high qualification, for he was keen on the reform of medicine. As will be shown presently, the character and type of the medical men recruited carried the burden of success.

The Academy's money was crucial, and bit by bit it was extracted. This process is recorded in the minutes of the Academy meetings, complete with the reluctance of Academy members to give up any money. Andreas von Gundelsheimer, no friend of the Academy and Stahl's predecessor, had forced 1,000 thaler from the Academy for the setting up of the *theatrum anatomicum*.[71] Christian Maximilian Spener, the son of the Pietist Philipp Jacob Spener, had held dissections there.[72] In 1714 the king made him a professor of anatomy, but Spener died that year. The next years leave some doubt as to the Academy's honesty in spending money for practical medical or even intellectual projects. From the minutes of the Academy we find that Stahl, on 7 October 1716, has induced the king to ask for the 1,000 thaler for medical purposes. The Academy blocked this request as long as possible. The conflict was resolved in such a way that the Academy did pay out the money, but under the condition that the *theatrum anatomicum* (building and teaching) would be under its jurisdiction.[73] This was in 1717. Stahl aquiesced, but was angry enough to add (and this throws some light on his opinion of the old-guard physicians in the Academy) that he had certainly not wanted the money for himself.[74] His project had been to use some of the money to pay for the return and salary of Caspar Neumann,[75] an excellent chemist and pharmacist who was studying in London, and whom Stahl wanted for the *Hofapotheke* in Berlin. In 1719 Neumann was back in Berlin and in office as *Hofapotheker*. Neumann had earlier connections with Halle, with both Hoffmann and Stahl, and Stahl appreciated Neumann's formidable knowledge of chemistry. In 1721 Neumann was accepted into the Academy.

The financing of medical improvements eased as the king became more adamant about having what he wanted. The Academy could no longer back out of its support of the anatomical theatre. Neumann

71 Ibid., pp. 183ff.
72 Ibid., pp. 193ff.
73 AAW I, I, XIV, Nr. 2 (the Academy tried to block funds, 1716–17; accepted obligations for anatomical theatre and teaching; but reminded again of the financial obligations it had incurred as late as 1723!). A. Harnack, *Geschichte der Akademie*, pp. 228ff.
74 AAW I, XIV, Nr. 2. Bl. 98–9 (letter of Stahl dated 8 Nov. 1717).
75 Ibid., for Neumann's biography see A. Exner, 'Der Hofapotheker Caspar Neumann (1683–1737)' (PhD Diss., Berlin, 1938).

had been paid for from other sources. Thereafter, in the 1720s, the advance in medicine should not be sought so much in institutional development, but rather – and this has been overlooked – in the way that the positions were being filled. Heinrich Henrici,[76] a colleague of Stahl's at the University of Halle about whom Stahl justly rather despaired, became professor of anatomy in 1719. He was replaced in 1723 by August Buddeus,[77] a much more competent man. Buddeus also had Halle connections. He belonged to the same family as the Pietist theologian Johann Franz Buddeus, with whom Stahl had written the *Observationes selectae*. He received his doctorate from Leiden in 1721, a necessary detour with respect to anatomical competence. He was appointed to the Academy (who also paid for him) in 1723 and was made director of the natural science/medical section (*physikalisch-medizinische Klasse*) in 1725. Caspar Neumann was already in the Academy. The famous chemist Johann Heinrich Pott (1692–1777) was added to the Academy in 1722 (also receiving support) and taught chemistry at the *collegium medico-chirurgicum*. Again it is possible to trace a leading figure back to Halle. Pott had begun his studies in Halle as a theology student, and it was Stahl's influence that turned him to chemistry.[78] He succeeded Neumann as *Hofapotheker* upon Neumann's death in 1737. As the official historian of the Academy writes about the third volume of writings the Academy finally produced (published in 1727), and which the medical men and chemists dominated: 'It was the school of Georg Ernst Stahl whose voice is here present.'[79]

Stahl's role cannot be over-emphasised: He was a major influence in extracting money; he had the king's ear, an influence of vital im-

---

76 For Henrici see W. Kaiser and K.-H. Krosch, 'Zur Geschichte der Medizinischen Fakultät der Universität Halle im 18 Jht.', in *Wissenschaftliche Zeitschrift der Martin-Luther Universität Halle-Wittenberg*, No. 5 (1965), pp. 358–60. What is not mentioned there is Henrici's capacity to avoid work. Stahl complains of being alone on the faculty except for A. Goelicke (Henrici is appointed, but absent): Zentrales Staatsarchiv, Dienststelle Merseburg, Ministerium des Innern, Rep. 52, Nr. 159 N3c Fasz. 26. The complaints about Henrici also occur in the minutes of the Academy – he is 'lazy' (AAW I, IV, 36 [minutes], pp. 34–5). But then, this was the claim of Krug von Nidda, who wanted money back for the Academy. Fate was unkind: von Nidda died 30 June 1719 and Henrici was appointed in his place (30 Nov. 1719) as director and as professor of anatomy.
77 Buddeus has been largely overlooked, but the Academy minutes show him to be an extremely conscientious man (AAW I, IV, 36, pp. 61ff). He matriculated in Halle on 25 May 1716. On 3 April 1725 he received the official appointment as professor of anatomy, Hoff-Rath, and Leib-Medicus. However he had been at the anatomical theatre since 1723 as the main teaching physician.
78 *Dictionary of Scientific Biography*, 'Pott, Johann Heinrich', with literature cited there.
79 A. Harnack, *Geschichte der Akademie*, vol. I/1, p. 236.

portance; he had the impatience of a hard-working man and the ethos of a Pietist from Halle; finally, he had institutionalised power as president of the *collegium medicum*. In 1724 he was joined by the man who was to suceed him in all these posts of medical power: Johann Theodor Eller.[80] Eller had studied under Stahl in Halle, after which, like Neumann, he spent some years in travel, visiting the major centres of medical learning (notably those in Holland). In 1721 he returned to German territory, becoming court physician in Anhalt-Bernburg, and city physician in Magdeburg, an area with close connections to Halle and Berlin.

Eller possessed a spirit akin to that fostered in Lutheran Pietist circles, which had also left its formative mark on Stahl and on the king. He had a profound commitment to use his life to stave off the wrath of God – what Francke called 'gegen den Riß stehen'. In 1727 Eller took on, in addition to his other medical involvements, the directorship of the Charité Hospital.[81] The Charité was a new foundation and its aims were consonant with the Prussian state's new and systematic concern for the poor and with its interest in medical proficiency. The classes to be cared for in the Charité were the poorest of the poor:[82] the diseased who had nowhere else to go, those suffering from venereal disease and prostitutes who were about to bear children. Eller was also a member of the *Armendirectorium*, the board charged with care for the poor, so he was well acquainted with these problems. But he strove for something else at the Charité, namely to establish clinical teaching. As he wrote in the book that presented the intentions and detailed plans for the Charité, the teaching at the *collegium medico-chirurgicum* was going well, the examinations and instruction at the *theatrum anatomicum* were launched, but what was missing was bedside teaching ('vor dem Krancken-Bette selbst') in which the student could be actually shown how to cure 'inner' and 'external' (meaning surgical) illness.[83] In an exemplary manner the daily details of such teaching and of patient care were worked out for the Charité. The food and the lodging, as well as the medical care, were better than in any other institution for the poor, and it was

80 A Koehler, *Die Kriegschirurgen und Feldärzte Preußens und anderer deutscher Staaten* . . . (Berlin, 1859), Theil I, pp. 145–56; W. Kaiser, 'Johann Theodor Eller (1689 bis 1760)', in *Zahn-, Mund- und Kieferheilkunde*, 64 (1976), pp. 277–87.
81 The best source is his own book on the Charité: *Nützliche und auserlesene Medizinische und Chirurgische Anmerkungen* . . . (Berlin, 1730); P. Diepgen and E. Heischkel, *Die Medizin an der Berliner Charité bis zur Gründung der Universität* (Berlin, 1935). (The introduction on the *collegium medico-chirurgicum* in this book is misleading.)
82 See Eller's description and M. Stürzbecher, *Beiträge zur Berliner Medizingeschichte*, pp. 123ff. 'Ueber die Patienten der Charité im Jahre 1731'.
83 J. T. Eller, *Nützliche und Auserlesene Medizinische* . . . *Anmerkungen*, p. 5.

difficult to get patients to leave. Even through the vicissitudes of later years the Charité survived as a teaching hospital with a wide intake amongst the poor. In the nineteenth century it established for medical science a leading position. Eller left the Charité in 1735 when he was appointed first court physician to Frederick William I in succession to Stahl.

The founding of the Charité Hospital with its provisions for teaching was a crucial addition to medical education. But let us return to the turbulent years of the *theatrum anatomicum* and the Academy of Science. We have shown how the financing through the Academy established the medical teaching there, that it was expanded in the 1720s, and that the medical men and chemists who were given posts were well-trained and competent. The lost thread of our fabric that must be taken up here is that of the *collegium medicum*. The point that has been missed so often and that has created great confusion is that, in essence, by 1723, when a new proclamation regarding medical teaching was in the making, the teachers at the anatomical theatre and the members of the *collegium medicum* were much the same men. All the important ones (except Stahl) were members of the Academy. In 1723 then, when a first draft of a new *Medizinal Ordnung* appeared,[84] (its main feature being the suggestion for a more stringent examination in medical learning), the Berlin medical teachers and the examining body were almost identical. It is therefore not surprising that with the official Edict of 1725,[85] regulating definitively the spectrum of qualifications for physicians and other medical practitioners, the *collegium medico-chirurgicum* was given both teaching *and* examining rights. The *collegium medico-chirurgicum* now provided the name for what had been institutionalised at the anatomical theatre for years. In effect these two institutions were conflated. But here another factor determined further developments: The expanded *collegium* became an instrument by which competence could be judged. It was, lastly, responsible for examinations and thereby set the seal of approval on anyone it sanctioned. This was particularly important if the practitioner, as surgeon or midwife, had no medical degree. It was also important for licentiates if there were questions as to competence. Since the creation of the *collegium medico-chirurgicum* was part of a reiteration and sharpening of the rules of medical practice (a royal edict), administrative bite was added.

84   M. Stürzbecher, 'Aus der Geschichte des Collegium medico-chirurgicum in Berlin', in *Medizinische Mitteilungen der Schering AG* (21. Jahrgang, 1960), p. 111, mentions this.
85   Reprinted in M. Pistor, *Das Gesundheitswesen in Preussen*, 2 vols. (Berlin, 1896–1898), I, pp. 4ff.

The creation of the *collegium medico-chirurgicum* with the Edict of 1725 also meant that surgeons were integrated with the 'learned' or university-based prestige of the internist, a development that in Prussia stemmed directly from the situation we have been at such pains to illustrate. The role of Frederick William's interest in the expansion of the Prussian army and the proportion in it of better qualified *Feldschärer* (army surgeons) cannot be discussed here.[86] Interestingly enough, however, the first set of teachers at the *theatrum anatomicum* were graduates of universities, not army or regular surgeons. The Edict of 1725 regulated medical life in Prussia for some time. Its major architects were none other than Eller and Stahl.[87]

When Eller died in 1760 a new generation was waiting in the wings. These men, too, were dominant personalities, but they worked and implemented their ideas within the established patterns of already prestigious institutions. The new king, Frederick II ('the Great') had assumed office in 1740. It was the era of a culturally Francophile king who treasured the Academy, but filled it with Frenchmen. He liked the arts and philosophy. Medicine, for him, was a practical discipline, one amongst others.[88] He did not have to interfere as much as his father had done. He inherited what had now properly become the capital of Prussia. Berlin mattered as a centre of medical science. When in 1810 the University of Berlin was officially inaugurated, it was built around the core of the medical teaching that already existed in fine functional order.[89] Surgeons and the old 'learned doctors' were on a par. Bedside instruction, with separate wards for gynaecology and venereal diseases, was well under way at the Charité. In effect, all the structural requisites for advanced teaching and for scientific exploration were at hand. Medicine and medical discoveries changed the face of the discipline, but its 'progression' rested on institutions formed by a different spirit. It had not really been the Enlightenment, that movement of secularised trust in man's capacity

86 In order to deal adequately with the literature on this subject, much of which goes back to works written in the late nineteenth century, one has to be very sceptical about the Prussian military 'myth'. Books tend to celebrate overmuch the 'technological creativity' attendant on Prussian militarism. Even Max Lenz, *Geschichte der Universität Berlin*, I, p. 39, sees the *collegium medico-chirurgicum* as primarily a military creation.
87 M. Pistor, *Grundzüge einer Geschichte der Preussischen Medizinalverwaltung*, p. 11.
88 A. Harnack, *Geschichte der Akademie*, I, pp. 269ff, shows how, when the Academy was restructured (1743–6) under Frederick II, the gentlemen and scholars of which it was now comprised (a 'true Academy') wished to exclude the medical men, who were 'only professors at the anatomical-chirurgical college and members of the old Society'.
89 The 'college' was dissolved on 13 Dec. 1809. In 1810 the University of Berlin was inaugurated.

to vanquish the troublesome through reason, which had now reached its true zenith under a king, 'the Great', who admitted little in the realm of higher powers. Rather it had been those now shadowy people who had felt their own lives to be 'instrumental' in working for a more equitable kingdom (the *Waisenhaus*, the Charité, instruction for surgeons at the *theatrum anatomicum*) that had laid the foundations for this progress. It was Lutheran Pietism and its spiritual home, Halle, that had, so to speak, raised the fear of God for Prussia. On that foundation the reformers had banned secular glories: metaphysical speculation, the idle arts, the pomp and circumstance of court life. Stahl, Francke, Eller, Frederick William I and the rest had been pious men, driven by spiritual turmoil. 'Our soul is exceedingly filled with the scorning of those that are at ease, and with the contempt of the proud' (Psalm 123). In Frederick the Great's time Sans Souci was built, and when the University of Berlin was inaugurated it exemplified the new humanist learning and the rise of medical science. The Humboldt University and the Charité survive today as monuments to a time of classicism. The intellectual forces that created these institutions, however, were considerably less serene, and perhaps more interesting.

Acknowledgements

The archival research for this article was made possible through a scholarship granted by the International Research and Exchanges Board. I wish to thank the achivists of the Akademie der Wissenschaften, the Staatliches Zentralarchive, Dienststelle Merseburg, the Universitätsarchiv Halle and the Archiv der Francke'schen Stiftungen for their very kind and helpful assistance.

8

The politics of health and the institutionalisation of clinical practices in Europe in the second half of the eighteenth century

OTHMAR KEEL

It is a generally accepted thesis in the history of medicine that the clinical practice of the last decades of the eighteenth century remained a *bedside* or *protoclinical* healing art and that clinical or hospital medicine was not, strictly speaking, constituted until after the French Revolution. It is, in addition, maintained that clinical or practical teaching institutions created in Europe in the course of the eighteenth century were little more than nosological theatres whose function was to illustrate the table of morbid or pathological essences. In sum, this thesis argues that all clinical research and training activities of the eighteenth century can be reduced to the model of the Boerhaavian clinic.

The institutional and conceptual framework of clinical practice, research and teaching (in different European countries) was not invariant or dependent upon the Boerhaavian model for the entire century but, on the contrary, evolved along several different lines. Although there were indeed major differences between the pre-Boerhaavian and Boerhaavian clinic and post-revolutionary hospital medicine, it can be shown that there was considerably less distance between the foreign, and to a certain extent French, clinical practices (in medicine, surgery, 'obstetrics', pharmaceutics, etc.), of the last decades of the eighteenth century and the hospital medicine of the early Paris clinical school than is generally supposed. This will be shown through an examination of the place held by the foreign and French institutional and conceptual models in the late eighteenth century in the constitution of the Parisian clinical *problématique* at the beginning of the Revolution.

I

Certain institutional and/or theoretical models of medical practice elaborated in France itself before the Revolution had great importance

in the formation of the Paris school *problématique*. This is well known.
One need only recall the importance of the anatomico-localist approach to disease of the eighteenth-century Parisian surgical school
and surgical institutions for the growth of the Paris school's anatomico-clinical medicine. Indeed, one need only mention such names as
Petit, Louis and Desault, or such institutions as the Academy of Surgery, the College of Surgery and Desault's school of clinical surgery at
the Hôtel-Dieu.[1] Or consider, at the end of the *ancien régime*, the
emergence of a tendency towards a practical observational medicine
within that sector of the medical corps typified by such practitioners
as Bordeu or, later, by Vicq d'Azyr and the organisers of the Royal
Society of Medicine[2] as well as hospital practitioners. Of course, it
would also be necessary to take into account the anatomico-pathological or anatomico-clinical work of such physicians as Lieutaud, Chambon de Montaux and Pujol de Castres or the work of medical practitioners interested in surgical diseases (Duverney, Winslow, Antoine
Petit).[3]

However, in addition to these models and often in combination

1   See C. A. Wunderlich, *Geschichte der Medizin* (Stuttgart, 1859), p. 244; O. Temkin,
'The Role of Surgery in the Rise of Modern Medical Thought', *Bulletin of the History
of Medicine* 25 (1951): 248–59; E. Ackerknecht, *Medicine at the Paris Hospital 1794–1848*
(Baltimore, 1967), p. 25; R. H. Shryock, *Histoire de la médecine moderne* (1936);
published in French, Paris, 1956), p. 107; M. J. Imbault-Huart, *L'école pratique de
dissection de Paris de 1750 à 1822 ou l'influence du concept de médecine pratique et de
médecine d'observation dans l'enseignement médico-chirurgical au XVIIIème siècle et au début
du XIXème siècle* (Thése Doc. ès Lettres, Paris, 1973), and 'Les chirurgiens et l'esprit
chirurgical en France au XVIIIe siècle', *Clio Medica* 15, no. 3/4 (1981): 143–57; P.
Huard and M. J. Imbault-Huart (eds.), *La médecine hospitalière française au XVIIIe siècle*
(Strasbourg, 1980); see Huard and Imbault-Huart, 'L'hospice du Collège de chirurgie
de Paris ou hospice Royal de chirurgie', pp. 109–24; A. Corlieu, *L'enseignement au
Collége de Chirurgie depuis son origine jusqu'à la Révolution Française* (Paris, 1890); P.
Huard and M. Grmek, *La chirurgie moderne: ses débuts en Occident. Seizième, dix-
septième, dix-huitième siècles* (Paris, 1968); P. Delaunay, *Le monde médical parisien au dix-
huitième siècle* (Paris, 1906); T. Gelfand, *Professionalizing Modern Medicine: Paris
Surgeons and Medical Science and Institutions in the Eighteenth Century* (Westport,
Conn., 1980). See also C. Daremberg, *Histoire des sciences médicales*, 2 vols (Paris
1870), II, pp. 1241–96; Huard, 'L'enseignement médico-chirurgical', in R. Taton
(ed.), *Enseignement et diffusion des sciences en France au XVIIIe siècle* (Paris, 1964), pp.
171–236; Othmar Keel, 'Cabanis et la généalogie de la médecine clinique' (PhD
thesis, McGill University, 1977), 465ff. and 481ff.
2   See, e.g., F. Vicq d'Azyr ('Anatomie pathologique', *Encyclopédie méthodique:
Médecine* [1790], II, pp. 236–612), who insists on the importance of pathological
anatomy for medicine. Let us not forget that even Corvisart, *docteur régent* of the
Paris faculty, was a clinician from the old régime, trained before the Revolution in
accordance with the anatomico-clinical model designated by such names as
Auenbrugger, Morgagni, Stoll and J. P. Frank and under the tutelage of Desault,
Portal, A. Petit, Vicq d'Azyr and others.
3   See Imbault-Huart, *L'école pratique de dissection*, and P. Huard and M. J. Imbault-
Huart, 'La clinique parisienne avant et après 1802', *Clio Medica*, 10, no. 3 (1975): 173.
Consider, too, the contributions of Vieussens, Sénac, L. Rivière, J. J. Wepfer and
Heberden for an idea of the medical-localist clinic in Europe before the Revolution.

with them, there were foreign models whose impact was as great if not greater on the development of the Paris school's theoretical and practical *problématique*. True, some of the foreign physicians and surgeons have achieved the status of 'precursors' of the Paris school. But, when they have, it is only as exceptional cases or isolated antecedents whose work, it is presumed, was destined to be ignored, misunderstood or forgotten in their own countries, because their medicine was the prisoner of a conservative or archaic problematic, nosological and Hippocratic, which blocked the scientific potential of innovations such as those, for instance, of Auenbrugger or Morgagni. Hence, the latent phase between Auenbrugger and Corvisart or Morgagni and Bichat: It seems that not only did the clinic make no progress in the intervening fifty years, but it regressed until the arrival of the Parisian clinicians and the dissolution of the Hippocratic approach.[4] It appears that a medicine content to contemplate symptoms blinded the nosologists and retarded the productive exploitation of the potentialities of Auenbrugger's and Morgagni's anatomico-clinical approach. Or so it must seem when, for example, it is affirmed that, without Laennec, Morgagni would not have resurfaced.

I do not agree with such an analysis. In fact, in many countries the anatomico-localist approach was consolidated in the eighteenth century after Morgagni's work, and the work of many foreign physicians and surgeons was very important for this consolidation. Moreover, foreign practitioners opened the way for the Paris clinicians and the institution of the anatomico-localist or 'surgical' approach to internal disease.

The Paris clinicians quite explicitly recognised the foreign practitioners who had preceded them and cited their work as models for the constitution of an anatomico-clinical approach. Thus, for example, in 1818, Pierre Rayer, himself a former student of the Paris School, wrote: '*A veritable revolution* has occurred in Nosology. This revolution was prepared by the writings of Schenk, Bartholin, Bonet, Morgagni, etc. . . . Pathological anatomy has proved that almost all continuous or intermittent fevers are *symptoms of material organic lesions*.'[5]

4 See, e.g., M. Foucault, *The Birth of the Clinic*, trans. A. M. Sheridan (London, 1973), p. 126: '. . . the clinic, a neutral gaze directed upon manifestations, frequencies, and chronologies, concerned with linking up symptoms and grasping their language, was, *by its structure*, foreign to the investigation of mute intemporal bodies; *causes and locales* did not interest it: it was interested in history not geography. Anatomy and the clinic were not of the same mind: . . . it *was clinical thought that for forty years prevented medicine from hearing the lesson of Morgagni!'* My emphasis.
5 P. Rayer, *Sommaire d'une histoire abrégée de l'anatomie pathologique* (Paris, 1818), p. 160, n. 3. My emphasis.

In support of this, Rayer cited as examples the work of clinicians who, for the most part, were foreign. These included "J. P. Frank's *Practical Medicine;* Tissot for his *Historia epidemiae biliosae,* Lausanne, 1755; Finke, *De morbis biliosis,* 1776; and Roederer and Wagler, *Tractatus de morbo mucoso,* Göttingen, 1783'.[6] He also cited, in this regard, Torti,[7] Sarcone,[8] Reil,[9] Stoll[10] and others.[11] Rayer continued, 'The knowledge of inflammation has become more exact and the number of these diseases has augmented considerably as they have become better known.'[12] According to the author, this had been the result of work done first by Stoll and Reil and, later, by Pinel and Broussais. Let it be noted, however, that amongst foreign clinicians contributing to the understanding of inflammation, Rayer omitted such authorities as John Hunter,[13] James Carmichael Smyth,[14] Matthew Baillie[15] and Aloys Vetter,[16] a student of Frank's. Rayer wrote further on that 'we have been led to doubt the existence of nervous diseases without material lesion of the organs which are their site, while, at the same time, scalpel in hand, a large number of hitherto unknown alterations have been demonstrated.'[17] Here Rayer cited only foreign workers as examples. He listed, in effect, 'Morgagni, Voigtel, Autenrieth, Soemmering, Groding, Kelch, Marshall, Haslam'.[18] He then explained: 'The untold advantages drawn from pathological anatomy in the study of haemorrhages and diseases

6 Ibid., p. 160.
7 See F. Torti (1658–1741), *Synopsis therapeutice specialis* (1712).
8 See M. Sarcone (1732–97), *Istoria ragionata dei mali osservati in Napoli nel corso dell'anno 1764* (Naples, 1764).
9 See J. C. Reil (1759–1813), *Memorabilia clinica medico-practica,* III (Halle, 1790–3), and *Ueber die Erkenntniss und Kur der Fieber* (Halle, Berlin, 1799–1815).
10 See M. Stoll (1742–88), *Ratio medendi in nosocomio practico Vindobonensi* (Vienna, 1779–90), and *Aphorismi de cognoscendis et curandis febribus* (Vienna, 1786).
11 *Sommaire,* p. 161.
12 Ibid.
13 See O. Keel, 'La pathologie tissulaire de J. Hunter', *Gesnerus* 37 (1980), 1/2: 47–61; and 'J. Hunter et X. Bichat: les rapports de leurs travaux en pathologie tissulaire', *Actes du XXVIIe Congrès International d'Histoire de la Médecine* (Barcelona, 1981), II pp. 535–49; 'Les conditions de la décomposition analytique de l'organisme: Haller, Hunter, Bichat', in *Les Idéologues;* special issue of *Les Études Philosophiques,* no. 1 (1982): 37–62.
14 See O. Keel, *La généalogie de l'histopathologie: Une révision déchirante.* Philippe Pinel, lecteur discret de J. C. Smyth (1741–1821). Préface de Georges Canguilhem. Librairie Philosophique J. Vrin (Paris, 1979).
15 On Baillie, see O. Keel, 'La formation de la problématique de l'anatomie des systèmes selon Laennec', in *Laennec. 1781–1826. Revue du Palais de la Découverte* (special issue on Laennec), 22 (Aug. 1981): 189–207.
16 See A. Vetter, *Aphorismen aus der pathologischen Anatomie* (Vienna, 1803), pp. 29–49, 91–303. Note that Vetter uses Baillie's and Soemmering's work.
17 *Sommaire,* p. 161.
18 Ibid.

known as organic by some authors – that is, diseases called surgical and the *innumerable* class of organic lesions *of the modern nosologist* – are generally accepted and of such simple exposition as to require no further discussion'.[19] At this point Rayer referred to yet another series of largely foreign authors (e.g. Richter, Abernethy and Scarpa) and then continued:

> It seems to me that we have yet to understand the extent to which, at the end of the eighteenth century, pathological anatomy diminished the physician's taste for all theory, no matter how brilliant. The vast number of facts collected about organic alterations, the exactitudes of their description, the publication of many general treatises and the large number of excellent monographs, the beautiful illustrations with which the anatomists embellished their works, the application of chemistry to the study of pathological hygrology which has become an experimental science; the special research undertaken in pathological physiology has assured the *eighteenth century a place of prime importance in the history of morbid anatomy.*[20]

But, as Rayer had already shown, many of these accomplishments were due to foreign physicians and surgeons. How, one might ask, can it be maintained that the anatomico-localist or anatomico-clinical approach of the Parisian school *gestated* only in the hands of the eighteenth-century Parisian or French surgeons?[21] The clinical *problématique* was produced through the interaction of an institutional and conceptual framework whose specific coordinates are not reducible to Parisian surgery, but must include *European surgery* and, *equally important, European medicine* (including French before the Revolution).

II

What kind of foreign institutional organisation served as a model for the Parisian clinic if by institutional organisation the new forms of medical practice, research and training such as those erected within the transformed or partly medicalised hospitals and/or institutions are to be understood?

The constitution of a clinico-localist approach to disease required

19 Ibid. My emphasis.
20 Ibid., pp. 124–5; my emphasis. See also P. L. Entralgo, *La historia clínica* (Madrid, 1950), chap. V, and Keel, 'Cabanis'.
21 As it has been claimed. See Imbault-Huart, *L'école pratique* and 'Les chirurgiens', Huard and Imbault-Huart, 'La médecine hospitalière', Gelfand, *Professionalizing Modern Medicine*.

hospital or institutional structures (free hospital teaching, private amphitheatres, etc.) for the observation of a significant number of patients and for dissection. It is also known that these conditions were indispensable for the replacement of the Hippocratic art of passive observation of the symptoms of a single individual by the diagnosis through anatomico-clinical correlation based on frequency. Moreover, these conditions were indispensable for the emergence of a therapy based on statistical considerations and the development of a pathological anatomy. The foreign models used in the erection of the institutional and pedagogical framework made the hospital the new 'laboratory' of medical science. In other words, the medicalisation of the hospital in the sense that the hospital became the new centre of medical practice and research, thus overlapping practical surgery (which was already hospital centered), was made possible by a practical problematic or a clinical technology. This *hospital problématique*, by creating the institutional conditions for a medical–surgical interaction, permitted the constitution of the fundamental doctrine of the Paris school, that is an anatomico-localist or 'surgical' approach to disease.

Although foreign models for the Parisian clinical school have been recognised, until now they have been recognised only as accessories. The realisations of these models have, in fact, been largely overlooked. For example, Boerhaave's clinic at Leiden or the clinics at Vienna and Edinburgh are consistently recalled as foreign models. These clinics began, as is known, with a small number of patients – about a dozen. According to many authors, such clinics functioned as a sort of nosological theatre wherein the students were presented with a concrete and empirical illustration of the different essential species of the nosological table.[22]

Now, were it only that which the Paris school had taken as a foreign model, it would be fair to say that this model had little impact and that the Paris school quickly went beyond this protoclinical model or nosological theatre in its creation of a veritable hospital medicine based on the observation of a large number of patients. Ackerknecht, for example, has written that Boerhaave's twelve beds in Leiden cannot be compared with the twenty thousand inmates of the Parisian hospitals in 1790.[23] It would also be fair to state, with

22 See, e.g., Foucault, *Birth of the Clinic*, pp. 58ff.
23 *Medicine at the Paris Hospital*, p. 15. Note, however, Tenon's figure of 20,000 *pensionnaires* includes all residents helped by the hospital and not just the ill. The number thus eludes comparison. According to Coste 'Hôpital', in Alard, Alibert, Barbier et al. (eds.), *Dictionnaire des sciences médicales*, 60 vols. (Paris, 1812–22), 21, p. 493), in 1806, there were 3,580 occupied beds in the Parisian hospitals (not including the hospices). See also Ackerknecht, ibid., pp. 18ff.

Foucault, that as regards the Hippocratic clinics of foreign countries, the Paris school created, through a radical epistemological rupture, something completely new: true clinical medicine for which the hospital was now the central structure. All the same, it is difficult to accept such a thesis for there are levels other than that of the protoclinical at which the foreign models functioned for the Paris school and within which they gained their importance.

The important model was, in fact, not the university clinic or university hospital by itself, but a set of models derived from the partial medicalisation of the hospitals and their transformation into centers of medical practice and practical or clinical training, which, in the beginning, was rarely university based. The progress of this process of partial medicalisation of the hospitals accelerated the realignment of medicine and surgery that itself became a model.

Originally, the medicalisation of hospitals in Austria, Germany, Italy, England and elsewhere, and the consequent transformation of the conditions of medical practice, research and training, was incited and sustained by social, political and ideological conditions of considerable purview.[24] Starting in the second half of the eighteenth century, the field of medicine underwent an important transformation in different European countries. Diverse reforms or innovations converged towards a common objective: the promotion of a practical or observational medicine. This concerned not only medicine itself, but also surgery, 'obstetrics' and pharmaceutics. Observational medicine

24 This and the following paragraphs summarise themes more amply developed in my 'Cabanis'. On the relationship between mercantilist ideas and the public health reform programs or the medicalisation of society in such different countries as Germany, Austria, France and England, see G. Rosen's many articles in *From Medical Police to Social Medicine* (New York, 1974). On the relations between the public health movement, the development of the hospital system and the use of these institutions for the purposes of training and research, see M. C. Buer, *Health, Wealth and Population in the Early Days of the Industrial Revolution* (London, 1926). For France, see 'La médicalisation en France du XVIIIe au début du XIXe siècle', *Annales de Bretagne et des pays de l'Ouest*, 86, no. 2 (1979), and J. P. Goubert (ed.), 'La médicalisation de la société française 1770–1830', *Historical Reflections* 9, nos. 1, 2 (1982). For medicalisation in Austria and Germany, see E. Lesky, *Österreichisches Gesundheitswesen im Zeitalter des aufgeklärten Absolutismus* (Vienna, 1959) and Jan Brugelmann, 'Observations on the Process of Medicalization in Germany', in Goubert (ed.), pp. 131–52. On medicalisation in England, see E. G. Thomas, 'The Poor Law and Medicine', *Medical History* 24 (1980): 1–19, who has studied, within the framework of the Poor Law legislation, the institution of a sanitary control of the population by the parishes in collaboration with the hospitals, infirmaries or dispensaries (pp. 3–6). For a general discussion of the relationship between medicalisation and the emergence of 'modern' medicine, see O. Keel and P. Keating 'Autour du *Journal de Médecine de Québec*: programme scientifique et programme de médicalisation', in R. A. Jarrell and A. E. Roos (eds.), *Critical Issues in the History of Canadian Science, Technology and Medicine* (Ottawa, 1983), pp. 101–34, esp. 119ff, and Keel, 'Cabanis'.

required a practical or clinical training to be articulated, according to diverse modalities, with hospital or institutional experience (ambulatory services, dispensaries).

This new institutional or hospital-clinical training was realised in several ways. In some countries – Austria, Scotland and, later on, France – the decisions were made by local or central political authorities who localised the training, from the beginning, with the official context of a reformed university teaching. Elsewhere the implementation of practical training was often conducted outside the context of university teaching within a less official framework (such as the hospitals and/or private schools or even a new form of apprenticeship centered around hospital or clinical experience).[25]

The various reforms of medical training can be related to specific economic, socio-political and ideological conditions. Varied doctrines and policies (populationism, mercantilism, cameralism, neo-mercantilism) of the seventeenth and eighteenth centuries rendered demographic growth one of the bases of commercial and economic prosperity as well as a foundation of state power and military security. Population growth was considered one of the conditions of the production and enlarged reproduction of the work force, as well as a determinant of the size and importance of military force. Population growth also guaranteed the potential fiscal resources necessary for the expansionist policies of the monarchies and states of the time.[26]

A policy of demographic expansion has, as an obligatory corollary, a programme of public health, or medical police as it was sometimes referred to, since the health of the population was a regulatory parameter of the conservation and enlarged reproduction of the demographic mass.[27] A programme of public health comprised several

25 On the private schools and their relations with health care institutions in England, see Z. Cope, 'The Private Medical Schools of London 1746–1914', in F. N. L. Poynter (ed.), *The Evolution of Medical Education in Britain* (London, 1966), pp. 89–109. See also the references in n. 44, this chapter, and Buer, *Health, Wealth, and Population*, pp. 116ff. On W. and J. Hunter's schools and those prior to theirs in London, see G. C. Peachey, *Memoir of William and John Hunter* (Plymouth, 1924), and R. Porter's essay in this volume, chap. 1.

26 Although the physiocrats were generally opposed to mercantilist principles, they incorporated, in their own way, the populationist thesis: G. Weurlesse, *Le mouvement physiocratique en France*, 2 vols. (Paris, 1910), II, p. 268. The 'populationist' credo was propounded in numerous political, administrative and medical treatises in the eighteenth century. See, e.g., M. Didelot (*Instruction pour les Sages Femmes*, 1770): 'A State is only as powerful as it is populous . . . as the hands that work and those that defend are numerous.' Cited in E. Badinter, *L'amour en plus: Histoire de l'amour maternel, XVIIe–XXe siècle* (Paris, 1980), p. 147.

27 C. Hannaway has made this point for the French case in 'From Hygiene to Public Health: A Transformation in Western Medicine in the Eighteenth and Nineteenth Centuries', in T. Ogawa (ed.), *Public Health* (Tokyo, 1981), pp. 117–18:

interdependent lines of action. In addition to an extended series of measures for the improvement and control of the public's health, certain objectives referred specifically to medical training. Of considerable importance was the reform of the hospitals through medi-

'Not until mid-century did the government envisage a continuing involvement in issues affecting health and begin planning a more systematic response to epidemics. The precipitating factors for the new approach were the coming into prominence in government circles of administrators with strong physiocratic views and massive outbreaks of the animal disease, rinderpest. The basic philosophy of the physiocrats was that the land and its products were the primary sources of wealth for a state. From this perspective, a healthy vigorous population of humans and animals was necessary for a vigorous agricultural economy and all factors which threatened this equation required State attention.' On populationist doctrines and policies in eighteenth-century France, and their implications for public health, see W. Coleman, 'L'hygiène et l'état selon Montyon', *Dix-Huitième Siècle*, no. 9 (1977): 101–8. On physiocratic policy, public health and the population, see H. Mitchell, 'Rationality and Control in French Eighteenth Century Medical Views of the Peasantry', *Comparative Studies in Society and History* 21 (1979): 82–112, esp. 89–90. See also, 'Politics in the Service of Knowledge: The Debate over the Administration of Medicine and Welfare in Late Eighteenth-Century France', *Social History* 6, no. 1 (1981): 185–207, esp. 199ff. On the origins of a national public health programme in late eighteenth-century France, see D. Weiner, 'Le droit de l'homme à la santé – une belle idée devant l'Assemblée constituante: 1790–1791', *Clio Medica* 5, no. 3 (1970): 209–25, and L. J. Jordanova, 'Policing Public Health in France, 1780–1815', in Ogawa (ed.), *Public Health*, pp. 12–32. On public health welfare and medicalisation programmes in eighteenth-century France, see the following classics: J. P. Desaive, J. P. Goubert, E. Le Roy Ladurie, J. Meyer, O. Muller, J. P. Peter, *Médecins, climats et épidémies à la fin du XVIIIe siècle* (Paris, 1972); J. P. Peter, "Les mots et les objets de la maladie. Remarques sur les épidémies et la médecine dans la société française de la fin du XVIIIe siècle', *Revue Historique* 246 (1971): 13–38; J. P. Goubert, *Malades et Médecins en Bretagne, 1770–1794* (Rennes, 1974), also 'The Extent of Medical Practice in France around 1780', *Journal of Social History* 10 (1976–7): 410–27. On the relationship between welfare policy and health policy in France, see also C. Bloch, *L'assistance et l'état en France à la veille de la Révolution* (Paris 1908), and O. Hufton, *The Poor of Eighteenth-Century France 1750–1789* (Oxford, 1974). Foucault (Foucault [ed.], *Les machines à guérir* [Paris, 1979]), has shown that in eighteenth-century France it was a health policy based on 'the abundance of the population, always defined as the origin of wealth and power' (p. 10) that induced, amongst other things, the medicalisation of the hospitals; see pp. 7–17. With regards to the studies just mentioned, Rosen's work offers the advantage of making a comparative approach possible. Strange as it may seem, most of the studies done on medicine, the public good and politics or the state in France never use the comparative dimension to understand what was happening in other countries with regards to the relations between politics, the state, society and medicine. What about programme and policies of medicalisation in countries other than France? If those who study France do not compare it with other countries, is it because they do not want to, because of specialist scruples or because they believe nothing has ever happened outside France? Rosen, on the other hand, has long provided the elements for an outline of a comparative approach. True, he did not himself develop such an analysis but he studied, in succession, different countries on the question of politics and medicalisation. Thus, for France, see Rosen, *From Medical Police to Social Medicine*, 'Mercantilism and Health Policy in Eighteenth Century French Thought', pp. 201–19 and 'Hospitals, Medical Care and Social Policy in the French Revolution', pp. 220–45. For Germany, Austria and Italy, see pp. 120–41, 'Cameralism and

216 *Othmar Keel*

calisation and the institution of a network of establishments (infirmaries, dispensaries, health and prevention centres) whose function
was to be the supervision of the population's health.[28] These new
health structures were also to serve as training centres for health care

the Concept of Medical Police'; pp. 142–58, 'The Fate of the Concept of Medical
Police, 1780–1890'. For England, see 'Medical Care and Social Policy in Seventeenth
Century England', pp. 159–75; 'Economic and Social Policy in the Development of
Public Health', pp. 176–200. In my thesis ('Cabanis') I undertook a comparative
analysis drawing a parallel between France and the different countries constituting
the Austria of the time (including, e.g., Lombardy) and I outlined a further parallel
between the former and Germany and England (see pp. 17ff, 160ff, 507ff). My
problematic is different from that of the authors mentioned here in that I tried to
show that in most eighteenth-century European countries, through a certain iso-
morphism, different health programmes and policies contributed not only to a
relative medicalisation of health care structures but also (and Rosen does not
mention this) to the modern clinical medicine. See also Keel, 'La place et la fonction
des modèles étrangers dans la constitution de la problématique hospitalière de
l'Ecole de Paris', *Actes du Colloque de l'Académie Internationale d'Histoire de la Médecine*
(Paris, 1982); also in *History and Philosophy of the Life Sciences* 6 (1984), 41–73.
28 On the medicalisation of the hospitals and/or other health care institutions in
post-1750 Europe, see Keel, 'Cabanis', chap. 5, 9–11. On hospitals and health care
structures in England, see F. N. L. Poynter (ed.), *The Evolution of Hospitals in Britain*
(London, 1964). See also U. Tröhler, 'Klinisch-numerische Forschung in der brit.
Geburtshilfe 1750–1820', *Gesnerus* 38 (1981): 1/2: 69–80, and 'Britische Spitäler und
Polikliniken als Heil- und Forschungstätten 1720–1820', *Gesnerus* 39 (1982), 1: 115–
32. On medicalisation in Europe, see A. Imhof, 'The Hospital in the 18th Century:
For Whom? The Charité Hospital in Berlin, the Navy Hospital in Copenhagen, the
Kongsberg Hospital in Norway', *Journal of Social History* 10, no. 4 (1977): 448–71. On
the voluntary hospitals in England, see the detailed studies of the hospital archives
and registers carried out by J. Woodward, *To Do the Sick No Harm; A Study of the
British Voluntary Hospital System to 1875* (London, 1974); H. Burdett, *Hospitals and
Asylums: Their Origin, History, Construction, Administration, Management and Legisla-
tion*, 4 vols. (London, 1891–3), and B. Abel-Smith, *The Hospitals, 1800–1948* (London,
1964). See also G. B. Risse, 'British Voluntary Hospitals in the Eighteenth Century:
For Better or Worse?' (unpublished paper), and J. V. Pickstone and S. V. F. Butler,
'The Politics of Medicine in Manchester, 1788–1792: Hospital Reform and Public
Health Services in the Early Industrial City', *Medical History* 28 (1984): 227–49. For
medicalisation in different countries, see the more global studies of D. Jetter,
Geschichte des Hospitals, 5 vols. (Wiesbaden, 1966–82), and *Grundzüge der
Krankenhausgeschichte* (Darmstadt, 1977). On the general problem of the medicalisa-
tion of European hospitals, see E. Lesky (ed.), J. P. Frank, *A System of Complete
Medical Police* (Baltimore, 1976), esp. 'Medical Science and Medical Educational
Institutions in General' (pp. 283–324); 'Medical Institutions in Particular' (pp. 325–
64); 'Medical Institutions of Learning; the Examination and Confirmation of Medical
Practitioners' (pp. 325–63). For the problem of the medicalisation of eighteenth-
century hospitals and its relation to urbanisation, see G. Rosen, *From Medical Police
to Social Medicine*, 'The Hospital, Historical Sociology of a Community Institution',
pp. 288ff; J. Imbert, *Les hôpitaux en France* (Paris, 1958); J. D. Thompson and G.
Goldin, *The Hospital: A Social and Architectural History* (London, 1975). For the
medicalisation of the Paris hospitals and in particular the Hôtel-Dieu at the end of
the eighteenth-century, see L. S. Greenbaum's studies: 'Jean-Sylvain Bailly, the
Baron de Breteuil and Four New Hospitals of Paris', *Clio Medica* 8 (1973): 261–84;
'Tempest in the Academy. Jean-Baptiste Le Roy, the Paris Academy of Sciences and
the Project of a New Hôtel-Dieu', *Archives Internationales d'Histoire des Sciences* 24

personnel. For example, the national, economic and 'populationist' preoccupations as well as the pedagogical preoccupations that led to the institution of new hospital structures were already present in Britain by 1720 in the movement to found a hospital at Edinburgh. As D. Hamilton has noted,

The first moves towards a hospital in Edinburgh came with the appearance of an anonymous pamphlet in 1721, probably written by the Monros, calling for a hospital. The motives, as far as can be judged from the pamphlet, were charitable, *economic and educational:* 'As men and Christians we have the strongest inducements and even obligations to this sort of charity . . . That humanity and compassion naturally prompt us to relieve our fellow creatures when in such deplorable circumstances as many are reduced to, naked, starving and in utmost distress from pain and trouble of the body and anguish of the soul: that as relief of these is a duty, *so it is no less advantage to the nation, for as many as are recovered in an Infirmary are so many working hands gained to the country:* that *students of physic and surgery might* hereby *have rather a better and easier opportunity of experience* than they *have had by studying abroad, where such hospitals* are, a great charge to themselves, *and a yearly loss to the nation:* And as a Proof of the whole, they *appealed to* the good *effects to the infirmaries in all other Civilised Nations.'*[29]

(1974): 122–40; ' "Measure of Civilization", the Hospital Thought of Jacques Tenon on the Eve of the French Revolution', *Bulletin of the History of Medicine* 49 (1975): 43–56; 'Hospitals, Scientists and Clergy in Eighteenth-Century France', *Episteme* 10 (1975): 51–9; 'Health-care and Hospital-building in Eighteenth-century France: Reform Proposals of du Pont de Nemours and Condorcet', *Studies on Voltaire and the Eighteenth Century* 42, Transactions of the Fourth International Congress on the Enlightenment, II (1976): 895–930. See also Foucault (ed.), *Les machines à guérir;* cf. D. Weiner (ed.), *The Clinical Training of Doctors, An Essay of 1793, by Ph. Pinel* (Baltimore, 1980). For the medicalisation of French hospitals, see M. Jeorger, 'La structure hospitalière de la France sous l'Ancien Régime', *Annales: Economies Sociétés Civilisations* 32 (1979): 1025–51: 'French hospital structure may thus be read in three ways: as an ancient reality, dominated by the concern for an undifferentiated charity, as a deep reality of the eighteenth century marked by its social protection role, as a future reality which is already taking form, *that of the guarantor of national health'* (my emphasis). For the medicalisation of hospitals in different countries, see, Keel, 'Cabanis'.

29 D. Hamilton, *The Healers: A History of Medicine in Scotland* (Edinburgh, 1981), pp. 122–3. My emphasis. Quoted also in A. L. Turner, *Story of a Great Hospital: The Royal Infirmary of Edinburgh (1729–1929)* (London, 1937), pp. 39–40, and Woodward, *To Do the Sick No Harm,* p. 21. A. Monro (*primus*) is considered the author of this text. This passage is also found in another text by Monro: *An Account of the Rise and Establishment of the Infirmary* (Edinburgh, 1730). From the seventeenth century on, populationist preoccupations led to the formulation of health programmes implicating the institution of medicalised hospital structures serving the ends of clinical

A second element of the program was often the reform of the health 'professions' through the organisation of new forms of apprenticeship or knowledge acquisition including the training of sanitary personnel capable of implementing an efficient health policy and able to neutralise illegal, uncontrolled and 'harmful' therapeutic practices. This training was to be articulated about a practical pedagogical form with an accent on direct 'clinical' experience acquired through contact with patients in the new health structures: hospitals and/or private schools, ambulatory services, maternity hospitals, dispensaries and home visits.

According to the promoters of demographic-sanitary policies, the hospital, once reformed or medicalised, would be an essential part of a programme of prevention and of the re-establishment of the health

training and practice. According to Petty: 'Now suppose that in the King's dominions there be 9 millions of people, of which 360,000 dye every year, and from whom 440,000 are borne. And suppose that by the advancement of the art of Medicine, a quarter part fewer dye. Then the King will gain and save 200,000 subjects per annum, which valued at 20 L. per head, the Lowest price of slaves, will make 4 millions per annum benefit to the Commonwealth. *Now I consider that the thorough and profound search into the natural and entire state of animals by anatomy and into their depraved and vitiated estate by the comparative and contrasted observations in hospitals, may in 100 years advance the art of medicine as above said. Therefore it is not the Interest of the State to leave Phisitians and Patients (as now) to their own shifts'* (The Petty Papers: Some unpublished writings of Sir William Petty, edited from the Bowood Papers by the Marquis of Lansdowne [London, 1927]. My emphasis). The foregoing is quoted in Rosen, *From Medical Police to Social Medicine*, 'Medical Care and Social Policy in Seventeenth Century England', pp. 165–6. See also pp. 172–3, where Rosen shows how this economic, demographic policy was a condition for the development of the eighteenth-century English hospital movement. The English movement constitutes the counterpart of the Continental medical police movement although on a different basis (limited government activity articulated with private initiative and cooperative action). On the social, political and ideological conditions of the eighteenth-century English hospital movement, see also Buer, *Health, Wealth and Population*, and Woodward, *To Do the Sick No Harm*, esp. 1–23. Of course, many variants of eighteenth-century health policy accented the conservation of subjects and productive forces. See, e.g., S. T. Anning, *The General Infirmary at Leeds*, 2 vols. (London, 1963–66), who cites the first annual report: 'There are many useful and industrious Manufacturers and Labourers who, whilst they are in Health, are able to provide well for the present Subsistence of themselves and their Families, but with all their economy can make no great provision against the time of sickness . . . Now, when any of these are by sickness, or Accidental Hurt, unfit for work, they are commonly unable to procure any medical assistance: Whereas, by the advantage of an Infirmary, many of them will probably soon be restored to the strength and Capacity of Labour.' Anning comments: 'A result happy not only for the patient but also for his employer'; vol. 1, pp. 3–4. The *problématique* of the reproduction of productive forces was to be reinforced by the context of the development of urban demographics, the development of manufacturing and commercial activities and the development of colonial and military activities. This problematic could, moreover, be easily combined, in different ways with the concomitant practices determined by philanthropic, self-help, religious and other ideologies. It was also possible to displace the mercantilist problematic towards a problematic that did not accept the *dirigiste* or statist framework but remained, nonetheless, preoccupied with the conservation of subjects and productive forces.

of the collectivity. The transformed hospitals were to be not only the best equipped centres for the control of disease through concerted action on a large scale but also the most important sites for practical training of the agents responsible for the supervision of the public's health. The acquisition of experience and the 'tangible' knowledge of Enlightenment philosophy were to be possible in the hospital. It was only in the hospital, according to the proponents of such policies, that one might acquire the training and the practical experience necessary for the production of practitioners able to supplant the charlatans undermining the health of the population and, consequently, the security and prosperity of the state.

The health-demographic-policy *problématique* implicating the medicalisation of the hospitals through the implantation of clinical institutions was revived and proposed as a model for France by C. G. Würtz in his *Mémoire sur l'établissement des écoles de médecine pratique à former dans les principaux hôpitaux civils de la France à l'instar de celle de Vienne* (Paris, Strasbourg, 1784):

> And what an advantage for Paris, for France, and for all the subjects of the realm if, in this city, we were to give to our art the same possibilities of improvement which, so far, have been accorded surgery and the veterinary arts. Why should we not be equally interested in filling the void that has prevented this city from being the most important in all Europe for the exercise of clinical practice as it is the Athens of all the other pleasant and useful sciences.
>
> The presence of foreigners would be marked; good medical observations multiple, our art more extensive, stronger, *a larger number of citizens saved and, in consequence, the state enriched; health and life would be revived in many provinces which, not finding the necessary help in their doctors, are given over blindly to the ignorance of charlatans. I believe that Government [la Politique] has heretofore overlooked an important principle [ressort] of population in neglecting the means of conserving the subjects of the king. Perhaps the project that I have just proposed would be one of the most efficacious.*
>
> Would not the execution of this project be greatly facilitated by the many hospitals established in this city and the provinces? It would only be a question of appointing two Professors in some of these hospitals, one for theory and the other for practice.[30]

---

30 *Mémoire*, pp. 35–6. Würtz presented this paper in 1781 to the Société Royale de Médecine of which he was a member. Vicq d'Azyr refers to it in his *Plan de constitution pour la médecine en France* (Paris, 1790), p. 158.

Within the logic of demographic-health policy then, the hospitals were necessarily the centres of medical practice and training. Moreover, for sympathisers with these doctrines, it was also clear that the hospital in its entirety had to be exploited in terms of observation, research and clinical training. This meant the penetration of all sectors of the hospital and not just the restricted material available in the clinical school, where there were but few beds. In their eyes, the clinical schools had only a propaedeutic function. Training and research were to have the entire hospital as their domain.[31] The hospital was valued as a centre of clinical training initiating students into a concrete form of clinical experience through contact with the most practical branches of the medical arts such as surgery or obstetrics. Health policy promoters saw the hospital as a site whose empirical-practical problematic (surgery, anatomico-localist approach, and so on) would infuse medical science and where, in return, medicine would enrich the practical disciplines with the scientific basis they lacked.[32]

The medicalisation of the hospital is perhaps best understood by considering that the eighteenth century saw a very partial and very unequal transformation of certain institutions of social regulation and public assistance in different European countries into therapeutic and medico-scientific institutions. There was, of course, before the end of the eighteenth century a medico-scientific presence in public assistance and social control institutions. Nonetheless, during the eighteenth century, the health and medico-scientific function became much more important. This is not to say that the latter function supplanted the regulatory or social assistance function within the hospital or general assistance system. In this respect, the medicalisation of the hospital system remained quite uneven well into the nineteenth century, especially in France.[33]

31 Keel, 'Cabanis' Chaps. 9–10, and 'La place'.
32 Ibid.
33 Some authors (see Ackerknecht, *Medicine at the Paris Hospital*, p. 17), maintain that the Revolution medicalised the hospitals by separating the sick from the poor and that this was the condition for the clinical 'revolution'. However, consider J. Léonard's analysis of the hospitals in the first decades of the nineteenth century in his *La médecine entre les savoirs et les pouvoirs* (Paris, 1981): 'The hospital, the hospice, the asylum – which sheltered the poor, the injured, the fevered, the impotent, the alienated, lost children, the homeless, the aged, the outcasts, the beggars, and crippled soldiers – were freed with difficulty from their former function as social regulators and their monastic or carceral reputation. These establishments which may have constituted exemplary sites of scientific observation and human devotion, bore constant witness against medicine and surgery. Public opinion gave them no confidence; peasants and workers showed them open aversion. It would be unjust to hold the physicians and surgeons responsible for certain odious or archaic characteristics of the hospital, for they were often the first and sometimes the only

There were, however, beach-heads in the eighteenth century in the sense that certain zones were medicalised to the extent that a distinction between the ill and the 'watched' or assisted was already quite advanced. These institutions were already being exploited as areas for the production and reproduction of medical knowledge.[34] It should also be noted that a good number of institutions, although unmedicalised with regards to inmate selection (they contained heterogeneous categories of pensioners: the sick, the healthy, the deserving poor, the handicapped, the poverty-stricken), served nonetheless as an important terrain for observation, experience and

ones to denounce these traits and their advice was often ignored by the administrators – prudent contributors, finicky accountants, privileged through money (merchants, bankers, industrialists, landowners) or authority (high-level functionaries, lawyers, ecclesiastics) – who saw these monuments of suffering as *indispensable social refuges rather than veritable health care centers* which inflicted upon the different socially dependent categories the austerity which seemed to them equivalent to their failure. Foul food, crumbling surroundings, rotten remedies, such were the leitmotiv of the doctors' complaints. In spite of the existence of workhouses and orphanages and the maintenance of beggars' prisons where reclusion was coupled with forced labour, *the hospitals and the hospices continued to shelter for better or for worse countless units of human wreckage* . . . Contagion proliferated on the vermin of the straw beds. Two patients in the same bed could still be seen. *It was not unusual for orphans or for the "insensed" to attend operations which were carried out in the middle of the common room.* Even in normal times, the classical distinction between the injured and the fevered was far from exhausting the variety of individuals hospitalized. Promiscuity added to the hospital hell: it was not known where to place the incurable or the chronics; the convalescent, the blind and the deaf mutes sometimes camped out amidst the contagious; the venereally diseased – when they were not completely excluded – were placed with those who had skin diseases. Too many beds placed too close together and wrapped with sinister curtains; dirty floors covered with sawdust; negligent and bawdy nurses; cold, airless rooms; barely drinkable water, etc., according to hygienists, the whole was detestable. Enormous *caravanserails* of misery, *the hospitals and hospices of the large cities were monstrous figures: the Paris Hôtel-Dieu with its 1400 beds was one of the worst death-houses in France;* the Salpêtrière, with 360 sick-beds, 800 mad, and 3900 incurables offered a hallucinating spectacle; the general hospice at Rouen sheltered 200 individuals and employed only two surgeons and three interns. The large surgical services were announced from afar by a putrid odour and, during operations, by screams and cries. The nightmare of a hundred moaning invalids! *A museum of pathological curiosities assembled for the edification of the students!'* (pp. 98–100; my emphasis). Nonetheless, even in these unfavourable conditions, the hospitals and even the most disadvantaged hospitals like the Hôtel-Dieu or the Salpêtrière managed to function as the 'observatories' or 'laboratories' of clinical science. It should be mentioned that from this point of view, a certain number of hospitals in Austria, Germany and Great Britain were more medicalised both in the eighteenth and nineteenth centuries than the French hospitals, which doubtless represented an advantage for the development of the clinic. On this point, see Keel, 'Cabanis' and 'La place'.
34   On this point, see Keel, 'Cabanis', chaps. 9–10, and for France, see J. P. Goubert, 'La médicalisation de la société française à la fin de l'Ancien Régime', *Francia* 8 (1980): 253ff.

training for medical personnel who, over the years, occupied an increasingly important place.

In the same vein, although it is true that the direction and control of hospital institutions rarely fell with the purview of a medical directorship,[35] the fact that religious orders or lay administrators (local élites or functionaries, subscribers and philanthropists) imposed an order that did not necessarily correspond with a medical regime (whence, for example, the conflicts between the nuns and doctors[36] over the handling of the patients – laicisation is a long and uneven process[37] – or between doctors and religious or lay hospital administrators over the ultimate ends of the hospital) does not negate the fact that even within these unfavourable conditions, many hospitals, including the least medicalized (in France, for example, the *Hôpitaux généraux* received pensioners who were not ill in contrast to the Hôtel-Dieu, which in principle accepted only those who were)[38] served

35 In some countries, in the last decades of the eighteenth century the direction of the hospitals had already been handed over to physicians. This was particularly the case in the absolutist states of central Europe. For example, Dr J. Quarin was named director of the Allgemeine Krankenhaus (2,000 beds) by Joseph II when the hospital opened its doors in 1784. Dr J. Nelly followed as director in the period 1791–5 and was replaced by Dr J. P. Frank in 1795. See Keel, 'Cabanis', chap. 9; B. Grois, *Das Allgemeine Krankenhaus in Wien und seine Geschichte* (Vienna 1965), pp. 11–12. In Lombardy, at Milan, the physicians directed the Ospedale Maggiore where P. Moscati (1739–1824) was the director in 1785. P. Pecchiai, *L'Ospedale Maggiore di Milano nella storia e nell'arte* (Milan, 1927), pp. 337–45, and 'I medici Direttori dell'Ospedale Maggiore di Milano,' in *L'Ospedale Maggiore* II (1914), 801–4. See also E. Lesky, *Einführung zur Nachricht an das Publikum über die Einrichtung des Hauptspitals in Wien (1784)* (Vienna, 1960).
36 See L. S. Greenbaum, 'Nurses and Doctors in Conflict. Piety and Medicine in the Paris Hôtel-Dieu on the Eve of the French Revolution', *Clio Medica* 13, 1/2 (1979): 247–67. See also D. B. Weiner, 'The French Revolution, Napoleon and the Nursing Profession', *Bulletin of the History of Medicine* 46 (1972) 274–305. On the resistance of the religious personnel to the medical personnel, see pp. 280ff. See also Colin Jones, 'Professionalizing Modern Medicine in French Hospitals', *Medical History* 26 (1982): 341–9.
37 See, in particular, O. Faure, 'L'hôpital et la médicalisation au début du XIXe siècle: l'exemple Lyonnais (1800–1830)', in *Annales de Bretagne et des pays de l'Ouest* 86, no. 2 (1979): 277–90. Cf. pp. 280, 286. See also L. Boulle, 'La médicalisation des hôpitaux parisiens dans la première moitié du XIXe siècle', in Goubert (ed.), *Historical Reflections* 9, nos. 1, 2 (1982): 33–44. Boulle has shown that as late as 1820–30, the process of laicisation was only relatively successful: 'Health care is carried out under the direction of the nuns. They direct the distribution of the food and medicaments. The history of the hospitals, impregnated with christian charity, explains the clearly confessional character of the establishments . . . The sisters have the upper hand vis-à-vis the healers and the servants who are in direct contact with the patients' (p. 39). See also M. Candille, 'Les soins en France au XIXe siècle', *Société française d'histoire des hôpitaux* 28 (1973): 33–79, and Léonard, *La Médecine*. On the importance of the nun's position in the hospital starting with the Consulat, see Léonard, pp. 52ff. See also Weiner, 'The French Revolution . . .'.
38 On this point, see M. Jeorger, 'La structure hospitalière', pp. 1026ff.

partially as clinical institutions. These institutions, in spite of the obstacles, were foci of medical observation, practical experience and training or apprenticeship. This was the result of the increasing occupation of important functions by medical personnel within the hospital system.

Many conflicting but not mutually exclusive functions coexisted within the hospital system: religious, social welfare, social control, medical, scientific and pedagogical. The fact that the hospitals were relatively unmedicalised as regards, for example, general administration[39] and unlaicised support personnel or completely unmedicalised as regards nursing personnel and daily-life activities was no obstacle to the progressive insinuation of a medical regime via therapeutic needs and the incremental development of a medico-scientific and sanitary function in the interstices of other functions in the system.[40] The hospitals were consequently able to develop as centres of medical knowledge or 'laboratories' for the constitution and transmission of this knowledge before becoming medicalised in other respects.

Foreign models had the greatest importance for France with regard to the medicalisation of the hospitals or their transformation into the 'laboratories' of medicine. The important model in this respect was that of the British hospitals such as those in London and other cities.

39   This is still the case for the beginning of the nineteenth-century in France. See O. Faure, 'L'hôpital', p. 283, regarding Lyon: 'We must insist on the meagreness of the results. *The hospitals remained, above all, asylums even though there appeared from within those concerns and those sectors which were more medicalised.* This cohabitation may be explained by the attitude of the groups working within the hospitals. The hospital administrators, whether they were the co-opted men of the Old Regime or members of the social élite, saw the hospital as a social regulator. This vision led them to reject all novelty and to maintain their absolute authority at any price. They refused many initiatives coming from more enlightened authorities who, for reasons of public order and without calling into question the fundamental ends of the hospital, wished to use the hospitals for the diffusion of medicine within the population and to bring the hospitals into conformity with the rules of hygiene. For the latter, the physicians represented an important relay with regards to internal transformations' (my emphasis).

40   As Faure (ibid., p. 299) has pointed out: 'To examine the relations between the hospital and medicalisation is to respond to three questions: what were the novelties which helped to change the hospital into a health care centre? To what extent did recourse to the hospital represent one of the ways in which society is medicalised? What role did the hospital play in the general process of medicalisation: training of medical personnel, distribution of medicines and outdoor care, participation in the struggle against smallpox?' The first question is of particular interest in this essay. On this point, for the first decades of the nineteenth century, the assessment is the following: 'Did the personnel become more competent and did their role widen? Was the hospital space rearranged with a view towards promoting hygiene and avoiding contagion? Were there new remedies and new therapies. *In these sectors, novelties and anachronisms coexisted*' (my emphasis).

These, it should be noted, were at least as important in this regard as the Royal Infirmary in Edinburgh. For example, in the *Plan de constitution pour la médecine en France*, which became the charter of the Paris school, Vicq d'Azyr presented the English hospitals as the model to be followed if the French institutions were to become centres of research and training in medicine, surgery and anatomico-pathology. According to Vicq d'Azyr: 'The teaching project exposed herein can only be carried out within the hospitals for it is with the eyes rather than the ears that students must learn in this area of study.'[41] After having exposed his plan for hospital teaching in rural areas, Vicq d'Azyr explained: 'This is more or less the English usage: one finds *in each hospital* a teaching-room, operating and dissection rooms. In Paris itself, at the Hôtel Dieu, there is a magnificent set-up for surgery. The same may be said for Rouen.'[42] If we are to believe Vicq d'Azyr, then it must be admitted that there was, to a certain extent, both inside and outside France, clinical practice in the hospital before the institution of a formal academic clinical teaching during and after the Revolution.

The apparent paradox is that with few exceptions (i.e., Edinburgh, Oxford, Cambridge)[43] clinical teaching in British hospitals and infirmaries existed before the emergence of academic clinical schools or the institution of clinical chairs in the university faculties. A similar situation obtained in France where certain institutions proposed by Vicq d'Azyr for clinical training in surgery (Hôtel-Dieu in Paris, in Rouen) also existed outside the university framework.

It is evidently not the university hospital that served here as a model for the institution of clinical medicine. Vicq d'Azyr clearly had in mind the delegation of clinical teaching to physicians and surgeons working in the Paris hospitals or in the provinces. In both cases he referred to English and certain French models none of which had any university affiliation. In this respect it might be noted that in London, the idea of a non-university clinical medicine was perpetuated well before the beginning of the nineteenth century. In fact, in the *Discours*

41 *Plan de constitution pour la médecine en France* (Paris, 1790), p. 161.
42 Ibid., p. 164. Cited in Gelfand, 'The Gestation of the Clinic', *Medical History* 25 (1981): 177. See Keel, *La généalogie*, pp 51–7, 102–15.
43 On the institution of a clinical school at the Radcliffe Infirmary in connection with a clinical chair, see A. H. T. Robb-Smith, 'Medical Education at Oxford and Cambridge Prior to 1850', in Poynter (ed.), *Evolution of Medical Education* pp. 44ff. See also A. G. Gibson, *The Radcliffe Infirmary* (Oxford 1926). Oxford students completed their clinical training at London or Edinburgh (Robb-Smith, ibid.). Since the beginning of the eighteenth century, Cambridge students attended St Thomas's Hospital in London and continued to do so after the opening of the Addenbrooke's hospital in 1766. See Poynter, 'Medical Education in England since 1600', in C. D. O'Malley (ed.), *The History of Medical Education* (Berkeley, 1970), pp. 238ff.

préliminaire sur l'histoire des cliniques, written in 1824, Auguste Gauthier described the situation as follows:

In London, there is neither a university nor an establishment for medical instruction. Rather, for about the last 50 years, the physicians of many hospitals are authorised by the government to give courses on the many branches of medicine [note the specialisation]. They receive no fixed emolument from the State; their courses are paid for by the students and forms their salary. Many of them teach *clinical medicine and surgery* with distinction, particularly at Guy's Hospital, St Thomas's, St Bartholomew's and several others.[44]

44 The discourse is at the beginning of V. von Hildenbrand, *Médecine pratique,* trans. A. Gauthier (Paris, 1824), p. XXXIV. Many sources enable one to pick out the beginnings and the development of medical and surgical clinical teaching in the hospitals or infirmaries of London and England in the second half of the eighteenth century and especially in the last thirty years. See F. N. L. Poynter (ed.), *The Evolution of Hospitals in Britain* (London, 1964), and in particular, C. Newman, 'The Hospital as a Teaching Center', pp 187–205, esp. pp. 196–201: 'That is why medical schools in England all came to be associated with, and were often started by hospitals, whereas elsewhere it is more the rule that medical schools were started by universities and universities actually founded and maintained hospitals to provide facilities for medical teaching. In England, it was more common for the medical men in a big town to start a medical school in the local infirmary, and for the medical school by its success to encourage, and by its presence to form the nucleus for the starting of a university' (p. 200). See also W. H. McMenemey, 'The Hospital Movement of the Eighteenth Century and its Development', in Poynter, *Evolution of Hospitals,* p. 65: 'The profession quickly recognized the use of hospitals for teaching and also the value of those intangible assets which went with a hospital appointment. The pupils paid fees and, when duly fledged, recommended to their chiefs patients who could afford a consultation'. See also F. N. L. Poynter, 'Medical Education in England since 1600', in O'Malley (ed.), *History of Medical Education,* pp. 235–49, esp. 238–40. See also H. C. Cameron, *Mr. Guy's Hospital (1726–1948)* (London, 1954), pp. 79–96, 145ff., 167–80. Cameron's book reproduces the primary sources that show that clinical teaching fell within the larger teaching framework, which included theoretical sections such as anatomy, chemistry and materia medica. As J. Peterson has pointed out in *The Medical Profession in Mid-Victorian London* (London, 1978): 'The eighteenth-century hospitals had been the informal site of medical education with surgeons bringing their hospital apprentices with them to learn at the bedside and in the operating theatre. *Physicians-in-training had come, paid a fee for hospital practice, and walked the wards, observing patients and physicians at their work.* From the late eighteenth century, individuals surgeons – and *sometimes physicians – began offering courses of lectures within the hospital walls.* Out of these casual beginnings came the early Victorian establishment of the medical schools' (p. 157, my emphasis). As can be seen, the hospital is the framework for practical teaching (clinical) and theoretical teaching not only in surgery but also in medicine. True, surgical pupils predominated at the London hospitals, but nevertheless, since about the 1770s, hospitals provided a 'whole course of lectures for the improvement of pupils in chirurgical and medical knowledge'. See Peachey, *Memoir of William and John Hunter,* p. 300. See also E. M. McInnes, *St Thomas' Hospital* (London, 1963), chap. VII, esp. pp. 74–82. See also A. E. Clark-Kennedy, *The London: A Study in the Voluntary Hospital System,* 2 vols. (London, 1962–63), I, pp. 165ff; J. Thornton, 'The Medical College from Its Origins to the End of the Nineteenth Century', in V. C.

Gauthier's information was derived from Joseph Frank's journal of his medical tour of England and France in 1803 published the following year.[45] Another observer had already written at the turn of the century: 'In England, *in all the great hospitals*, lessons on *practical medicine and surgery* are given. The most interesting are those of St Bartholomew's, St Thomas's, Guy's and the London.'[46]

According to the philanthropist John Howard (*An Account of the Principal Lazarettos in Europe . . .*, London, 1789), the capacity of London hospitals in the eighteenth century was as follows: London Hospital (120 beds); St Bartholomew's Hospital (428 beds), Middlesex Hospital (70 beds), St Thomas's Hospital (440 beds), Guy's Hospital (304 beds), St George's Hospital (150 beds).[47] Coste, in an account of London hospitals in 1779 and 1786, gives the following figures: St Thomas's: 460 beds; St Bartholomew's: 400 beds; the Hospital for French Protestants and their Descendants: 200 beds; Westminster In-

Medvei and J. Thornton (eds.), *The Royal Hospital of Saint Bartholomew, 1123–1973* (London, 1974), pp. 43–77, esp. 50ff. For the clinical practice of physicans of Bart's see Franklin in Medvei and Thornton, pp. 126–85. On the development of medical teaching in eighteenth-century hospitals and infirmaries see Woodward, *To Do the Sick No Harm*, p. 25: 'The standard of medical education rose dramatically with the advent of the voluntary hospital movement.' Cf. A. Chaplin, *Medicine in England during the Reign of George III* (London, 1919), pp. 137–8. See also W. B. Howie, 'Medical Education in 18th Century Hospitals', *Scottish Society for the History of Medicine Report of Proceedings* (1969–70): 27–46, esp. 37–42. W. F. Bynum, 'Health, Disease and Medical Care', in G. S. Rousseau and R. Porter (eds.), *The Ferment of Knowledge* (Cambridge, 1981), makes the following comment, which is convergent with my arguments here: 'But the historiography of formal medical education is still in a rather primitive state except for the famous centres, and much more could be done on *the extent to which hospitals not attached to universities were used in teaching*', p. 239, my emphasis. This applies not only to England but also to other countries in the eighteenth century. It will be necessary to study how hospitals unaffiliated with universities served not only teaching purposes but, perhaps still more, the ends of research and the production of knowledge. See also Keel, 'Cabanis', and *La généalogie*, pp. 51–7, 102–15.

45 Joseph Frank, *Reise nach Paris, London, und einem grossen Theile des Ubrigen Englands und Schottlands ins Beziehung auf Spitäler . . .* (Vienna, 1804–5), pp. 210ff.

46 See A. Flajani, *Saggio filosofico intorno agli stabilimenti scientifici in Europa appartenenti alla medicina* (Rome, 1807). Translated in part by L. Odier: *Extraits d'un ouvrage du Dr. A. Flajani sur les établissements publics relatifs à la médecine* (Geneva, 1811). Odier, p. 32; Flajani, p. 29. Flajani also writes, 'As there is no university in London there is, strictly speaking, no clinical school. But, *in all the hospitals*, lessons are given on the diseases present. So it is that at Guy's Hospital, which is one of the best, the three physicians that direct it, Drs. Babington, Curry, and Marcet, alternatively give *excellent clinical lessons*, two months each, from the first of November to the end of April. Rounds are every day at 11 a.m.' (my emphasis). For clinical practice outside London, see E. M. Brockbank, *The Foundation of Provincial Medical Education in England and of the Manchester School in Particular* (Manchester, 1936); on Manchester, pp. 37ff; on Birmingham, pp. 117ff; on Leeds, pp. 119ff. See also Tröhler, 'Britische Spitäler, pp. 119ff.

47 Howard, pp. 131–7.

firmary: 210 beds; Guy's: 430 beds; St George's: 270 beds; the London Hospital: 160 beds; Middlesex Hospital: 150 beds.[48]

One can easily see that towards the end of the eighteenth century, London had at its disposition, as did Paris, an important health infrastructure that served in a large measure for clinical practice. As is evident in a letter from John Hunter to the governors of St George's Hospital, the hospital in London in the second half of the eighteenth century was easily construed as a field of research and as rich terrain for the acquisition of knowledge: 'When I solicited to be appointed one of the surgeons to St George's Hospital, it was not with a view to augment my income, either immediately by the profits of the hospital or in a secondary way by increasing my practice, but *to acquire opportunities of extending my knowledge that I might be more useful to mankind.'*[49] Doubtless, one may be sceptical of Hunter's self-appreciation. Nonetheless, the appeal to such an argument at least indicates that at the time, it was readily admitted that the hospital was a framework for the production of knowledge.

The hospital served, moreover, not only as a site for observation and research but also as a training centre. It is claimed that during his tenure as a surgeon at St George's Hospital, Hunter trained over a thousand students. Joan Lane gives an indication of the importance of training at St George's Hospital in the period 1770–9 in her essay 'The Role of Apprenticeship in Eighteenth Century Medical Education':[50] 'During the period 1770–79, at St George's, John Hunter had 449 pupils, John Gunning had 103 and the three other surgeons there had 284 between them, a total of 836 pupils!'[51] Already in 1757, there were more than 100 pupils. As Lane has noted 'With the development of twenty-six civilian provincial hospitals in Hunter's lifetime, many more training facilities were available for post-apprenticeship instruction.'[52] These facilities were, in addition, combined with other opportunities for research and/or clinico-pathological training given by other institutions such as the private anatomy schools and the museums or pathological anatomy collections.

---

48 Coste, 'Hôpital', in Alard et al. (eds.), *Dictionnaire des sciences médicales*, vol. 21 (1817), pp. 367–544. For the London hospitals' capacity in 1779 and 1786, see pp. 504–6.
49 Letter (28 February 1793) quoted in E. Finch, 'The Influence of the Hunters on Medical Education', *Annals of the Royal College of Surgeons* 20 (1957): 219. My emphasis. Quoted also in Jessie Dobson, *John Hunter* (Edinburgh and London, 1969), p. 332, and Peachey, *Memoir of William and John Hunter*, p. 150. Cf. the essay by Gelfand, Chap. 5, this volume.
50 Chap. 3, this volume.
51 Ibid. See also, Peachey, *Memoir of William and John Hunter*, pp. 150.
52 Chap. 3, this volume.

Baillie, for example, explained in the preface to his *Morbid Anatomy of Some of the Most Important Parts of the Human Body* (1793) that his research in pathological anatomy was made possible by the following three conditions: (1) a physician's post in a large hospital, (2) a teaching post in an anatomy school and (3) the regular use of William Hunter's collection of pathological preparations.

> My situation [Baillie wrote] has given me more than the *ordinary opportunities* of examining morbid structures. Dr. Hunter's collection contains a *very large* number of preparations exhibiting morbid appearances, which I can have recourse to at any time for examination. Being physician to *a large hospital*, and engaged in *teaching anatomy*, I have also very frequent opportunities of examining diseases in dead bodies.[53]

It was, therefore, not only the hospital but also the anatomy school that presented frequent occasions for the study of disease within cadavers. In other words, the hospital was not the only site or the only structure to permit the formation of knowledge of the anatomico-localist, anatomico-pathological and anatomico-clinical type.

This raises a very important point. The 'anatomy' school (such as William Hunter's and Baillie's school, and many others) covered practically the whole domain of medicine: Much more than surgery was taught. As Peachey has noted, the course given in Hunter's school included 'the whole *medical* curriculum with the exception of chemistry, materia medica and experimental philosophy'.[54] The syllabus was to teach students 'all the arts of examining diseases'.[55]

Clearly, a school that permitted the observation of many diseases and the performance of a large number of dissections could only favour an interaction between medicine and surgery and thus form a localist, anatomical or "surgical" point of view. The syllabus insisted upon the value of a quantitative approach to pathological facts: the school allowed one to observe a large number of diseases, to practice numerous dissections and surgical operations and to make many pathological preparations illustrating the diseases.[56] It may be said that in such a school one cultivated not only anatomy and surgery, but also physiology and medicine. There was, thus, a form of *de facto* unification of the different branches of the medical arts. Given that this school remained open for many years, many students were trained.

---

53 In A. E. Rodin, *The Influence of Matthew Baillie's Morbid Anatomy. Biography, Evaluation and Reprint* (Springfield, Ill., 1973), p. 70. My emphasis.
54 See Peachey, *Memoir of William and John Hunter*, p. 128.
55 Syllabus of the course given by W. Hunter and W. Cruikshank (September 1782 issue of *European Magazine*), quoted in Peachey, ibid, p. 130.
56 Ibid.

So it was with John Hunter's private teaching, which trained several hundred students.[57] These generations of students were trained within a *problématique*, one of whose leading characteristics, *the interpenetration of medicine and surgery*, has been explicitly described by Hunter's student, J. Abernethy (1764–1831), in his Hunterian Oration (1819):

> Medicine is one and indivisible, it must be learnt as a whole, for no part can be understood if learnt separately. The physician must understand surgery; the surgeon, the medical treatment of disease. Indeed, it is from the evidence afforded by external disease, that we are able to judge of the nature and progress of those which are internal.[58]

The medico-surgical clinical training acquired in the private schools (anatomy schools, hospital lectures or teaching, and so on) was, more often than not, combined with practical experience obtained not only in the large London hospitals but also in the smaller health-care units such as the infirmaries, the dispensaries and the maternities. One way in which private lessons and hospital training were combined was that prevalent at St George's Hospital: 'As to the attendance of our pupils on lectures, they have to go for their anatomy to Windmill Street – for their midwifery to Queen Street, Golden Square, for their Chymistry, Materia Medica and practice of physick to Leicester-Fields.'[59]

In other cases, a professor might combine his private school teaching with his hospital teaching or he might give both theoretical lessons and practical clinical training: John Hunter once did so. Students were then able to follow private teaching and a course of practical training under the aegis of the same teacher.

Private medical schools like William Hunter's or, later on, John Hunter's, existed outside the hospitals, functioning, at the same time, in connection with them. To these private schools must, however, be added the schools that were set up within the framework of the London hospitals. A contemporary hospital surgeon (1793) explained the emergence of these schools:

> From the year 1780 to the present period schools for *surgery and physick* with the different professors have been established at Guy's and St. Thomas's . . . which wisely uniting for the common good, give the pupils belonging to either, *the oppor-*

57 Finch, 'Influence of the Hunters', p. 219; G. Qvist, *John Hunter, 1728–1793* (London, 1981), p. 25.
58 Quoted in Finch, 'Influence of the Hunters', p. 223. My emphasis.
59 Surgeons' letter (27 May 1793) to the committee appointed to examine the laws relative to the surgeons' pupils and to consider the best method of improving their education. Quoted in Peachey, *Memoir of William and John Hunter*, p. 302.

tunity of attending upwards of 700 patients. That a 2nd school
has been established at St. Bartholomew's on nearly the same
plan, with *the opportunity of attending near 500,* and even at the
London where they have not so many beds for patients as
ourselves.[60]

As can be seen, these non-university hospital schools of clinical
medicine and surgery had at their disposal considerable observational
material.

It is clear that for such students as M. Baillie, Abernethy and A.
Cooper, London presented exceptional possibilities for the acquisition of a complete medical education. Baillie was able to combine
training as a student of William Hunter's at the Windmill Street
school with hospital training at St George's under the direction of
John Hunter and a complete series of lectures or theoretical courses
on the different branches of the medical arts. And from the 1780s,
teachers like Baillie and Abernethy did in turn train many pupils in
medicine as well as in surgery.

In fact, the importance of the London hospitals for the clinic was
recognised by S. G. C. Bruté, who wrote in his *Essai sur l'histoire et les
avantages des institutions cliniques* published at Paris in year XI (1803)
that 'the large hospitals, such as St Bartholomew's, St Thomas; the
Middlesex and St George's, have opened abundant sources of instruction to the students'.[61]

As Bynum has noted, according to the *Medical Register* published in
1783 by Samuel Foart Simmons, there were 161 medical posts in the
London hospitals, infirmaries and dispensaries.[62] This included 78
posts for the 148 physicians and physician-midwives, 53 posts for the
220 surgeons, and 30 posts for the 600 apothecaries. This implantation of medical practitioners in the hospitals and dispensaries allowed
the latter to become teaching centres.[63]

Other specialised hospitals were used for observation, research
and, to a certain extent, teaching. These institutions received patients
suffering from smallpox, venereal diseases and mental illness. There
were, moreover, ten maternity hospitals.[64]

Although the dispensaries accepted fewer patients than the large
hospitals, they also served research and training needs within an
anatomico-localist point of view in medicine. Thus, Chaplin has writ-

60 Surgeons' reply to Hunter's address (1793), quoted in Peachey, ibid., p. 291. My
emphasis
61 Bruté, p. 169. See also Keel, *La généalogie,* pp. 51–7, 102–15.
62 Chap. 4, this volume.
63 Ibid.
64 Ibid.

ten: 'A particular interest attaches to the "Public Dispensary" in Carey Street, for it was there that Robert Willan and his pupil Thomas Bateman prosecuted their researches in Dermatology, and gave to the world the first attempt to classify skin diseases from an anatomical standpoint.'[65]

I have previously indicated that, beginning in the second half of the eighteenth century (and sometimes earlier), hospitals or infirmaries in England (and elsewhere in Europe) were becoming centres of practical (clinical) research and training in medicine and surgery before the existence of university clinics.[66] The clinical teaching given by a university professor at the Royal Infirmary in Edinburgh before 1750 was therefore an exception to the rule. Lawrence rightly notes that it was twenty-two years after the foundation of the Edinburgh medical school when Rutherford gave his first clinical lecture in 1748.[67] There is, moreover, a difference between a clinical lecture and clinical

---

65 *Medicine in England*, p. 22.
66 Keel, *La généalogie*, pp. 51–7, 102–15; Keel, 'Cabanis'.
67 Chap. 6, this volume. On the anatomical, localist or 'surgical' approach to disease and on the interpenetration of medicine and surgery at Edinburgh, especially with the Monros, see Lawrence, ibid., and Keel, *La généalogie*, esp. pp. 72–3, 77–84, 108–10; see also Keel, 'La formation . . .', pp. 195–6, 205–6. On Monro's (*secundus*) praise of pathological anatomy and stress on physical diagnosis in his teaching, see Lawrence, chap. 6, this volume: 'The most obvious feature of Monro's teaching is his strongly developed concept of local disease, and the associated idea of invasion along the planes defined by topographical anatomy . . . Monro clearly seems to have performed far more post-mortem examinations than did his predecessors.'' In fact, Monro's anatomical and localist orientation enabled him to consider disease at the tissue level and not only at the organ level. (See Keel, *La généalogie*, and 'La formation . . .') Monro (*tertius*) could claim that his father (*secundus*) was, with Hunter and J. C. Smyth, one of the founders of general anatomy. See Keel, 'Les conditions . . .', p. 56, n. 25. Lawrence (chap. 6, this volume) points out that 'corpses for anatomy were less frequent in Edinburgh than London, but *there were wax models in abundance*' (my emphasis). Monro even tried to apply Auenbrugger's new technique of percussion, which clearly shows his 'interest in establishing clinical correlation with local internal pathology' (Lawrence, ibid.). On the 'modern' aspects of Cullen's and Gregory's teaching, see Lawrence, this volume, as well as on the 'puzzle' of Cullen's nosology: 'Finally, it [nosology] was intended not as a finished product, but as a structure within which *to study pathological anatomy* and pursue nosography. Cullen wanted disease species to be defined ultimately by the results of *many* post-mortems.' This point is developed in C. J. Lawrence 'Medicine as Culture: Edinburgh and the Scottish Enlightenment' (PhD thesis, University of London, 1984): 'Cullen particularly praised Morgagni's work as being the correct approach to nosology.' Cullen attacked humoral theory as contradicted by the clinical practice (Lawrence, ibid.). In fact, Cullen's solidism largely preceded Pinel's and served as its model. Moreover, Lawrence (ibid.) points out that 'the publication of Morgagni's work in 1769 (English translation) seems to have given new encouragement to the enterprise of pathological anatomy in Edinburgh'. On the quantitative approach to disease in Edinburgh, see Lawrence, this volume. The use of statistical methods by Edinburgh-trained physicians as well as by other British physicians and surgeons has been studied in U. Tröhler,

instruction. Although there were no clinical lectures in Edinburgh
before 1748, clinical instruction had been given since the opening of
the Royal Infirmary in 1729. As Turner recalled, 'Since the opening of
the Little House in 1729, clinical instruction had been given by the
physicians and surgeons attending in rotation for short periods.'[68]

Thus, even in Edinburgh, the Infirmary was the site of clinical
practice, research and training in medicine as well as in surgery before the institution of clinical lectures by university professors. Nonetheless Alexander Monro (*primus*), for example, university professor
of anatomy and surgery, was able to contribute to clinical instruction
by virtue of being one of the six ordinary surgeons attached to the
infirmary since its opening[69] and with whom students received practical instruction.[70]

Irvine Loudon in 'The Origins and Growth of the Dispensary
Movement in England'[71] notes that the number of admissions to the
London general hospitals lay somewhere between 20,000 and 30,000
at the end of the eighteenth century and that the number admitted to
the dispensaries was about 30,000.

Five new hospitals were founded in London between 1720 and
1745: Westminster (1720), Guy's (1724), St George's (1733), London
Hospital (1740) and the Middlesex Hospital (1745).[72] Moreover, between 1770 and 1792, sixteen dispensaries were opened. Elsewhere,
within the framework of the voluntary hospitals and dispensaries
movement, thirty-two hospitals and infirmaries were opened between 1773 and 1798.[73] From the beginning, the new possibilities for
clinical research and the study of disease offered by these institutions
were quickly exploited.[74]

'Quantification in British Medicine and Surgery 1750–1830; with special reference to
its introduction into therapeutics' (PhD thesis, University of London, 1978). See also
Tröhler, 'Klinisch-numerische Forschung', 'Britische Spitäler'.
68 *Story of a Great Hospital.*
69 Turner, ibid., p. 57.
70 Ibid., pp. 58–9.
71 *Bulletin of the History of Medicine* 55 (1981): 324. Cf. R. Porter, *English Society in
the Eighteenth Century* (London, 1982), p. 302. In England in 1800, the 'voluntary
general hospitals' had approximately 4,000 usable beds, half of which were in
London. See Abel-Smith, *The Hospitals*, pp. 1–4, and Woodward, *To Do the Sick No
Harm*, p. 36. On this point, see also Bynum, chap. 4, this volume. In fact, in 1800
the hospital structure in Great Britain was even larger: Abel-Smith's calculations
include only England and Wales. The Royal Military Hospitals and the Marine
Hospitals had a considerable number of pensioners. For example, the Haslar
hospital had a 2,000-bed capacity in 1761. See C. C. Lloyd, 'Naval Hospitals', in
Poynter (ed.), *Evolution of Hospitals in Britain*, p. 151.
72 Loudon, 'Origins and Growth of Dispensary Movement'; Porter, *English Society*;
Woodward, *To Do the Sick No Harm*; Buer, *Health, Wealth and Population*, pp. 126–50.
73 Loudon, ibid.; Woodward, ibid.; Buer, ibid.
74 Loudon, ibid.; Porter, *English Society*; Woodward, ibid., pp. 24–6; Buer, ibid.

Still other institutions such as the military and marine hospitals served as foci for clinical observation and the transmission of knowledge in eighteenth-century England. Hence, in addition to the clinical schools such as the one at Edinburgh, a whole range of institutions (civil hospitals, military hospitals, maternity hospitals, charities, ambulatory services, dispensaries, private schools) served as a terrain for research and training.[75]

Many new institutions founded within the framework of the voluntary hospital movement presented the additional advantage of being rather more medicalised than the older institutions in that the former were reserved for the ill (for the worker unable to pay for health care) to the exclusion of such categories as the destitute, the unemployed and beggars, who had their own institutions (poor-house, workhouse, pest-house, almshouse). The system of letters of recommendation[76] needed for entry into the hospital and dispensaries permitted one to effectively select the ill from amongst the numerous categories for which the health care structures had been instituted. The term 'hospital' may therefore be legitimately applied to the British medical institutions of the closing decades of the eighteenth century, contrary to Ackerknecht's belief that such entities arose only in Paris after the Revolution: 'The Paris hospital of our period was, in its conception and organization, no longer a medieval receptacle of all miseries. It had eventually become a medical institution and thus served as a cradle of the new medicine.'[77]

With respect to medical institutions and practices, P. Huard and M. J. Imbault-Huart, in their article on Tenon's trip to England, have noted that English medicine continued to fascinate the French well

---

See also Chaplin, *Medicine in England*, pp. 22ff, and Tröhler, 'Britische Spitäler', pp. 118ff.

75 On the marine hospitals and/or hospital ships as centres of clinical experience, see Keel, *La généalogie*, pp. 103–4. Cf. U. Tröhler, 'Towards Clinical Investigation on a Numerical Basis: James Lind at Haslar Hospital 1758–1783', *Proceedings of the XXVII International Congress of the History of Medicine* (Barcelona, 1981), I, pp. 414–19. See also Tröhler, 'Britische Spitäler'. See also Lloyd, 'Naval Hospitals', in Poynter (ed.), *Evolution of Hospitals*, pp. 150–2. C. Lloyd and J. Coulter, *Medicine and the Navy (1200–1900)*, 4 vols. (Edinburgh and London 1961), III, pp. 187–261. On the military campaign hospitals, see Neil Cantlie, *A History of the Army Medical Department*, 2 vols. (Edinburgh and London, 1974), I, pp. 102ff. On the maternity hospitals as a field of clinical practice, see Buer, *Health, Wealth and Population*, pp. 141ff. A. Gunn, 'Maternity Hospitals', in Poynter (ed.), *Evolution of Hospitals*, pp. 77–101; H. R. Spencer, *The History of British Midwifery from 1650 to 1800* (London, 1927), pp. 73ff.

76 On the system of subscribers' recommendation letters, see Woodward, *To Do the Sick No Harm*, chap. 5, esp. pp. 38ff.

77 Ackerknecht, *Medicine at the Paris Hospital*, p. 22. I. Waddington, 'The Role of the Hospital in the Development of Modern Medicine: A Sociological Analysis', *Sociology* 7 (1973): 211–24.

after the end of the eighteenth century.[78] In the same vein, writing of the hospital situation in England at the turn of the eighteenth century, Flajani, an on-the-spot observer, affirmed in his book on European clinical and medical establishments that 'In England, the hospitals have attained a degree of perfection rarely attained in other countries'.[79]

III

There would appear to be a false trail that, according to Huard and Imbault-Huart, amongst others, leads from a *médecine facultaire* in the middle of the eighteenth century to a hospital medicine that, beginning in 1794 in France, reconceptualised the clinic in terms of large numbers. This thesis is always based on the same argument: There

78 See P. Huard and M. J. Imbault-Huart, 'Le voyage de Jacques Tenon (1724–1816) en Grande Bretagne (1787) et ses conséquences', *Proceedings of the XXIII International Congress of the History of Medicine*, 2 vols. (London, 1974), I. On English hospitals taken as a model for France, see also L. S. Greenbaum, 'The Commercial Treaty of Humanity, La tournée des hôpitaux anglais par J. Tenon en 1787', *Revue d'Histoire des Sciences* 24, no. 4 (1971): 317–50. Medicalisation is more advanced in the English hospitals: There were 'four times as many nurses' (p. 329); the state of cleanliness should be a model for France (pp. 329, 344); the mode of administration is better (p. 330). The English hospitals like those at Plymouth are a model for the distribution of the patients and patient-care specialisation: '15 pavilions, isolated (10 for the patients and 5 for the services), aerated, each containing 100 patients in six rooms, each room devoted to a particular type of disease . . . , have made the hospital, from a scientific point of view, a model "for all Europe" '; p. 341. The second part of the third report of the Académie des Sciences hospital commission, published 12 March 1788, is devoted to the internal order of the new hospitals 'in conformity with British practice'. The greatest number of specifications in this second part comes directly from Tenon. The report makes no mystery of the admiration for England; p. 342: 'The number of beds is reduced to 30 per room ("the English experience has confirmed our principle")', p. 342. 'In addition, the report foresees the creation of an English dispensary in the Parisian parishes where patients receive the free services of a physician, a midwife, a surgeon, and an apothecary'; p. 343. Yet another model was 'that of the installations devoted to the teaching of surgery and anatomy within the hospital itself'. For the English model, see Greenbaum, pp. 346–7: 'The English experience thus had a considerable influence on his life's work, hospital construction according to scientific principles.' Tenon's hospital reform ideas are truly situated within the framework of the mercantilist problematic: 'In his letter to George III which accompanied his *Mémoires*, Tenon defined the principle of governmental responsibility with regards to illness and poverty. Force and national prosperity may only be obtained through the protection of a large population's health. This is king's business.' See also Greenbaum's other articles, n. 28, this chapter.
79 See Odier, *Extraits*, p. 62, and Flajani, *Saggio*, pp. 85, 209ff. Flajani shows that numerically the clinical framework in the English hospitals was more important than in the French hospitals. For a given number of patients there were, in England, more physicians and surgeons (who were also clinical instructors or teachers) than in France. See p. 231 and table I.

were only a few beds in the eighteenth-century clinical schools; this
was the result of the 'structure' of the clinical thought of the time.
Recall Huard and Imbault-Huart's judgement: 'The old distrust of the
nosologists for the hospital which corrupted the essence of disease
made them wish for very small clinics (12 beds for Stoll and de Haen).
The new hospital medicine, on the contrary, demanded a large
number of beds for the study of lesions.'[80] The same form of argu-
mentation can be seen at work in Gelfand:

> Eighteenth-century authors considered the selection of a small
> number of patients to be a principle of critical importance for
> clinical instruction. Boerhaave's figure of six male patients and
> six females was often followed. See Georg Christoph Wurtz,
> *Mémoire sur l'établissement des écoles de médecine pratique à former*
> *dans les principaux hôpitaux civils de la France à l'instar de celle de*
> *Vienne* (Paris, 1784), p. 17. Wurtz described the clinical teach-
> ing conducted by Maximilian Stoll, de Haen's successor at
> Vienna. Ibid., pp. 17–27. W. Turnbull (trans.), *A Treatise on*
> *chirurgical diseases and on the operations required in their treatment,*
> *from the French of Messrs. Chopart and Desault* (London, 1797), I,
> 16ftn., mentioned that the Edinburgh infirmary selected about
> 25 or 30 patients out of a total of about 200 and placed them
> in separate wards.[81]

To show the inadequacy of this thesis we will begin with Edinburgh itself. (We will return to Vienna later.) In 1757 the Edinburgh
Royal Infirmary clinic contained 30 beds of a total of 100. When the
Infirmary opened in 1729, it contained only 6 beds. By 1745 the hospital contained only 34 beds. However, within several years, the
number quadrupled: Around the middle of the century then, the
situation had changed radically and Edinburgh was provided with
the hospital infrastructure necessary for a clinical medicine based on a
relatively large number of patients. Indeed, the link with the model of
the Boerhaavian clinic was broken. From 1750 there was a regular
increase in the number of beds assigned to the clinic: 10 beds in 1750,
15 in 1751, 20 in 1752, 29 in 1757. The clinic's beds remained at about
this level for the remainder of the century. The general hospital population of the Royal Infirmary (which had a 228-bed capacity in 1748)
grew regularly in the second half of the eighteenth century: more

80   P. Huard and M. J. Imbault-Huart, 'Concepts et réalités de l'éducation et de la
profession médico-chirurgicale pendant la Révolution', *Journal des Savants* (April–
June, 1973): 136, n. 25.
81   T. Gelfand, 'The Hospice of the Paris College of Surgery (1774–1793), a Unique
and Invaluable Institution', *Bulletin of the History of Medicine* 47 (1973): 375.

than 110 patients in 1758, more than 120 in 1768 and approximately 200 from 1775 onwards.[82] For purposes of comparison, let us consider the Parisian Hôpital de la Charité (where Corvisart's clinic was to be installed), which in 1788 had not more than a 208-bed capacity. In the first years of the nineteenth century, it contained not more than 230 patients. At the same time, the Edinburgh Royal Infirmary had 250 patients. Such an infirmary was certainly big enough to carry on clinical research. Remember that it was in a hospital (Necker) of only a 136-bed capacity that Laennec produced his fundamental work in clinical diagnosis.

At Edinburgh as at Vienna, bedside instruction was not given only in the clinical wards. Other wards were used for instruction and hospital physicians other than professors gave clinical instruction. As A. L. Turner wrote, 'While instruction in medicine at the bedside, *as originally practised in the ordinary wards, continued to be conducted by physicians attending in rotation*, teaching the clinical lectures remained for many years in the hands of the professors to whom the special wards were assigned for that purpose.'[83]

Similarly, as Turner has noted, practical teaching in surgery was given both by the 'surgeons in ordinary' and by the 'professors of the university'.[84] In his comparative study of European hospitals, Flajani gave a description of the system in operation at Edinburgh from the beginning in which the different parts of the hospital served practical teaching purposes. According to Flajani, the ordinary physicians of the Edinburgh Royal Infirmary 'visit their patients every day at noon and, like the clinical professors, keep a daily journal in order that the *students admitted to these visits* may read it'.[85] Moreover, like the clinical professors, the ordinary professors received an annual fee of three guineas from each student.[86]

It was not only in Great Britain but also in other European countries that, in the last decades of the eighteenth century, the field of clinical research and training (in medicine, surgery etc.) was extended to the entire hospital and ceased being restricted to a small ward with a few beds. Hence, we also learn from Flajani that there were no separate wards for teaching at Berlin. All patients in the hospital (the Charité), which had a 700-bed capacity (1,000 beds at the end of the eighteenth century), were considered research and training material. Here, then,

82 Turner, *Story of a Great Hospital*, pp. 134–49.
83 Ibid., p. 138. My emphasis.
84 Ibid., p. 142.
85 Odier, *Extraits*, p. 91.
86 Ibid.

was a large-scale clinic.[87] Note that before the inauguration of Berlin University in 1810, the Charité was a non-academic hospital.

According to Gauthier's history of the clinic, medical practice in Copenhagen was analogous to that in Berlin. In 1758, King Frederick V had established a large hospital in the capital. From the beginning, clinical training was undertaken throughout the hospital. The first physician and not a faculty professor was charged with training the students, maintaining the journal of observations, and doing the autopsies. As Gauthier notes, Bang, the first physician, published in 1789 a work entitled *Praxis medica*, 'which is based on observations collected over a period of many years of practice and of which the number of patients' stands at more than twenty thousand'.[88] Can this be pre-Boerhaavian or Boerhaavian bedside medicine? Furthermore, in 1761 a maternity clinic was created in Copenhagen, and this establishment was presented as a model by the physician J. B. Demangeon in a book published in Paris in year VII (1799) entitled *Tableau historique d'un triple établissement réuni en un seul hospice à Copenhague*.

In eighteenth-century Italy one finds – varying according to city and hospital – sometimes one, sometimes the other, sometimes both

87 Flajani, *Saggio*, pp. 14, 83. For other hospitals and clinics in Germany in the second half of the eighteenth century, see Flajani, p. 15: Tübingen, Halle, Erlangen, Würzburg, Kiel, Marburg, Bamberg, etc. See also D. Jetter, 'Die ersten Universitätskliniken Westdeutscher Staaten', *Deutsche medizinische Wochenschrift* 87 (1962): 2037–42. For Berlin, see A. Imhof, 'Hospital in the 18th Century': 'Stimulated by the famous clinic of H. Boerhaave (1668–1738) in Leiden, Joh. Th. Eller (1698–1760) built the Charité-Hospital into the *largest* clinic in Germany'; p. 458. My emphasis. For the relations between cameralist health policy, the development of the hospital system and the beginnings of clinical institutions, see Jetter, *Geschichte des Hospitals: Westdeutschland von den Anfängen bis 1850*, 5 vols. (1966), I, 93–182. See also Keel, 'Cabanis', chap. 9. Cf. E. Heischkel, 'Medizinischer Unterricht im 17 und 18. Jahrhundert', *Deutsche Medizinische Rundschau* 3 (1949): 292–6; Heischkel, 'Die Poliklinik des 18. Jahrhunderts im Deutschland', *Deutsche Medizinische Journal* 5 (1954): 223–5. Imhof describes the Berlin Charité Hospital in the years 1731–42 as follows: 'The Charité Hospital was *at the same time* a military hospital, a hospital for poor sick people, and a hospital for the aged and the infirm with a *capacity of 400 beds; it was simultaneously a clinical training center.*' 'Hospital in the 18th Century', p. 451. Here too the hospital provided many services simultaneously: military health services, medical care health services, public assistance services and pedagogical services. On the importance of Morgagni's paradigm and the practice of dissection for physicians and surgeons of the eighteenth century at the Charité Hospital see P. Diepgen and E. Heischkel, *Die Medizin an der Berliner Charité bis zur Gründung der Universität* (Berlin, 1935), pp. 50, 75. On Berlin see J. Geyer-Kordesch's essay in this volume, chap. 7. For clinical training in the German hospitals, see also Puschmann, *History of Medical Education*, trans. E. H. Hare (London, 1891). On the quantitative or statistical approach to disease of the Charité physicians, see Diepgen and Heischkel, ibid., pp. 35, 50.
88 Gauthier, *Discours préliminaire*, in Hildenbrand, *Médecine pratique*, p. XXIX. J. B. Bang (1747–1820), *Selecta diarii nosocomii Fridericiani Hafniensis* (1789).

models of clinical training, that is, either a clinical training given directly in the ordinary wards or a training given in special wards but complemented with visits to the other wards. In the large urban hospital, clinical science and training were brought to bear on the entire hospital.[89] The large hospital clinical centres are constantly invoked in the writings of Parisian physicians. Padua, Genoa, Rome, Bologna, Milan, Turin, Florence, Naples and Pavia are repeatedly cited as models. As is well known, French doctors had ample opportunity to examine the functioning of these clinical hospitals before, during and after the Italian campaigns.[90] Not surprisingly, then, in 1792 R. N. D. Desgenettes proposed the Italian hospitals as models for clinical practice in his 'Observations sur l'enseignement de la médecine dans les hôpitaux de la Toscane, lues à la Société royale de médecine de Paris dans sa séance du 15 mai 1792':

The Société Royale de Médecine has proposed as the subject of a prize the following question: determine the best means of teaching practical medicine in a hospital. It has, at the same time, invited all physicians cognizant of presently existing clinical schools to submit their observations. The programme indicates as models for the contestants the clinical schools of Leyden, Edinburgh, Vienna, Göttingen, Milan, Pavia, Erlan-

89 See A. Pazzini, *L'ospedale nei secoli* (Rome, 1958). See also L. Belloni, 'Italian Medical Education after 1600', in C. D. O'Malley (ed.), *History of Medical Education,* pp. 105–20. For the history of clinical practice in Italian hospitals, see Gauthier, *Discours préliminaire,* pp. XX–XXI, XXXIff. (Padua, Rome, Pavia, Genoa, Florence, Pisa, Sienna, Milan, Turin, Naples, Bologna). A very detailed general survey of clinics and hospitals in different Italian cities can be found in L. Valentin, *Voyage en Italie,* 1st ed. (Paris, 1826). See also Flajani, *Saggio,* pp. 1–12, 81ff, 206, 220, 239. For the Milan hospital school see P. Pecchiai, *L'ospedale maggiore di Milano . . .* (Milan, 1927); L. Belloni, *La scuola ostetrica milanese* (Milan, 1955). See also E. Coturri, 'Le scuole ospedaliere di chirurgia del granducato di Toscana (secoli XVII–XIX)', *Minerva Medica* (1958): 2072–122. There was university or university-linked clinical teaching quite early in Italy. From at least the sixteenth century, such teaching existed, notably at Padua. See L. Munster, 'Die Anfänge eines klinischen Unterrichts an der Universität Padua im 16 Jahrhundert', *Medizinische Monatsschrift* 3 (1969), and J. J. Bylebyl, 'The School of Padua: Humanistic Medicine in the Sixteenth Century', in C. Webster (ed.), *Health, Medicine and Mortality in the Sixteenth Century* (New York, 1979). In 1764 the Venetian senate established a new plan for the chair of clinical medicine (which was to be held at the hospital). G. dalla Bona was the first occupant. See Gauthier, *Discours préliminaire* n. 44, this chapter, pp. XX–XXI, XXX–XXXI. A Comparetti, *Saggio della scuola clinica nello spedale di Padua* (Padua, 1973). See also the excellent paper by J. J. Bylebyl, 'Commentary on L. Premuda, The Influence of the Nineteenth-Century Vienna School of Italian Medicine: The Roles of Padua and Trieste', in L. Stevenson (ed.), *A Celebration of Medical History* (Baltimore, 1982), pp. 200–11.

90 See Ackerknecht, *Medicine at the Paris Hospital,* p. 28: 'Italian authors were also of considerable influence . . . Many physicians, including Broussais, went to Italy with the French armies'.

gen, Genoa, about which, well known works have been published. *There also exist other institutions* which, although *perfectly well directed, are less well known;* such is the case, for example, of *the principal hospitals of Tuscany, where the different branches of the healing arts are taught in a theoretical and practical manner.*[91]

Bylebyl has shown, in an important paper, the importance of university clinical teaching in Italy, but he also quite judiciously points out that practical training was assured within a parallel framework: 'Indeed, for the leading physicians of the large cities, whether or not they also lectured on medicine, it appears that no sharp distinction was made between practice and teaching.'[92] Clearly, one must not underestimate the influence of the university clinic in Italy or elsewhere for the emergence of hospital medicine. In this respect, one need only consider the clinics at Rome, Padua, Pavia and Austrian Lombardy. Nonetheless, those hospitals with weak links or no links at all with the university constituted a vast framework that was both spatially and chronologically necessary for clinical or hospital medicine. As can be seen from the following passage from Morgagni, eighteenth-century physicians were clearly aware that the hospital generated anatomico-clinical knowledge and had since the sixteenth century:

(When I reflect) on how much greater an opportunity hospitals offer for the observation of rare diseases, but especially *of the more common ones*, the more regret I feel for the ancient physicians, who necessarily lacked this (opportunity), because hospitals were first established only shortly before the time of Justinian . . . And if from the time of their institution it had been permitted *to use hospitals to study diseases, both in living patients and through the post mortem*, one can imagine how much progress medicine would have made over the following ten centuries by considering *how much it has accomplished since around the beginning of the sixteenth century when these two modes of investigation began to be permitted.*[93]

Bylebyl adds the following commentary: 'Thus Morgagni had a clear conception of hospital research as a distinct and important historical phenomenon, *but he regarded it as an invention of the sixteenth*

91 In Bacher (ed.), *Journal de Médecine, Chirurgie et Pharmacie*, (May 1792), vol. 91, pp. 233–4. My emphasis.
92 Bylebyl, in Stevenson (ed.), *Celebration of Medical History*, p. 201.
93 Quoted in Bylebyl, ibid., p. 202. My emphasis. See also J. B. Morgagni, *The Seats and Causes of Diseases Investigated by Anatomy*, 3 vols., trans. B. Alexander (1769; reprint, New York, 1960), I, p. XXXI.

century rather than of the eighteenth.'[94] Summarising the clinical training conditions of physicians in Italy since the sixteenth century, Bylebyl explains:

> As part of this *broader practical orientation,* Italian physicians were, by the later part of the sixteenth century, already quite accustomed *to using hospitals as places of medical teaching and research,* both clinical and anatomical. This included not only having the students visit hospitals together, with their teachers, *both to see patients and to witness dissections,* but in some cases, young doctors would *go through a period as an assistant hospital physician* before entering into private practice.[95]

We have shown that the aforementioned hospitals, infirmaries and dispensaries did serve as models for Paris. Indeed, was it not an informal clinic at the levels of practice, research and teaching that developed in most of the non-university Parisian hospitals at the beginning of the Paris school? As has been observed, occupying a hospital post or having the responsibility for a hospital service could be more important than having a clinical chair for the large number of hospital clinicians who had no university post.

What has been said so far concerning various countries applies equally to Austria. It was not only the university clinic but, in a more general way, the new hospital structures that served as a model for Paris. In the preface to his treatise on practical medicine (*Ratio medendi in nosocomio practico Vindobonensi,* Vienna, 1779–90, 7 vols.), Stoll (1742–87) explicitly maintained that the clinical school had only a propaedeutic function and that following this training, the entire hospital was to serve both for experience and as a means of teaching. Concerning the medical reform carried out by A. Störck (1731–1803), head of the Vienna medical faculty, which began in 1774, Stoll wrote:

> This great man, born for the good of science, his country and those who govern it, has since undertaken a great number of improvements facilitating clinical study. He has transferred the hospital to a more fitting site by reuniting it with the Holy Trinity in whose locale it is contained. There, a *great throng* of patients places within the grasp and within the sight of the physician the choice of *all diseases.* The students have, in addition, the advantage that when they have learned enough from the restricted number of patients contained in the hospital clinic they can be presented with a *much larger field in which to perfect their practice. They may then be let into the large wards,*

94 Bylebyl, in Stevenson (ed.), *Celebration of Medical History.* My emphasis.
95 Ibid. My emphasis.

which daily contain all species of disease. Somewhat like new soldiers prepared by a few light skirmishes for more serious battle, these students, having studied the character of diseases on several patients, can be further *instructed by seeing a large number;* and by practising at their own expense, they form a certain practical judgement and obtain a singular faculty of discernment, indispensable qualities for whoever wishes to practise medicine with success and for which reading alone will never give.[96]

Störck's reform, by making the entire hospital domain the object of clinical training, consolidated a hospital medicine based on a large number of patients. At Vienna's Trinity Hospital the large number of patients arriving at the ambulatory services was exploited for both experience and training:

The provident care of our illustrious president has again produced resources of great importance for the acquisition of the facility needed for the exercise of this difficult art. In effect, as many individuals are afflicted with infirmities which do not render them bed-ridden, we receive them daily, at fixed hours, at a particular place in the hospital where their diseases are displayed and, ordinarily, we furnish them with medicines without charge which they use at home. *Now, as every year hundreds arrive looking for help, do not those who attend the multitude of sick-poor have an excellent opportunity to obtain complete instruction in the practice of medicine in all manner of disease?*[97]

Since 1775, and even before, medical training in Vienna was organised in terms of a large number of patients: Hospital services other than the clinic served as a field of experience for the students, and in addition, clinical training was given in these other departments:

So that there be nothing left to desire, even to the mind most desirous of knowledge, we give, in addition, in the same establishment, by order of our illustrious president, other practical lessons as a sort of complement to clinical medicine

96 M. Stoll, *Médecine pratique*, French translation by O. Mahon (with notes by Pinel, Mahon, Baudelocque) (Paris, year IX; 1801) I, pp. XXII–XXIII. My emphasis. Cited in Keel, 'Cabanis', p. 422. It should be noted that A. de Haen, like Stoll later, already had at his disposition (in addition to the clinical and the hospital beds) a large number of patients from the dispensary at the municipal hospital. See E. Lesky, 'The Development of Bedside Teaching at the Vienna Medical School', in O'Malley (ed.), *History of Medical Education*, p. 223. See also note 99.
97 Stoll, *Médecine pratique*, pp. XXIII–XXIV. My emphasis. Cited in Keel, 'Cabanis', p. 424.

independently of the fact that this part of the teaching is given every day at the public college before a large audience. The art of midwifery is demonstrated to *medical students* by Raphael Steidele, professor of surgery and a very experienced man in this respect. He begins with the help of very ingenious mannequins that he has invented for this purpose and, finishes *in a definitive manner, at the bedside of pregnant women.* Thus, those not content with theory alone and wishing to be trained in the practice of this art, have ample opportunity to do so. The same professor gives *daily instruction,* with great dexterity and distinguished talent, to *numerous students in the practice of surgery, anatomy, and surgical operations. As many cadavers as are necessary are supplied to those who particularly wish to cultivate anatomy and to practice the art of dissection.*[98]

Before the opening of the Allgemeine Krankenhaus (1784), and the Imperial Academy of Medicine and Surgery in 1785, there was only one official or university clinical school.[99] However, varied services in the different hospitals constituted the framework for a medical practice that it would be difficult to qualify as Boerhaavian bedside medicine. This practice would be more aptly termed first-stage hospital medicine,[100] the second stage being the more systematised hospital medicine in the years following 1815 in Paris and elsewhere.

The hospital services formed the framework for a type of medical observation that scanned a large number of patients: In effect, these

---

98 Stoll, pp. XXIV–XXV. My emphasis. Cited in Keel, 'Cabanis'. In 1774, within the framework of A. Störck's reforms, an extraordinary chair of surgery was created at Vienna and conferred on R. J. Steidele (1737–1823), surgeon and obstetrician. Steidele was to teach surgeons and midwives and to maintain a surgical clinic for the former at Trinity Hospital. See Keel, 'Cabanis', pp. 425, 462. See, also Lesky, *Osterreichisches Gesundheitswesen,* pp. 85, 208.

99 This university clinical school based at Trinity Hospital was built upon two chairs: clinical medicine and clinical surgery (1754), which began in the municipal hospital and was transferred to the Trinity Hospital in 1776, and clinical surgery, founded in 1774 and based from the beginning at Trinity Hospital. See Keel, 'Cabanis', pp. 425ff.

100 For these points and those that follow see Keel, 'Cabanis'. See also E. Lesky, 'L. Auenbrugger, Schüler Van Swietens', *Deutsche Medizinische Wochenschrift* 84 (1959): 1017–22, and Lesky, in O'Malley (ed.), *History of Medical Education,* pp. 217–34, and *Die Wiener medizinische Schule im 19. Jahrhundert* (Graz-Cologne, 1965), as well as Lesky's numerous other major studies on Viennese and Austrian medicine of the eighteenth and nineteenth centuries. See also R. A. Kondratas, 'Joseph Frank (1771–1842) and the Development of Clinical Medicine' (PhD thesis, Harvard University, 1977). It should be noted that one of the elements of Störck's reform, *Instituta facultatis medicae Vindobonensis* (Vienna, 1775), pp. 39ff, gave students in surgery the possibility of *completing their clinical training through surgical practice in the Viennese hospitals.* Cf. Keel, 'Cabanis' p. 425, and Lesky, *Osterreichisches Gesundheitswesen,* p. 84.

hospitals received, on average, between 150 and 300 patients. Here discoveries such as Auenbrugger's percussion, which presupposed the examination, physical diagnosis and dissection of a significant number of patients, were possible. Klemperer wrote in this respect:

The discovery of this new method depended of course on the positivistic principle of localizing disease in organ alterations and Auenbrugger was inspired by this idea. Vienna of the 18th century with the Boerhaave disciples Van Swieten and de Haen in *full charge of all medical affairs gave every opportunity to the performance of autopsies and they were done in well administered hospitals where full-time physicians attended to their duties which included necropsies. This organization of hospitals was an important factor contributory to the advancement of clinical-anatomic investigations, a point stressed by Morgagni* in his letter to Scheiber.[101]

In Viennese hospitals, the first statistical analyses (de Haen, Stoll), the first hospital therapeutic experiments, the generalisation of the practice of dissection (again, in large numbers) – in short, the emergence of an anatomico-clinical medicine – were possible.[102] Rayer wrote in this respect: 'Van Swieten had established hospitals in Vienna where this science [pathological anatomy] was cultivated with as much ardour as the price of its study was valued.'[103] Rayer continued:

Diseases which present both vital and sensible organic lesions are singularly enlightened by pathological anatomy. This science confirmed and often rectified clinical observations, changed presumptions into certitudes, focused, in an irrevocable way, the mind of the physician on the site of the disease. Antoine de Haen rendered incontestable these truths in his learned lessons *Ratio medendi in nosocomio practico* (Vindobon., 1756–1773) destined to enlighten certain aspects of the history and treatment of disease. This example has been followed illustriously by Störck, Collin, Stoll, his followers.[104]

These tendencies were, of course, accentuated with the creation of the Allgemeine Krankenhaus where medical observation focused on an even larger hospital population.[105] On its opening in 1784, the large Viennese general hospital contained 2,000 beds, and all the

101 Klemperer's introduction to the facsimile ed. of Morgagni, *Seats and Causes of Diseases*, p. VII. My emphasis.
102 See Keel, 'Cabanis', chaps 5–6, 8–11. See also E. Lesky, 'L. Auenbrugger, Schüler van Swietens'. For the anatomico-clinical approach of the first Vienna school, see E. R. Long, *A History of Pathology* (London, 1928), pp. 102ff.
103 *Sommaire*, p. 86.
104 Ibid., p. 91. See also Entralgo, *La historia clínica*, pp. 207–19.
105 See Keel, 'Cabanis', chap. 9.

hospital services were used from the beginning for clinical research and training even though there was founded within the hospital itself a university clinical school with a restricted number of beds.[106] In 1817, in the article 'Hôpital' in the *Dictionnaire des sciences médicales*, Coste again proposed the Viennese institution as a model for France: 'The general hospital at Vienna . . . is far too similar to what has been hoped for and what has not been completely executed in France, for the many advantages joined in its position, construction and well organised divisions not to have determined my choice in its favour.'[107]

This is how clinical training functioned when Coste, accompanying the Napoleonic armies, visited the hospital in 1805 after the victory at Austerlitz:

The art of healing is taught in a theoretical and a practical manner at this hospital; one of the pavilions in the first quadrangle has been given over to the school for dissections; it is in the *wards themselves that the professors show the students the observations to be collected according to the nature of the disease. In serious or extraordinary cases as well as during major operations, all the professors and practitioners are on hand to give advice and the students profit greatly from these occasions for their own instruction. Independently of this resource common to all parts of the hospital, there are, at the centre of the great quadrangle, special wards given over to the clinics.*[108]

In addition to the general hospital, Emperor Joseph II had created the Imperial Academy of Medicine and Surgery for the training of military physicians and surgeons. Founded in 1785, at the instigation of the king's first surgeon, the Italian Brambilla, this institution was to

---

106   See Keel, ibid. See also, E. Lesky, 'Das Wiener allgemeine Krankenhaus, seine Gründung und Wirkung auf Deutsche Spitäler', *Clio Medica* 2 (1967): 23–37, and 'Johann Peter Frank als Organisator des medizinischen Unterrichts', *Sudhoffs Archiv für Geschichte der Medizin und der Naturwissenschaften*, 39 (1955): 1–29. When the Viennese general hospital opened in 1784, the university practical school contained twelve beds corresponding to the chair of internal medicine held by Stoll and another room with twelve beds corresponding to the chair of surgery held by Steidele. See D. Jetter, *Geschichte des Hospitals. Wien von den Anfängen bis um 1900*, 5 vols. (Wiesbaden, 1982), V, p. 52. To this might be added the obstetrical service, which served as a clinical school for the chair in obstetrics. Beginning with J. P. Frank's (1745–1821) arrival in Vienna in 1795, the number of beds for the medical clinic rose to twenty-four and those for the surgical clinic to forty. See Keel, 'Cabanis' p. 434, and Lesky, 'Johann Peter Frank', pp. 20ff.
107   Coste, in Alard et al., *Dictionnaire*, p. 423, '*Motifs de la préférence donnée aux exemples pris chez l'étranger*'.
108   Ibid., p. 472, my emphasis. See also Lesky, *Die Wiener Medizinische Schule*, pp. 52ff.

promote the unification of medicine and surgery. The Academy was placed beside the large Gumpendorf military hospital, which had a 1,200-bed capacity. Parallel with the training given at the general hospital, the establishment provided complete medical and surgical training that was as practical as it was theoretical. Here again, within a non-university framework, clinical research and training were carried out on a large number of patients. Such would be the case in Paris before, during and after the Revolution. Nevertheless, in Vienna both an internal and an external clinic were already established at the Gumpendorf military hospital in 1781 even before the opening of the Academy.[109]

In 1784 the general hospital at Vienna officially opened its obstetrical clinic. It is important to note that at the maternity, clinical training dealt with all patients. In other words, the maternity was already constituted as a large clinic replete with internships.[110] Johann Boër (1751–1835), the clinician in charge of the maternity, dissected the bodies of women who died during childbirth and every year published the establishment's mortality statistics. These statistics were calculated year after year and their abundance helped Semmelweis make his famous discovery.[111]

The Viennese hospital structures, like those in other European countries, offered a model to be followed presenting as they did health care units of a significant size and hospital services specialised according to the type of ailment (internal, external, chronic, acute, etc.). This differentiation of services favoured the institution of specialised clinics. Thus, as early as 1812 a specialised ophthalmological clinic was opened at the Vienna General Hospital by Professor Beer.[112] The already quite specialised hospital services presented homogeneous material and offered a serial analysis of different cases, which favoured a 'statistical' approach to diagnosis and treatment. Moreover, as dissection was practised systematically at the Viennese hospitals even before the opening of the General Hospital, the existence of differentiated health care structures, on the one hand, and dissection centres, on the other, made possible an anatomico-clinical

109   See Keel, 'Cabanis', chap. 9, pp. 435ff.
110   See Keel, ibid., and Lesky, *Wiener Medizinische Schule*, pp. 72–8ff.
111   See Keel, 'Cabanis', chap. 11, pp. 564ff, and Lesky, *Wiener Medizinische Schule*, p. 211.
112   See Keel, 'Cabanis', p. 613, and Lesky, *Wiener Medizinische Schule*, pp. 79–86. Lesky shows that Beer's Viennese ophthalmological clinic served as a model for all countries. Many future foreign professors of clinical opthalmology were trained here. See ibid., p. 82.

246 *Othmar Keel*

approach based on the analysis of numbered frequencies.[113] In addition, the existence since 1796 of centralised dissection rooms at the General Hospital, where more than 600 autopsies were performed annually, permitted the comparative analysis of different types of pathological formations.[114] The institution of the specialised function of prosector also contributed to the development of pathological anatomy.[115] It is hardly surprising that in these conditions, one of the first specialised works in pathological anatomy appeared in Vienna in 1803: Aloys Vetter's (1765–1806) treatise.[116]

IV

Even in France, contrary to what is ordinarily thought, hospital medicine was not 'born' with the institution of a kind of academic clinical teaching (for example, the three well-known *écoles de santé* instituted by the law of Frimaire, 1794: Paris, Montpellier, Strasbourg). The clinical schools appeared after the hospital had already become, albeit partially and in unequal ways, the new framework of medical practice, research and training. The demands of practice and research within the framework of hospital medicine forced the instauration of institutionalised, but not necessarily official, modalities for the transmission of knowledge. As Huard has recalled: 'The teaching created by Desbois de Rochefort [predecessor and "patron" of Corvisart] at the Charité hospital was the result of *private initiative*, outside the framework of *official teaching*.'[117] In France, therefore, an essential part of clinical training took place outside the official university

113 'Cabanis', chaps. 5, 9, 11, and Lesky, 'Development of Bedside Teaching', pp. 224ff. Lesky writes: 'Moreover, we must not forget that when, in 1790, Vicq d'Azyr (*Nouveau plan de constitution pour la médecine en France*, Paris, 1790), suggested that clinical instruction should be instituted at Parisian hospitals, he confessed to having been impressed by the model of Vienna, and especially, that of Pavia, which we know was patterned after Vienna.' See also Lesky, 'Die pathologische Anatomie in Wien vor Rokitansky', in *Carl von Rokitansky, Selbstbiographie und Antrittsrede* (Vienna, 1960), pp. 21–2, and 'Leopold Auenbrugger, Schüler van Swietens', See also T. Vetter, 'A. R. Vetter (1765–1806): Un pionnier de l'émancipation anatomo-pathologique', *Clio Medica* 3 (1968): 'Following its founding by van Swieten (the Vienna School), de Haen, Störck, and Stoll accorded particular attention to organic lesions'; p. 225.
114 See Keel, 'Cabanis', pp. 432ff, and pp. 612ff; Lesky, *Wiener Medizinische Schule*, pp. 97ff.
115 Keel, 'Cabanis'. See also Lesky, 'Die pathologische Anatomie', pp. 22ff.
116 *Aphorismen aus des pathologischen Anatomie*. 'Vetter is, without doubt, the only person in Europe who, at 36 years of age, had performed thousands of autopsies' in T. Vetter, 'A. R. Vetter (1765–1806)', pp. 225, 230. One might compare Vetter with Hunter, Baillie, Soemmering, Bichat, Dupuytren and others.
117 Huard, in Taton (ed.), *Enseignement et diffusion des sciences*, p. 182.

framework. It should be recalled, moreover, that practical or clinical training, not only in surgery but also in medicine, was under way not only in civil hospitals but also in the marine and military hospitals, which played an important role in this respect before the Revolution.

In his *Observations sur les hôpitaux*, P. Cabanis points out that his mentor, J. B. Léon Dubreuil (1748–83), 'had founded several years before his death . . . a practical school in the marine hospital at Brest'.[118] Dubreuil was also involved in founding of the clinical school in the marine hospital at Toulon. And in the *Coup d'oeil sur les révolutions et les réformes de la médecine*, Cabanis intimates that, before the Revolution, Dubreuil's initiatives were supported by the government through Maréchal de Castries, the minister of the navy:

> I described in the same book (*Observations sur les hôpitaux*) the attempts made by my dear mentor, the virtuous Dubreuil, under the auspices of the Maréchal de Castries, then minister of the navy. I recalled that the two clinical schools at Brest and at Toulon were the fruit of these attempts and that the services they provided furnished me the proof of the justice of the views that guided their formation.[119]

As Delaunay more generally states: 'The clinical instruction that the faculties so parsimoniously dispensed to their students, seems to have been much more developed in the nosocomial military milieu even though surgical instruction naturally predominated.'[120] Delaunay notes that before the creation of the specialised military health service, the surgeons major were forced to give a yearly course in anatomy and surgical operations. Starting with the reform announced in the code of 1 January 1747, the physicians gave yearly medical courses in the military hospitals.[121] The regulations of 22 December 1775 added hospital-amphitheatres (at Lille, Metz and Strasbourg) for instruction to the aforementioned courses and stipulated in article XIII that 'each year of study must include a practical and clinical course on the prevalent diseases of the troops in the army and in the garrison'.[122] The students had to attend not only the medical and pharmacy courses but also the surgery courses. We are here, it might be noted, on the road to the unification of the different branches of the healing arts. The

118 C. Lehec and J. Cazeneuve (eds.), *Oeuvres philosophiques*, 2 vols. (Paris, 1956), I, p. 24.
119 Ibid., II, p. 219.
120 P. Delaunay, *La vie médicale aux XVIe, XVIIe et XVIIIe siècles* (Paris, 1935), p. 84.
121 Delaunay, ibid.. With regard to clinical practice in military milieux before the Revolution, see D. Vess, *Medical Revolution in France, 1789–1796* (Gainesville, Fla., 1975), pp. 25ff, and Imbault-Huart, *L'école pratique de dissection de Paris*, pp. 121ff.
122 Delaunay, *La vie médicale*, and Vess, *Medical Revolution in France*, p. 27.

first physician taught practical medicine; the second physician taught theoretical medicine and physiology.[123] The amphitheatres were abolished in 1780, but were re-established on 2 May 1781 with the addition of two more at Brest and Toulon. In 1788 they received the title of auxiliary hospitals. The teaching was placed under the supervision of the physician-inspectors of the departments.[124]

As regards the civil hospitals, the following facts should demonstrate that teaching was under way before the Revolution and independently of the Faculty of Medicine. 'As of 1774 [writes Imbault-Huart in connection with the École Pratique], the *Collège de Chirurgie* had its *Hospice de Perfectionnement* where it dispensed clinical instruction. It went from 10 beds in 1774 to 30 beds in 1783.'[125] There is no need to recall that at this point, the Collège de Chirurgie was independent of the Faculté de Médecine. L. Desbois de Rochefort (1750–86) began medical clinical instruction at the Charité in 1780 and was succeeded by Corvisart, who had been his assistant, in 1786. Similarly, starting in 1787 Desault instituted clinical surgical instruction at the Hôtel-Dieu: He had began this course of instruction in 1783 while he was still at the Charité. M. Wiriot has consequently written of the innovations in clinical training during the Revolution:

> Of the three clinical courses provided for, two existed already: the course of clinical medicine at the Charité, then called Hospice de l'Unité, where Corvisart had taken over from Desbois de Rochefort, and the course in clinical surgery at the large Hospice d'Humanité (i.e. Hôtel-Dieu) run by Desault. *What existed was not changed; a state of fact was made official:* Corvisart and Desault were named, respectively, professors of internal and external medicine.[126]

It should be stressed that it was about ten years before the hospital reforms of the Revolution and thus before the opening of the Paris Clinical School (1794) that Corvisart began, following Auenbrugger

123 Delaunay, ibid., p. 85.
124 Ibid.
125 Imbault-Huart, *L'école pratique de dissection de Paris*, p. 121; Huard and Imbault-Huart, in Huard and Imbault-Huart, eds., pp. 109–24. See also Gelfand, 'Hospice of the Paris College'.
126 *L'enseignement clinique dans les hôpitaux de Paris entre 1794 et 1848* (Paris, 1970), p. 31. My emphasis. See also C. Coury, *L'enseignement de la médecine en France des origines à nos jours* (Paris, 1968): 'The last 20 years of the 18th century were marked by the considerable development of hospital clinical teaching and its new orientation. *Inspired by foreign examples*, audacious precursors *outdistanced the official reforms by fifteen years.* This period no longer belonged to an outdated system: through anticipation, it inaugurated the renewed teaching of the beginning of the XIXth century'; p. 105. My emphasis.

and Stoll, to apply percussion and to teach physical diagnosis at the hospital. Hence, the *ancien régime* hospitals were able to provide the possibility of combining, as did Corvisart, the anatomico-clinical approach of the physicians (Morgagni, Auenbrugger, Stoll, etc.) with the 'surgical' localist approach to disease of surgeons like Desault (one of Corvisart's teachers) or of the Hunterian school.

As of the second half of the eighteenth century, and sometimes before, the hospital had become the centre of surgeons' practice and training and, to a lesser degree, the same may be said for physicians. From about 1720, the Hôtel-Dieu was already sufficiently 'medicalised' if we take medicalisation to mean the increase of medical personnel at the hospital and not the stringent purification of the hospital institution in the sense that the religious framework was replaced by a medical regime, which was surely not the case. Since 1720, in effect, there were positions for 100 surgeons: 74 *externes*, 12 surgeon *commissionnaires*, and 12 aides or *internes*. At the head of the corps was the *gagnant-maîtrise*, who obtained his *maîtrise* following six years of hospital service, and a head-surgeon who was a master of the Collège de Chirurgie.[127]

Surgeons could therefore work and learn at the hospital or within a clinical climate more than the medical students. It is not surprising, then, that in his plan for the constitution of French medicine, Vicq d'Azyr proposed the surgeon's hospital training as one of the models for the reform of medical education:

It would be easy to admit students as interns into the hospital, give them room and board, without any new expense or the addition of any new buildings. At the same time, instruction would be facilitated. In the practical sciences, one cannot learn if one does not participate. Now, the students admitted to the hospitals would participate in the treatment of the patients; they would care for them, they would live among them. This resource, already available to surgery, should be made available to the other branches of medicine . . . as Chambon and Doublet have proposed in their papers on this subject read before the Société de Médecine.[128]

Drawing support from these sorts of facts, Gelfand has argued that

127 C. Coury, *L'Hôtel-Dieu de Paris. Treize siècles de soins, d'enseignement et de recherche* (Paris, 1969), pp. 75ff. See also Coury, *L'enseignement de la médecine*, p. 104; M. Fosseyeux, *L'Hôtel-Dieu de Paris au XVIIe et au XVIIIe siècles* (Paris, 1912), pp. 400ff.
128 *Plan de constitution pour la médecine en France*, p. 63. Cited in Gelfand, 'Gestation of the Clinic', p. 77.

the gestation of the clinic took place not within academic medicine but within the (Parisian) profession of surgery.[129] In fact, in his haste to assure the Parisian surgeons a primary role in the 'gestation' of the clinic, Gelfand has ignored the contribution of British medical institutions and practitioners, particularly the surgeons (not to mention surgeons of other countries, e.g., Italy, Germany, the Netherlands and Spain). In a recent book review, for example (see his review of Keel, *La généalogie de l'histopathologie* [Paris, 1979] in *Annals of Science*, 38 [1981]: 248–9), he maintained that in the period under consideration, there was no 'medical [clinical] efflorescence in Britain' and that 'London itself had only a few teaching hospitals'. It should be noted, however, that in the present volume, Gelfand has since examined the English scene and now claims that 'London emerged as the world centre for clinical learning during the second half of the eighteenth century . . . ultimately eclipsing [its] neighbors across the Channel'!

In any event, there are difficulties. It is not true that medical students in France had no possibility of attending the hospitals. Of course (as Vicq d'Azyr remarked), there were no interns in medicine as there were in surgery. Nonetheless, there was practical training in medicine in the hospitals.[130] As Delaunay has written:

> Only students with 'licence' had to follow rounds in the hospital. However, the hospitals were more accessible than we have been led to believe: Jean Verdier's reports (he attended the clinic at the Charité in 1756), those of the Alsatian Dolde (1748) and the Swede, Thurnberg, who attended the Hôtel-Dieu and the Charité during their stay in Paris, teach us that there were not only surgery students in the hospitals.[131]

129 Gelfand, ibid., p. 177.
130 See Coury, *L'enseignement de la médecine*, part I, chap. VI, p. 103: 'Although, totally independent of the Faculties, at the level of administration, the hospitals usually recruited their doctors from amongst the regent physicians. Nonetheless, *the hospitals in the large urban centers were important centers of professional training*, and were reserved, in fact, for the physicians or surgeons working within the establishment; the latter constituted, to a certain extent, *their own school* which functioned according to the modalities of a restricted corporation'. (My emphasis).
131 Delaunay, *La vie médicale*, p. 83. See also, Coury, *L'enseignement de la médecine*, p. 73: 'The students were not obliged to undergo any training period or any exercise; at most, some Faculties forced future practitioners to submit to practical training at the hospital or with a local practitioner. This was the case in Montpellier since the 13th century and in Paris since the 14th century where certain masters were already supervising their students' clinical training . . . Several worthwhile attempts were made using the examples of Leiden, Edinburgh and Vienna. In 1729, the Strasbourg Faculty organised *genuine clinical medicine teaching at the hospital*. Students in Aix-en-Provence had been able to attend *lessons in clinical medicine at the Saint-Jacques Hospital* since the 17th century; those in Avignon obtained *the same facilities at the Sainte-Marthe Hospital* in the middle of the 18th century. At Angers, in 1718, under the impetus of Dean Pierre Hunaud II (1664–1728), the *Saint-Jean*

Already in the first half of the eighteenth century, the *Délibérations de l'Hôtel-Dieu* (31 August 1729, 4 April 1740) noted the presence of medical students, a presence made known by conflicts with surgical students. As Delaunay has also noted, 'The archives of the "Hôtel-Dieu" are full of complaints by the sisters about the disorder caused by the presence of the young folks in the patients' rooms.'[132] It may

Hospital became a veritable annex of the Faculty. In 1760, the Montpellier hospital, Saint-Eloi, was able to accept twenty students in its clinical service. At the end of the 18th century in Paris, large numbers of students attended the Hôtel-Dieu and the Charité, *less through university obligation than to freely follow the teachings of such well known hospital workers as Desbois de Rochefort or Desault'* (my emphasis). See also, 'Extrait des Archives de l'Assistance publique, communication', cited by A. Laboulbène, *L'hôpital de la Charité de Paris 1606–1878* (Paris, 1878), p. 27: 'The last century saw Baron, Fontaine, Le Hoc, Belleteste, Bourdelin, and Majault at the Hôtel-Dieu and Verdelet, Malvet, Macquard, Thierry de Bussy and Desbois de Rochefort at the Charité *give clinical lessons* to a restricted number of students, it is true, but chosen by the head of the service himself from the student body.' My emphasis. See also Coury, *L'Hôtel-Dieu de Paris*, p. 95, and 88ff. For the medical clinic in eighteenth-century France, Imbault-Huart, *L'école pratique de dissection de Paris*, 1973, pp. 109ff.

132 Delaunay, *La vie médicale*, p. 82. See also Delaunay, *Le monde médical parisien au dix-huitième siècle* (Paris, 1906), pp. 21ff, and 'Délibérations de l'ancien bureau de l'hôtel-Dieu', in L. Brièle (ed.), *Collection de documents pour servir à l'histoire des hôpitaux de Paris*, 2 vols. (Paris, 1881–3), II, p. 8. Brièle also discusses the presence of faculty physicians. The minutes of the hospital for 1781 provide an idea of how the medical business functioned. The minutes contain a text signed by nine physicians that points out that all departments were visited twice daily and that 'what is more, it is worthwhile observing that from six until noon there is always a physician on hand at the Hôtel-Dieu ready to present himself where needed (which is not an infrequent occurrence)'; p. 102. The minutes of 1788 indicate that the physicians occupied an important position as regards the handling of the patients. The Bureau asked the physicians' opinion on (1) the displacement of the patients, (2) how to assure the filling of patients' food prescriptions, (3) how to assure that the light meals given to patients were given in different rooms, (4) how to dilute the wine, (5) the changing of pregnant women's diets, (6) other changes of diet, (7) the reduction of the costs of drugs, (8) whether or not a third priest was need, and (9) how to get rid of incurables. See also *Professionalizing Modern Medicine*, pp. 100ff, and 'Gestation of the Clinic', pp. 173ff. Gelfand tends unduly to minimise the importance of the hospital as the site of clinical research and training for physicians as opposed to surgeons. It is true that in hospitals or infirmaries, surgeons could be more numerous and somewhat more permanent than physicians, but this does not imply that the physicians' hospital practice and training were negligible elements in the constitution of the clinical *problématique*. So much the more, since the latter permitted medicine and surgery to interact within the hospital framework. In addition, the other categories of hospital personnel – the apothecaries, the obstetricians, the 'nursing' staff – should not be forgotten as, like the surgeons, they too formed a permanent presence at the hospital. Even with the sometimes conflictual relations created by their presence, the different categories of hospital personnel, through their interaction, were constitutive of a clinical experience that was in no way reducible to surgical practice. Gelfand, in 'A Clinical Ideal: Paris 1789', *Bulletin of the History of Medicine* 5 (1977): 397–411, grants a reduced role to physicians like Chambon de Montaux in the constitution of the clinic's institutional space just before the Revolution, but goes on to reiterate that in his judgement, the clinical training of physicians did not exist in the eighteenth century. This judgement is not

be said that medical students were merely tolerated at the time. So they were. And so they remained for a long time. The growth of medical operatives within the hospitals never came about without resistance from the traditional authorities (religious subalterns, administrators) who controlled and directed the institutions. The surgeons themselves were confronted with resistance before, during and after the Revolution.

Outside Paris, in Caen, Montpellier, Strasbourg, Lyon and elsewhere, clinical training in medicine and not only surgery was well under way in the hospitals long before the Revolution.[133]

only inadequate as regards France, but worse still, it is extended to all of Europe: 'One must remember that hospital lessons of any kind were an innovation for French medical education in 1789. Intensive clinical residence training did not yet exist anywhere in Europe for physicians.' (p. 411). See also nn. 86, 88, 125, 129, 130, and 133 in the present volume.

133 *Delaunay, La vie médicale*, p. 83. See also n. 130. See also Imbault-Huart, *L'école pratique de dissection de Paris*, pp. 121ff. For Lyon, See J. P. Pointe, *Histoire topographique et médicale du Grand Hôtel-Dieu de Lyon* (Lyon, 1842), p. 345: '. . . although principally created as a work of charity, *always and in all countries, the large hospitals were, more or less, generally, used for teaching*, and in this respect as in others, the Lyon Hôtel-Dieu seems to have been the first to undertake this task'; p. 345. My emphasis. Pointe is referring to both medical and surgical training. See, by the same author, *Notice historique sur les médecins du Grand Hôtel-Dieu de Lyon* (Lyon, 1825): 'J. E. Gilibert, the Montpellier physician, became the hospital physician in 1734 . . . The care with which he ran his service *attracted a large number of students; this school trained many physicians* who, today, are so justly celebrated'; p. 36, my emphasis. See also pp. 45ff. Vicq d'Azyr (*Plan de Constitution*, p. 7) recognised that the medical system of the Old Regime had, all the same, permitted the training of good physicians although he thought the system could be improved: 'We do not deny the existence of some Faculties where diverse material is usefully and faithfully taught; there is no doubt that in spite of the corruption of some schools and the futility of others, *great physicians are trained*, but it is also beyond doubt that, within an improved scheme of things, a much greater number could be trained'. My emphasis. Moreover, Vicq d'Azyr admitted that hospitals could serve as a framework for training and research (in fact, they often already did). He merely pointed out that the teaching in the hospitals was not *public* and that it must be so, not only for medicine but *also for surgery*: 'In the largest hospitals, a *more specific* teaching should be authorised in the diverse departments . . . In these hospitals, there would be space for the maintenance of a certain number of students to whom the physicians and surgeons of these hospitals would give different courses of instruction. It would be sufficient to add a minor annual bonus to *the fees the physicians and surgeons already receive*. They would also receive a minor contribution on behalf of the students who would be given room and board . . . Notice, in this respect, that in the provinces, it is not a lack of hospitals for teaching that is at issue, but a lack of teaching in the hospitals. In practically all of the hospitals, there are *positions for students, paid health officers, a pharmacy, a herbal garden, and all the facilities needed for the pursuit of anatomy, surgery and instructive autopsies*. We have only to put these facilities to work' (p. 66, my emphasis). As Vicq d'Azyr previously noted, France did not lack physicians who often had hospital positions and who would have been able, with all the needed competence, to assume the function of *public* professors of practical medicine: 'It cannot be objected that the provinces lack the men necessary for such establishments: *The Société de médecine* is hardly ignorant of *all those* who would fulfil these functions with success. In addition to the savant professors of the

Clinical training was also given to medical students (as for surgical students) in other European countries. In Vienna, for example, even before Van Swieten's reforms (1754), students at a certain level were treated as *famuli* (interns or clinical clerks) at Trinity Hospital, where they assumed daily and nightly handling of the patients under the direction of the hospital physicians.[134] Posts for students in the hospitals had only loose connections with the university before Van Swieten's reforms:[135] It was therefore not so much a question of academic medicine though it was nonetheless within the field of medicine (as much as within the field of surgery) that the hospital became the centre of practice, training and clinical experience. Beginning with Van Swieten's reforms (1754), a more organic link was established between the hospital and the university, and it was henceforth within the framework of academic medicine (a reformed academic medicine) that hospital and clinical training – not only for physicians but also for surgeons – was inscribed.[136] The situation was consolidated by later reforms in Vienna: those of Störck in 1775;[137] those accompanying the creation of the Vienna General Hospital and Joseph's Academy of Medicine and Surgery in 1785[138] and, finally, Frank's reforms, which began in 1795.[139] Therefore, two different patterns in Vienna served as a framework for the growth of clinical medicine. In the first case, the training of physicians in the hospitals was undertaken outside the framework of academic medicine and, in the second case, within the

Montpellier university of medicine, do we not have at Dijon, M. Durande; at Nîmes, MM. Razoux and Baumes; at Caen, MM. Chibourg and le Canut; at Rouen, M. le Pecq; at Coutance, M. Bonté; at Moulins, M. Baraillon; at Besançon, M. Rougnon; at Nancy, M. Jadelot; at Lille, M. Boucher; at Valence, M. Daumont; at Toulon, M. Barberet; at Brest, MM. Elie de la Poterie and Sabatier; at Chartres, M. Mahon; at Lyon, M. Rast; at Saint-Brieux, M. Bagot, and *so many others* that may be taken at random from amongst the correspondents of the *Compagnie*' (p. 64, my emphasis).
134   See Keel, 'Cabanis', pp. 301ff, and Lesky, 'Development of Bedside Teaching', p. 221ff. For the fact that the conceptual and organisational framework of late eighteenth-century medicine filled, as did that of surgery (*foreign* and French – *not only* French!), and in conjunction with the latter, an important function in the genealogy of hospital medicine, see also Keel, 'La place et la fonction', *La généalogie* and 'Cabanis'. A few recent authors have, with reason, asked for a re-examination and a reassessment of this framework as traditional historiography has inadequately explored its positivity. See, e.g., Bynum, in Rousseau and Porter (eds.), *Ferment of Knowledge*, pp. 211–52. See also Tröhler, 'Klinisch-numerische Forschung', and 'Britische Spitäler'.
135   Keel, 'Cabanis', and Lesky, *Die Wiener Medizinische Schule*.
136   Keel, 'Cabanis', and Lesky, 'Gerard van Swieten, Auftrag und Erfüllung', in E. Lesky and A. Wandruszka (eds.), *Gerard van Swieten und seine Zeit* (Vienna 1973), esp. pp. 25–6.
137   See Keel, 'Cabanis' chaps. 9, 10.
138   See Keel, ibid., chap. 9, pp. 406ff, and chap. 10, pp. 453ff.
139   See Keel, ibid., chap. 9, pp. 434ff. chap. 10, pp. 453.ff; also Lesky, 'Johann Peter Frank'.

academic framework. However, in both cases, the growth of clinical medicine occurred not only within the field of surgery, but also within the field of medicine itself.

A long time ago, Puschmann, in his *History of Medical Education*,[140] pointed out, quite rightly, the inadequacy of the contention that doctors had no hospital training before the opening of clinical schools and that their training had been theretofore bookish. As some continue to maintain that the *gestation* of the modern clinic is to be found solely within the organisational and conceptual framework of Parisian surgery and neglect the importance of foreign medicine, French medicine and *foreign surgery*, it is appropriate to quote Puschmann's century-old remarks *in extenso*. (It will be noted that these comments are entirely concordant with the thesis advanced in this essay as well as in my previous work.)[141]

At most of the other German universities only policlinical institutions were to be found. *Efforts were made in some places to induce students to visit the hospitals where they might have the opportunity of observing patients. So, too, in other countries these methods of teaching had to suffice, in the absence of clinical teaching proper, that is to say lectures at the bedside. Education in the practice of the healing art was materially benefited by the very widely-spread custom of allowing the older students and the young doctors to work as practitioners for a considerable time in a hospital, where they were, by the leading doctors, made familiar with the requirements of practice.* In France and England, where this arrangement exists to the present day, members of the medical staff of hospitals often took pupils who paid stipulated fees for the practical instruction which they received. As J. HUNCZOVSKY states, such opportunities were afforded at St. Bartholomew's Hospital in London, in the Seaman's Hospital at Portsmouth, in the Hôtel Dieu at Paris, and at Rouen. In Italy a similar custom appears to have prevailed. LANCISI, after completing his course of medical studies, entered the S. Spirito Hospital at Rome in order to prepare himself for medical practice by further practical work of *several years' duration*. He recommended students of medicine to see *numerous* patients and to *visit the hospitals*, and he advised them to spend *several years* in this mode of study. Again, at the Trinity Hospital in Vienna, a number of students of *medicine* were constantly admitted in the capacity of *practitioners*. In the town

140 Trans. E. H. Hare (London, 1891); see esp. pp. 410–18.
141 See Keel, 'Cabanis' and *La généalogie*, pp. 54ff.

hospital at Bremen also the doctors in authority gave clinical instruction to the students who took part in the visits to the patients. *There is no doubt that arrangements of this kind prevailed at many hospitals.*

The archives of many an institution must contain important information upon this subject; it would be a thank-worthy task to collect and to complete the arrangement of such material, which, as yet, especially in the case of Germany, has been but very imperfectly done. *But the facts already adduced will be found sufficient to prove that the view reiterated in works on the History of Medicine even to weariness, that before the establishment of institutions for clinical teaching young doctors relied simply upon books and theoretical lectures for their technical knowledge, is incorrect, at least as a rule of general application. The circumstance that practical instruction at the bedside generally lay outside the curriculum of university study, and was not generally sought for until after the conclusion of such study and after promotion to the degree of Doctor, must have contributed to this mistaken view.* On the other hand it may frequently have happened that young Doctors of Medicine, possessed with a high sense of their new dignity, were unconscientious and daring enough to commence practice before they had acquired the practical skill which it demands; *but the majority recognized the necessity of practical training and visited the hospitals with this object in view, as is clearly shown in the numerous biographies and writings of the distinguished doctors of that period.*[142]

It is important to dispel any ambiguity that may result from the use of such expressions as appearance, birth or emergence of clinical medicine (or hospital medicine). Most authors use the appearance of university or academic clinical teaching in the hospitals as a criterion for the birth of clinical (or hospital) medicine. As a result, they equate the birth of the clinic with the institution of clinical chairs in France (the law of the fourteenth Frimaire, Year III) during the Revolution. However, even if this criterion is admitted, it is no less inadequate to have clinical medicine begin at the end of the eighteenth century. In fact, since about 1750, and certainly since 1770, a teaching of medicine within the hospital framework and linked to the universities was already under way in different parts of Europe (e.g., Padua, Vienna, Pavia and Edinburgh). As we have seen, this clinical medicine cannot be reduced to a *médecine facultaire* or a Boerhaavian-style protoclinic.

Moreover, university or academic medicine was only one of the

142 Puschmann, *History of Medical Education*, pp. 417–18. My emphasis.

forms within which clinical medicine emerged. In my opinion, clinical medicine also emerged in hospitals that had no official university teaching. In some cases, an unofficial medical education prevailed as when hospital physicians accepted medical students or young doctors, advanced pupils, clinical clerks and others who wished to complete their training or when, on his own private initiative, a university professor who was also a hospital physician introduced his students to the hospital. In other cases, it was non-university, private teaching such as that conducted by the London physicians, surgeons and apothecaries or Desbois de Rochefort, Corvisart and Desault in France before their teaching became official in 1794. In still other cases, it was non-university public education such as that given by the Académie de Chirurgie in Paris or the Josephine Academy of Medicine and Surgery in Vienna.

The hospital and/or the institutional structures (infirmaries, dispensaries, maternity hospitals, private schools tied to these structures) served as a framework for different types of clinical training (academic/non-academic, public/private, official/free, formal/informal). What is more important is that these structures had already become training sites (clinical observation of patients, therapeutic trials) and the loci of the accumulation of medical and surgical knowledge before clinical teaching (academic) was systematically under way. In other words, this hospital-type institutional system became the site of a new form of medical experience (clinical) and an instrument for the production and accumulation of knowledge and know-how for the physicians, surgeons, apothecaries, 'obstetricians' and others of the eighteenth century before becoming the site of university teaching and reproduction of this same knowledge and know-how. The chronological gap between the first event and the second varies according to country or town. The gap is smaller in Italy, Scotland, Austria and Germany than in France or, *a fortiori*, London.

Acknowledgements

The text is based on a translation from the original French by Peter Keating. For his invaluable help, at various stages of this work, I am grateful to him. Research for this paper has been partially supported by grants from the Killam Program, Canada Council, the Social Sciences and Humanities Research Council of Canada, and the Fonds national suisse de la recherche scientifique. Information was drawn from my 'Cabanis et la généalogie de la médecine clinique' (PhD thesis, McGill University, 1977) and from two research projects in progress, 'The Emergence of Hospital Medicine in Europe (18th–19th century)' and 'John Hunter's School and Medical Institutions in England'.

PART III. ANATOMY AND PHYSIOLOGY

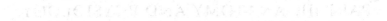

9

Vitalism in late eighteenth-century physiology: the cases of Barthez, Blumenbach and John Hunter

FRANÇOIS DUCHESNEAU

Vitalism has been taken as a general methodological stand in biological science. For vitalists, the phenomena of the living possess *sui generis* features that make them radically different from physical and chemical phenomena. Furthermore, such vital phenomena would manifest the existence and activity of a 'vital force' with specific dynamical and purposive faculties. At the beginning of our century, for instance, Hans Driesch (1867–1941) appealed to a vitalist concept of 'entelechy' to account for the regenerative processes of embryos of sea-urchins.[1] There have been many statements, especially from positivistically inclined historians and philosophers of science, stressing the sterility of vitalist principles in biological science, and more precisely in physiology. The main arguments have been as follows: (1) Resorting to vitalist principles would be no more than a verbal cover for lack of effective explanation; (2) it would hinder attempts to analyse phenomena down to their determining physico-chemical conditions; and (3) vitalist explanations would embody metaphysical accounts of purposive phenomena, unwarranted by statements of empirical laws.

As a matter of fact, such 'abstractive' strategies are seen to have culminated in the late eighteenth century, when they seemed to provide the theoretical basis for physiological investigations (even those of an observational or experimental kind). This is precisely the type of explanatory scheme that was to be found in the theories of Paul-Joseph Barthez, Johann Friedrich Blumenbach and John Hunter, the more representative 'vitalists' of that period. Their type of vitalism seems to have induced a trend towards radical antireductionism in the early nineteenth century, with the advent of various kinds of spiritualist or idealist biophilosophies, and more especially with the

---

1 See in particular, *Der Vitalismus als Geschichte und als Lehre* (Leipzig, 1905).

rise of *Naturphilosophie* in Germany. But according to the positivist methodological pattern, physiology moves away drastically from the vitalist speculations of the 1830s and 1840s. Thus, some of the major advances in nineteenth- and twentieth-century physiology might be viewed as theoretical reactions based on more rigorous empirical investigations and drawing apart from purely 'metaphysical' endeavours. Overall, the standard dual model would provide a cover for most of the radical discussions in subsequent physiological theory in a constant *va-et-vient* between vitalism and reductionism.

Happily enough, significant efforts can be traced in science itself to get away from that simplistic dual model, even amongst positivistically minded theoreticians.[2] In a more epistemological and historical perspective, I tend to feel that the connotations of 'vitalism' should be spelt into a variety of meanings according to the historical period and to the specific blend of methodological principles and ontological presuppositions involved in the historically situated theories. As an initial step towards disqualifying the dogmatic, all-encompassing, univocal meaning, I intend to establish the exact and limited meaning of 'vitalism' when used to designate Barthez's, Blumenbach's and John Hunter's respective ways of resorting to explanatory principles. In particular, my concern will be to examine the specifics of methodology connected with their so-called vitalist doctrines.[3]

I

Paul-Joseph Barthez (1734–1806) is generally considered to be a true representative of the medical traditions in force at Montpellier, where he took his medical degrees and was given a professorship in 1760. At first sight, his doctrine seems to gather elements from Stahl's animism (via Boissier de Sauvages), from Haller's theory of irritability and sensitivity as *vires insitae* in living organic structures (perhaps through Lamure and Tandon), as well as from the new doctrinal trend emphasised by Bordeu (himself trained at Montpellier) in his *Recherches anatomiques sur la position des glandes et sur leur action* (1752), and later known as organicism. I have come to the view that Barthez is not to be set in strict continuity with those influences. His physiology would not result from a combination of Stahl, Boissier, Haller and Bordeu, or from any of them specifically. On the contrary, it was

---

2 See, e.g., Claude Bernard, *Leçons sur les phénomènes de la vie commune aux animaux et aux végétaux* (Paris, 1878), pp. 46–50.
3 In the first two sections of this paper, devoted to Barthez and Blumenbach, I shall make selective use of material included in my book, *La Physiologie des Lumières. Empirisme, modèles et théorie* (The Hague, 1982).

to imply significant criticisms of those doctrines, and might be defined as a reaction to, and departure from, animism, Hallerianism
(assimilated in his views with a more general approach: solidism) and
organicism (as a kind of deviant solidism). A systematic survey of the
doctrine has to be premised for such consequences to become clear.

An initial statement is to be found in the *Oratio academica de principio
vitali hominis* (1773): It forms a short summary of the theses the *Nouveaux élémens de la science de l'homme* (1778; revised edition, 1806) developed. Between the *Oratio* and the first edition of the *Nouveaux
élémens*, the *Nova doctrina de functionibus corporis humani* (1774) sets two
objectives for adequate research. The first concerns the mechanical
use of organs. According to Lordat's summary:

> The second objective is to support a general thesis that the
> different parts of this work help demonstrate, namely that in
> all functions of the animal oeconomy, certain conditions pre-
> vent their being resolved into mere mechanical or chemical
> phenomena, as well as their being explained by simple vital
> reaction, such as conceived by solidists; but that the actions
> composing those functions are continually directed by a
> higher-order cause, which links, coordinates, adjusts them to
> an end, and induces on organs modifications needed to adapt
> them at all times [*dans tous les instants de la fonction*] to the
> actually required mode of action: such a cause should not be
> confused, following Stahl, with the thinking soul; and its way
> of acting should be expounded by converting into laws the
> general results of comparative facts.[4]

The *Nouvelle méchanique des mouvements de l'homme et des animaux*
(1798) expands the analysis on the mechanical use of parts.

The second objective, the main one for our purpose, sets up a kind
of research programme that the *Nouveaux élémens* (in both versions)
was to undertake to implement and justify. Barthez's main argument
is that functions show a specific autonomy of operation in the way
they utilise or modify structural conditions so as to maintain an adequate vital dynamism. A fundamental feature of this autonomy is the
orderly interplay of functions that can be assessed by correlating the
empirical data of physiological activities taking place under the conditions of life. An example is afforded by his analysis of sensitivity
(*sensibilité*).

Barthez opposes Haller's thesis that sensitivity is correlated with
consciousness at a *sensorium commune*, and depends upon a *machina*

4 Jacques Lordat, *Exposition de la doctrine médicale de P.-J. Barthez et mémoires sur la
vie de ce médecin* (Paris, 1818), p. 115.

nervosa connected with central receptive organs. Against Haller, one can argue from phenomena of irritation taking place in excised organs, for example viper or frog heads that have been recently removed. The irritating cause produces a functional activity analogous to that we can assign to sensitivity in the whole animal. Similar reactions must entail similar causes. There is no point in attributing irritability to a 'property concealed in the muscle fibres'; instead the action of sensitive forces should be regarded as an 'immediate cause of action for the motive forces in organs when they are solicited by irritating causes'.[5] There is also the case of polyps and mollusca, which have no nerves but are nevertheless 'very sensitive to the irritation of a stimulus that has been applied, and move in consequence of this irritation'.[6] Such an instance helps generalise sensitivity as a functional property belonging to all organic parts with more or less integration in dynamic processes. Polyps possess a sensitivity capable of regulating their own conservation, their heat equilibrium and so on. Since they have no sense organ, one must admit that states of diffuse and general sensitivity are possible.

Excised muscles evincing irritability should be assigned a 'local sensitivity' (*sensibilité locale*). It does not mean excluding the possibility that nerves can be sensitive; but they should not be viewed as the sole type of structure in which sensitivity can be exerted. Some observations support the same argument: Hard insensitive parts, for example tendons and tela cellulosa, become sensitive due to inflammation or lesion. Haller's law of equal ratio between sensitivity and the number and size of nerves is inexact, since parts without nerves, like the dura mater, can become very sensitive. Such empirical evidences show the relativity of Haller's thesis. Irritability is not to be rejected, but rather is to be integrated into a revised doctrine of organic sensitivity. There is no strict ratio between local sensitivity and resulting motions: Such a ratio (if one tried to state it) would prove very uneven between the various parts and highly variable for one and the same part. Sensitivity would involve various organs in various ways, according to the stimuli affecting them. Every organ seems to possess a specific mode of sensitivity (stimuli, for instance, act selectively on them); but on the other hand, one should conceive an integrated sensitive activity for the organism as a whole. Both aspects of sensitivity, general and specific, are correlated:

All the organs in a living animal body are probably capable of

5 *Nouveaux élémens de la science de l'homme*, 2d ed. rev. et considérablement augmentée. 2 vols. (Paris, 1806), I, sec. 101, p. 203.
6 Ibid., I, sec. 89, p. 181.

a general sensitivity that is common to them. They partake in it with the principal difference that it can be excited but seldom and slightly in some organs, and uncomparably more often in some others. The relative degrees of general sensitivity in the various parts of the animal body have not yet been determined, notwithstanding all the experiments undertaken.[7]

Under these conditions, sectioned nerves could be conceived as interrupting the conspiring activity of general sensitivity, while local sensitivity might be kept at a lower level of integration for a certain time. Or, to use Barthez's terms, it could mean an interruption in sympathy between the organ's nerves or even their fibrillar elements and the whole system of sensitivity, whose main instrument is the nervous network.

To analyse the functional and integrative aspects of sensitivity, Barthez resorts to the related notions of sympathy and synergy. Dating back to Hippocratic medicine, 'sympathy' meant a conspiring activity of the various organic parts in the phenomena of some given diseases. At the time of Boerhaave and Haller, there was a tendency to interpret sympathies as functional correlations due to either normal or pathological dispositions in the organic structures. On the other hand, 'synergy' was a notion used by Stahl and his school: Organic synergies are combinations of organic devices appropriated by the soul to exert impulses and effect control over the body for the sake of vital preservation.

In particular, Barthez breaks with mechanistic interpretations of sensitive and motive sympathies. For him, the autonomous correlation of the motive and sensitive forces forms the genuine dynamic unity of living body. 'Vital principle' is the name for this correlation of forces as autonomous of strictly structural dispositions. Doubtless, organic connections are implied in vital functions, but these connections appear in synergies. Barthez's meaning for synergies is a set of functional activities normally operated by means of complex organic devices. Synergies depend upon dynamic laws of the vital principle, but these laws are coupled with relatively stable organic processes:

By *synergy* I mean a conjunction [*concours*] of simultaneous or successive actions of the forces in various organs, so that these actions form by their harmonious or successive ordering, the proper type of a function of health or of a kind of illness (specifically characterising some organic structures); for exam-

7 Ibid., I, sec. 99, p. 197.

ple the generic type of an excretion or that of an inflammation.[8]

In such cases, the object of physiological enquiry is the order of
functional dispositions as they determine the agency of structures.
But this order is best expressed at a level higher than the 'organism of
functions', when confronted with phenomena manifesting vital activity beyond strict connectiveness with organic structure. Sympathies belong to such a class of phenomena: Phenomena show up as
sympathetic in so far as they outstretch the bounds of activities correlated with regular and stable organic dispositions.

However, the processes involved are not purely contingent; they
must conform to a specific functional lawfulness evidenced by regular
observable effects:

> The particular sympathy of two organs happens, when one
> being affected occasions obviously and repeatedly a corre-
> sponding affection in the other, without this sequence being
> possibly referred to chance, to the mechanism of organs or to
> a conjunction of actions conformable to the generic type of a
> function or affection of the living body.[9]

Barthez criticises the Stahlians for having focused only on synergies, which depend on an order of organic devices, while they
should have considered sympathies as paradigmatic for the analysis
of the subordinate effects of the vital principle. Connecting with this
position on laws of sympathies, two points are to be stressed. First,
true physiological analysis should aim not at causal explanations but
rather at translations of empirical data according to a system of *faits-
généraux ou faits-principes*:[10] Functional relations as evidenced in
sympathies, and subordinately in synergies, are presented as such
faits-principes. Second, in a physiology based on the notion of a vital
principle, statements of laws should not be considered as statements
of strictly necessitating conditions. Laws enunciating *faits-principes*
are somewhere between determinative and regulatory principles.
Barthez is prone to admit that his law-statements express a kind
of speculative plan reflecting not so much a constant order in the
phenomena taking place, as an ideal transcription of these, making
sense of the functional aspects, which seem irreducible to structuro-
mechanistic considerations.

The speculative character of his theory comes to the fore when he
distinguishes the system of the vital principle into two sets of forces:

8 Ibid., II, sec. 160, p. 8.
9 Ibid., II, sec. 156, pp. 1–2.
10 Ibid., II, notes, p. 15, n. 15.

'the forces which this Principle sets into action at every moment in all organs whether it be determined by fundamental laws or by foreign causes; and the radical forces, which it possesses potentially for maintaining the natural use of these acting forces'.[11] Organic activity can be triggered either by physical stimuli acting on living structures or by endogenous determinations to act. In both cases, the resulting 'motion' cannot show up as functional, adaptive, if it were not resulting partially or totally from specific forces overriding the dynamic dispositions of structures. Thus acting forces are connected to specific organic activities; they operate under proper circumstances and as a result of selective stimuli. An analysis of the notion of such forces reveals that (1) they do not involve any sufficient reason for the correlation and harmony between their several operations and (2) they do not involve any account for their substantive status as an integrated system of functional elements. Radical forces will afford both a *raison d'être* for the integrative activity of physiological (acting) forces and a *raison d'être* for the substantive character of the dynamical harmony and regulatory processes in the living body. Evidently, radical forces inherited some features of Stahl's notion of a *tonus*. That *tonus* was conceived as an intrinsic motion in parts enabling them to counteract tendencies to dissolution; it would form an immanent predisposing activity required for the support of living functions. But for Stahl, soul is the only true agent, and the *tonus* was viewed as a kind of specific mechanical disposition, serving a functional purpose, because produced and directed by a kind of 'infraconscious' *logos*. Barthez's view of radical forces is quite different. For him, the dynamic alternations in the exercise of functions and the constant modifications in physiological processes require that phenomenal or acting forces (i.e., forces identified by their apparent functional effects) be correlated with a substantive disposition to integrative programmatic activity: a kind of theoretical *raison d'être* for the combined processes in individual organisms. But such speculative entities as *radical forces* are constantly coupled with *acting forces*. They form the invisible face of a physiological 'Janus', with dynamic features that would serve to compensate the actual losses in functional activity and to re-equilibrate the system of the living principle.

The increases in radical forces, indirectly produced by an enacting of functions that conforms to health, require close attention. They always are in combined ratio with the degree of action that the acting forces develop in each main function within the animal oeconomy, and with the level of active

11 Ibid., II, sec. 233, p. 163.

relationships between all those functions that habit has set in the form of health proper to each individual.[12]

Physiological theory is supposed to account for the autonomy and activity of the living principle. And this means framing a theoretical representation of a system of specific forces to help interpret the *sui generis* empirical correlations of organic activity; this theoretical representation is to serve as the proper scheme for giving hypothetical anticipations of physiological laws. Hence the methodological specifications of Barthez's doctrine.

Barthez is an empiricist in that he believes that experimental causes should be considered only as general determinative factors in the course of phenomena. Using abstract terms to refer to such factors makes it possible to use inferences and computations so as to analyse phenomena systematically. Following Boissier de Sauvages's suggestions in the Prolegomena of *Nosologia methodica* (1763),[13] he refers to the analogy of such theoretical terms with the letters used in algebra:

> The names of *occult faculties* are useful to simplify the computation of phenomena [*calcul des phénomènes*], and to give it much more extension. These names being used as letters in algebra, no prejudiced opinion hampers the search for the proximate and immediate causes of facts. Thus one obtains much more easily and directly formulas or *general expressions of the analogies* of these facts.[14]

The algebraic x in physiological analysis would have a specific meaning and role. It would signify the heterogeneity between the laws of vital functions and those of inorganic nature, as well as between the laws of vital functions and determinations of the psychological agent. It would afford a new *combinatoire* of phenomena show-

---

12 Ibid., II, sec. 234, p. 166.
13 See *Nosologia methodica, sistens morborum classes, genera et species juxta Sydenhami mentem et botanicorum ordinem* (Amsterdam, 1763), Prolegomena sec. 210, and T. S. Hall, *Ideas of Life and Matter*, 2 vols (Chicago, 1969), II, p. 75: 'Sauvages deplored the tendency of modern thinkers to replace faculties, as supposed causes of vital phenomena, with such other agencies as subtle fluids (electricity was beginning to be suggested at this time as a *causa vitae*). Just as mathematicians when solving problems had long utilized unknown quantities, designated x and y for example, so, said Sauvages, physiologists should utilize faculties even when ignorant of their essential nature and of the way they evoke their effects. The algebraic analogy suggested by Sauvages was to play an important role in later physiological speculation. It raised the question, which was to be debated for more than a century, whether it was legitimate and useful – or, as some thought, illegitimate and dangerous – to make use in theory building of presumptive entities or agents whose essential nature was mysterious or whose reality was doubtful.'
14 *Nouveaux élémens*, I, nn. p. 16; see also, *Nouvelle méchanique des mouvements de l'homme et des animaux* (Carcassone, year VI – 1798), Discours préliminaire, p. ii.

ing the specific physiological connection involved, an intrinsic connection, and more fundamental than the order arising from anatomical, mechanical or chemical determinations. Indeed, the experimental cause is hypothesis, but it should be framed on the ground of an 'analytic computation of phenomena'.[15]

Barthez considers that scientific knowledge can develop only once an adequate principle or experimental cause has been posited. The experimental cause represents in common 'area of research' a type of complex phenomenon, set as heterogeneous if referred to laws derived from other experimental causes, presumably of a lower order. The abstractive experimental cause, expressing simply a given type of determinant for a specific order of phenomena, helps discard a priori hypotheses that would transgress the conditions of empirical explanation. Such hypotheses are uncertain and useless 'paraphrases'. On the contrary, if taken from facts relating to the experimental cause, analogical relations may unveil the 'secondary laws' of this cause, in other words, its general modes of operating; and they may be submitted to empirical control for confirmation. Framing these secondary laws, one might have to revise the system of experimental causes by effecting a synthesis of distinct sets of phenomena. Barthez's experimental cause makes it possible to locate in the phenomena significant facts, that is *faits-principes* serving as grounds for explanatory analogies.

Barthez contrasts the living principle to the principles of motion on the difference in complexity of its effects (laws). In hierarchical order, one finds the force of impulse, the forces of attraction, including those that produce magnetic and electrical phenomena, and forces of chemical or crystallographic affinities. Even though in each case the essential nature of the force is unknown, the phenomenal effects allow one to identify the laws of a specific dynamism. The more complex the effects, the more prone we are to admit an internal disposition to organise and integrate the resulting effects. But to postulate a micro-organisation to account for this disposition to organisation at the phenomenal level is to resort to a deceptive metaphor. No doubt, the correlation of complex phenomena in an organism supposes an internal interplay of forces, in contrast with the superficial (geometrical) activity of some more mechanical forces. Physiological functions are conditioned by an organisation more complex than that of crystals or metallic trees, but cannot be reduced to the microstructural elements of this organisation. With plants and animals, a vital

15 See *Nouveaux élémens*, Discours préliminaire, I, p. 14: 'It is by combining and computing well-observed facts relevant to each general cause or experimental faculty already identified, that one gets to discover the secondary laws of that cause.'

principle emerges, coeval with complex organic dispositions, but analysis shows it to possess strictly irreducible dynamic features: These consist in the system of vital motive and sensitive forces.

Consequently, Barthez denounces one of the postulates of the revised iatromechanism of Hoffmann or Boerhaave, assimilated by the new organicist trends, under cover of admitting 'vital properties'. This postulate defines solidism. From Baglivi to Bordeu and La Caze, through Haller and Whytt, 'the various solidists agree in subordinating the main phenomena of living body to sensitivity, irritability or an innate power of elasticity [*ressort*] in fibres'.[16] These various doctrines join in admitting that organic elements possess specific dynamical properties to produce sensitivo-motive spontaneity, properties that transcend the transmission and even conversion of motor effects strictly determined by physical stimuli. However, in accounting for such functional properties, solidists have to resort to micromechanical and/or microstructural hypotheses, and therefore to constructs that are arbitrary and inadequate in view of the regulative and integrative aspects of physiological activity. Instead, one must subordinate organic modalities to the 'essential determinations of the Principle of Life; which experience alone permits us to know, and whose laws transcend the laws of Physics and Mechanics'.[17]

Chapter 3 of the *Nouveaux élémens* raises the question of the ground for the living principle as a theoretical entity: 'Does the Vital Principle exist on its own or is it only a mode of the human body that makes it live?' In answering, Barthez uses the same type of philosophical stratagem Locke used to avoid siding with the materialists or with the spiritualists concerning the union of mind and body. Barthez states:

> It is indeed possible that, according to a general law set by the Author of Nature, a vital faculty endowed with motive and sensitive forces arises necessarily (in an independent way) in the combination of matter forming each animal body, and that this faculty contains the sufficient reason of the sequences of motions required for the animal to keep living. But it may also be that God joins to the combination of matter appropriate to forming an animal, a Principle of Life subsisting by itself and differing from man's thinking soul.[18]

The former alternative conforms to the organicist thesis. As a metaphysical solution, it is neither empirically proven nor invalidated by the methodological criticism Barthez had himself launched against

16 Ibid., I, p. 22.
17 Ibid., I, p. 25.
18 Ibid., I, sec. 36, p. 97.

solidism. But he does not believe such a view of the theoretical entity would prove heuristically profitable. By contrast, Barthez was to insist on facts suggesting the substantive autonomy of the vital principle: cases of destruction of the vital forces without apparent organic lesions, cases of integral activity being kept in spite of lesions, specific motions in states of violent stress (danger or irritation) and so on. But the main argument comes from the account of epigenetic phenomena. On the one hand, 'while organs get perfect and strong by degrees, the Principle of Life is perfect in its generative and vital functions from the very start in the formation of those organs'.[19] On the other hand, amongst various insects and animals, there seems to be a power to reanimate organic structures that are in a state apparently incompatible with vital activity (e.g., rotifers, volvoxes, tardigrades, tremellas). Even sleep and hibernation seem to require an energetic principle, distinct from structures, since these can be reanimated. Finally, the vital principle seems to act inconstantly if referred to structures: It shows phenomena of disappearance, reintegration and concentration for which the structural inherence of forces does not seem capable of accounting.

Nevertheless, Barthez keeps to methodological scepticism in regard to the nature of the vital principle: One must stay within the bounds of possible inference concerning the operative conditions of vital forces and the resulting order in phenomena; such inferences will give laws assignable to a specific principle of determination. The theoretical abstractions consistent with this methodology serve in ordering a given set of phenomena so as to show the appropriate laws determining them. They have meaning 'in so far as they serve to classify facts and to combine illuminating analogies'.[20] Such is the methodological character of Barthez's vitalism.

II

The main influences on Johann Friedrich Blumenbach (1752–1840) can probably be traced back to a combination of Hallerian and Wolffian theory. C. F. Wolff's *Theoria generationis* (1759; second edition, 1774) had restored epigenesis as a proper theory of generation and set a concept of *vis essentialis* as an epigenetic force, emerging in organic matter to promote the working out of more and more complex structures. Haller's model for physiology also influenced Blumenbach's views, especially concerning the plurality of physiological properties

19 Ibid., I, sec. 40, p. 104.
20 Ibid., I, notes, n. 18, p. 99.

to be connected with structural elements and systems of organs. But we shall focus on the essential concepts in Blumenbach's theory, which override the notions inherited from Haller or Wolff.

In his essay *Ueber den Bildungstrieb und das Zeugungsgeschäfte* (1781), Blumenbach frames a 'vitalist' interpretation of generation. His arguments are supported by further analysis in short papers, the more important of which are *De nisu formativo et generationis negotio nuperae observationes* (1787), and *Commentatio de vi vitali sanguinis* (1788). A revised edition of *Ueber den Bildungstrieb* was published in 1789. In regard to his theory of epigenesis, he attempted to reframe the Hallerian physiological theory in his *Institutiones physiologicae* (first edition, 1786). Some important theoretical elements were included in the later versions of his *Handbuch des Naturgeschichte* (first edition 1779–80). These texts enable us to complete the picture of his physiological system.

Wolff's *vis essentialis* is a power by which the nutritive material is distributed to the various parts of the plant or animal in formation. The *vis essentialis* would act to expand excrescences and monstrosities as well as the normal organism. But in explaining organic epigenesis, a sufficient reason should be provided to account for the production of a regular, harmonious structure: The expansion process should only be considered as a necessary condition for the formative process to take place. For instance, nutritive processes in the embryo can be considerably deficient. As a result, the formative principle will produce a dwarf organism but the type of organisation will remain unaltered. The *Bildungstrieb* as a projective force (inducing a regular structural pattern) needs to be distinguished from a mere vegetative force whose activity is more amorphous.

In Hallerian physiology, on the other hand, the main arguments against epigenesis were based on the principle that functional operations required complex structures in existence, even at the earlier embryonic stages.[21] Blumenbach's revision substitutes an architectonic force for an invisible structural disposition to act, as *ratio essendi* for the complex perceptible stages in succession, every phase evidencing an architectonic integration of the organism according to an immanent plan, the same throughout the whole sequence. According to a Newtonian model, forces refer to unknown internal dispositions of elements; following this pattern, Blumenbach transposes the sufficient reason for epigenetically derived complex structures into a spe-

21 On Haller's and Wolff's theories of generation, see Shirley A. Roe, *Matter, Life and Generation: 18th Century Embryology and Haller-Wolff Debate* (Cambridge, 1981), and Duchesneau, *La Physiologie des Lumières*, pp. 277–311, 313.

cific force. As attraction, *Bildungstrieb* or *nisus formativus* signifies a force whose determination consists in the constant empirical effects that correlate to it, even though the cause remains latent, as in the case of occult qualities. The set of phenomena assigned to the *Bildungstrieb* is the sequence of epigenetic events from the initial amorphism to the functional architectonic in the resulting organism. Not only do the phenomena of generation depend on this *nisus*, but by implication also those of growth, nutrition and reproduction in so far as they actualise a regular pattern. In the 1798 edition of his *Institutiones physiologicae*, Blumenbach notes:

1. I have used the term *nisus formativus* only to distinguish [this disposition] from the other orders of vital forces; by no means to explain the *cause* of generation, since I believe that it is buried in the utmost darkness, like the causes of gravitation and attraction, given that these consist in mere names which have been imposed on effects known a posteriori so to speak, in the same way as the *nisus formativus*.

2. I have chosen that term *nisus* mainly to express the vital energy of that disposition so as to distinguish it as clearly as possible from mere mechanical forces with which several philosophers have attempted in the past to link the matter of generation.

3. This doctrine concerning the *nisus formativus* focuses on one essential point, which by the way suffices to distinguish it from the plastic force of the ancients, from the force which the most deserving Wolff called essential, and from the other hypotheses of the same kind, namely that it consists in the conjunction of two explanatory principles on the nature of organic bodies, the physico-mechanical and the purely teleological.[22]

A good example of the proper function of the *Bildungstrieb* is afforded by nutrition. Taking lymph to be the nutritive material composing or recomposing the organic structures in an already formed organism, Blumenbach distinguishes two types of forces acting to assimilate it to parenchymas: on the one hand, 'a certain affinity . . . by which similar parts attract and assimilate homogeneous elements possessing affinity with them'; on the other hand, 'this *nisus formativus* which is to be held responsible for a just application of

---

22 *Institutiones physiologicae*, editio nova auctior et emendatior (Göttingen, 1798), sec. 587, n. *h*, p. 464. One should note that no. 3 is a reinterpretation by Blumenbach of his own methodology in the light of Kant's *Kritik der Urteilskraft*. Terminology aside, the features mentioned fit his initial theory of generation as well.

elementary and previously formless matter and for shaping it into a determinate figure'.[23] A fundamental architectonic power determines the typical structuration or restructuration once the structure is framed; as for assimilating forces, they emerge from the structure itself and correlate with the notion of a highly complex mechanism. Once we deal with all formed complex and functionally specialised parenchymas in a higher-order organism, tendency to regeneration in these parenchymas dwindles to the point of fading out: They become unregenerable.

> On the contrary, as I can infer from the many experiments I made to this end, this *reproductive force* in man and the other warm-blooded animals seems to have been given to almost none of the similar solid parts, which, besides contractility, possess some other kinds of vital force, namely irritability or sensitivity or finally proper life [*vita propria*].[24]

In other words, once the *nisus* has engendered a structure endowed with specific functional properties, it leaves the built-up architecture with more dispositional modalities to act for its conservation. There is an architectonic unity of potential relations between structures and functions in the *nisus* at the initial stage; the resulting specialised structures tend to lose the hegemonic character of the *nisus*, to the advantage of exerting selective functions. The contrast is not only between stages in the development of complex organisms, but as well between types of organisms, the lower-order organisms keeping more of the hegemonic *nisus* throughout their substance. Classifying architectonic phenomena in contrast with specialised functional operations depending on given structures enabled Blumenbach to reserve the concept of *nisus formativus* for the regular epigenetic features in organic life. His experiments on it focused on the *Conferva fontinalis* and the freshwater horned polyp, which show a clear disposition towards reintegrative adjustments when mutilated in a diversity of ways. On the other hand, he justified his views by a combination of empirical facts, conspiring phenomena so to speak, which tend to suggest this project-achieving force in fundamental organic processes. He therefore studied cases of pseudo-membranes, of preternatural bones and vessel-framing, as well as *partus monstrosi* and hybrid-forming genetic phenomena. He was convinced that the *Bildungstrieb* as an explanatory principle is some kind of conjectural notion that could be disqualified because of its speculative and metaphorical character, but he felt justified in resorting to it because such a

23 Ibid., sec. 463, p. 356.
24 Ibid., sec. 460, p. 355.

concept combines two sets of empirical references: On the one hand, it represents the data of epigenesis and structure forming; on the other, it affords an analytic expression for the functional combination of structures and processes one observes in the actualised organism. In a way, the validity of such an hypothesis consists in its capacity to relate distinctive features of organic life so as to unify anatomico-physiological and generative processes in a system. Blumenbach's theory is specific in the way it attempts to achieve such a synthesis.

In analysing Blumenbach's theory, T. S. Hall insists on the fact that a multiplicity of vital forces are called in as explanatory concepts. He notes that Blumenbach distinguished three kinds of vital powers, one for generation and growth, the other two for motility and sensitivity, with an additional category for the 'proper life' of each organ. This multiplicity of principles entailed some heterogeneity in the organic functioning, while Blumenbach argued for the interconnectedness of solids, fluids and vital forces in the organism, which forms a functional whole.[25] Specifically, what is the connection between the *Bildungstrieb*, which generates structures, and the other forces, which depend on specific structural dispositions? Resorting to the Newtonian model of explanatory unknowns does not suffice to account for Blumenbach's theoretical strategies.

An important aspect of the question relates to the way the typology of forces is achieved, by comparison with Haller's. Elasticity, as a physical property, as well as all properties pertaining to soul, is excluded. If we proceed empirically, we may identify certain physiological forces: The first is contractility (or cellular force), which resides in *tela cellulosa* and operates throughout the body. This principle accounts for phenomena Stahl had attributed to *tonus*, for example lymphatic absorption. Second, we get Hallerian irritability (or muscular force) and then sensitivity (or nervous force): Its seat is the nerve marrow; it operates 'as if the parts endowed with it were irritated by stimuli acting on them, while at the same time perceptions arise from them in the soul'.[26] The first two of those forces are termed 'common forces'. By the name 'proper life', Blumenbach identifies those forces by virtue of which only certain parts of our body fulfil the special functions assigned to them. Proper life is supposed to account for the appropriateness of a specialised structure to accomplish some functional operation of a set nature:

> There are in the human body some organs that so differ from all the others, either because of a particular structure or be-

---

25 Hall, *Ideas of Life and Matter*, II, p. 105.
26 *Institutiones physiologicae*, sec. 43, p. 35.

274 *François Duchesneau*

cause of a particular and quasi-abnormal motion or function, that they can hardly or not at all be explained by the laws of those common orders of vitality. Therefore, one must either change the features of those orders, form new ones, and set their limits, *or* till that be done, one may remove specific motions that characterise these particular organs, from the orders of general vital forces and distinguish them by the term *vita propria.*[27]

Instances can be given of proper life in the motions of the iris, of the Fallopian tube, in specific secretions and so on. Last, the *Bildungstrieb* must be set in a category on its own: 'This species of vital force, which solidifies the genital and nutritive humours, and which aspires from the start to organic nature, I have designated by the term *"nisus formativus"* as presiding over all generation, nutrition and reproduction in both organic kingdoms.'[28] The *Bildungstrieb* initiates an architectonic sequence involving the other vital forces.[29] Cellular force and proper life have no equivalents in Haller's theory. Hallerian properties take place in general but relatively complex structures. Cellular force belongs to the elementary texture of all organic parts. On the other hand, it affords a basis for the more complex functions, as it produces an elementary regulation throughout the organism, and maintains dynamic disposition in all structures. Proper life is also non-Hallerian in character. Secretions, for example, entail a diversity of processes (circulatory, lymphatic, nervous) and a diversity of structures. The coordinate, selective and timely effect requires some kind of regulative power to balance secretion and absorption and to adjust the system of organic dispositions. Blumenbach suggests that such processes refer to a principle capable of integrating lower-order organic operations as required by the function; these operations comprise the effects of other vital forces, namely contractility, irritability and sensitivity.

Even though irritability and sensitivity are Hallerian properties, they undergo a shift in meaning to fit Blumenbach's system. Sen-

27 Ibid., sec. 42, p. 33.
28 Ibid., sec. 38, p. 31.
29 See ibid., sec. 44, pp. 35–6: 'The order which I followed in presenting those various vital forces, is the same in which they manifest themselves in a man at birth and afterwards. In the first place, there needs have been an acting *nisus formativus*, before we can become certain enough of the very existence of the embryo. Almost immediately, in the jellylike body of the initial embryo contractility intervenes. Then, as soon as the muscular parts have been effected, irritability takes place in their very motive fibres. Then, in these few organs whose motion can be easily referred neither to contractility or to irritability, there is *vita propria*. Finally, in man after birth there is besides those forces also sensitivity.'

sitivity was considered as dependent on the network of nervous fibres connected with the cerebral sensorium commune; and the functional expression of sensitivity was supposed to be given in psychological awareness of sensitive impressions. Two significant modifications take place. First, Blumenbach admits that sensitivity can be functional independently of central brain activity: Some motions can be determined and directed by an integrative action at the level of the spinal marrow or even at that of some isolated nerves. Here, he sides with Whytt against Haller, but he rejects Whytt's pseudo-animism in pursuance of an organicist view that the degree of integrative action correlates with the state and nature of the organic dispositions. For instance, the regulative features depend on different structures in the cases of warm-blooded or cold-blooded animals.[30] Second, sensitivity now includes a function of reactivity that differs according to the level of structural integration involved: 'so that the nerves serve the purpose of sensation and convey the sensitive impressions which affect the body, to the sensorium, as messengers, and consequently either excite perception or by consensus occasion a determinate reaction'.[31] The examples he gives are the expanding and shrinking of the iris according to the stimulus of light on the retina, the effects of emotion and imagination on organic functioning, nervous 'sympathies' and the regulation of animal functions. Though Blumenbach does not seem to acknowledge Johann August Unzer's theory of the ganglion reflexes (cf. the latter's *Erste Gründe einer Physiologie der eigentlichen thierischen Natur thierische Körper*, 1771), he accepts Zinn's thesis that ganglions and plexus may serve to communicate nervous action and to organise some sensitive reactions. From a general viewpoint, sensitivity is called upon to play an integrative function over the various elements of the nervous network. Though Blumenbach admits of orderly correlation between structures and functions, this property seems to entail a plan for coordination that does not seem derivable from structures. Hence the specificity of sensitivity as a vital force.

Though Blumenbach is less explicit about irritability, there are reasons to suggest that he conceives of it less as a property of a given structure than as a force capable of achieving the integration of myriad processes. For instance, he maintains that the dynamic effects

---

30 See ibid., sec. 219, pp. 176–7: 'However, all the energy of the nervous system should not be held to depend solely on the encephalon, but also on the spinal marrow; there is even in the nerves themselves proper forces of their own, that suffice to agitate muscles; and the vascular cortex of these organs seems to feed and sustain such proper forces. In man, however, there are lesser forces of that type proper to nerves, and a major dependence of nerves on the encephalon itself, compared with other animals, specially cold-blooded ones.'
31   Ibid., sec. 220, p. 177.

caused by irritability complement one another in the various parts: They form a functional chain, for instance, in the vascular system. And so the integrative function of irritability is attributed to a principle that seems irreducible to structural conditions.

Blumenbach's vital forces seem relatively detached from the necessary conditioning of structures, which would apply to Hallerian properties. This being the case, what system, what epistemological model can fit them into a coherent physiological theory? Too easy a solution would be Hall's suggestion that vital powers could be indefinitely multiplied and diversified for the sake of deriving explanations. It seems more appropriate to examine Blumenbach's programme for a well-articulated physiology.

There is so to speak a 'regulatory idea' that may serve as a norm for systematising the theoretical concepts, namely the notion of an order of the phenomena dependent upon their integration in a functional system. This notion initiates a 'rational conjecture' appropriate for framing a physiological theory. For instance, in *De vi vitali sanguinis* Blumenbach suggests that no vital force can be postulated when the effect does not seem to relate functionally to maintaining or producing an orderly organic activity. The phenomena of vital forces (contractility, irritability, sensitivity, proper life, *nisus*) present this functionality, which seems not to apply in the case of fluids, except for those of generation.[32] Such a functionality is further manifested when we compare the effects of vital principles to the corresponding pathological phenomena. And so the forces assigned to the various organic devices are confirmed by the characteristic alterations in functional activity. Indeed, any analysis of vital functions can only be relative, because the phenomenal order results from a manifold of functional-structural conditions fitting in successive integrative levels.

> Not only do these four principles act and react on each other continually in the living human body. Fluids also act as stimuli on solids; and these solids by their vital force are so disposed as to receive the impulsion of those stimuli as well as to react on the fluids. Concerning the close harmony of the

---

32 See *Commentatio de vi vitali sanguinis* (Göttingen, 1788), p. 7: 'The function of the various orders of vital forces in the solids of our body, will become obvious to those who examine the matter carefully. Contractility in the cellular tissue (*cellulosa tela*) in general serves to push fluids inherent in the cavities of that tissue; irritability in the muscular fibre serves to actualise most motions, especially voluntary ones by means of muscles. Sensitivity in the nerve marrow serves to transmit the impressions of stimuli to a *sensorium*. In the uterus, the iris and in other parts of that sort, proper life is instrumental to achieving special functions. Blood as such does not seem to need any force, and this is generally the case with all animal humours, except when solidified by the *nisus formativus*, which can only be said of genital milk and plastic lymph.'

mind with its body, it will be enough to stress here that it extends much more widely than it could seem at first glance and on considering the matter superficially . . . From the infinite variety and change in the conditions relative to those four principles, it is easy to infer what a considerable *relativity* [*latitudo*] affects our notion of health.[33]

However, the balance between the various conditions adjusts continually and the organic devices involved co-ordinate their actions accordingly. Structures and forces in combination produce action and reaction effects that, though variable, remain typical of given functions. With Blumenbach, the epistemological model is characteristic in that vital principles are taken as if intervening on structures to induce functional effects, that is effects that combine holistically. The functional order in effects seems to be hypothesised in *sui generis* principles beyond the organic devices and stimuli, as if there were some addition of causal purposiveness to elements, structures and material conditions in interplay. This redundancy of goals on the means of organic activity is what Blumenbach conceptualises as a hierarchy of functional reasons 'embodied' in an architectonic principle (*Bildungstrieb*) and in derived principles (the common vital powers, or those proper to elementary or complex structures). The initial statements in the *Handbuch der Naturgeschichte* illustrate this very system. (1) Vital forces in the already formed organism are intimately connected with the organisation of the parts and with that of the whole they form. (2) The initial formation of the organism, according to the description of epigenetic phases, requires a cause comprising in itself the architectonic plan for individuals of such a species with the projected integration of parts in the resulting whole (that is an integration corresponding to the correlation of vital forces and organised structures). Hence (3) the *Bildungstrieb* acting on the matter to be organised differs from any *Bildungskraft* analogous to expansive forces in inorganic nature. (4) Because 'the conception of organised bodies as integrally involving purposiveness [*Zweckmässigkeit*]'[34] proves all purely mechanical accounts of the sequential formation of organised bodies to be inconsistent, the *Bildungstrieb* is conceived as a force answering to the specifics of an architectonic idea of structuro-functional integration, while at the same time describing a process of organic formation:

The term *Bildungstrieb*, like the terms designating all the other sorts of vital forces, cannot offer more explanation than mere-

---

33 *Institutiones physiologicae*, sec. 76, p. 56.
34 *Handbuch der Naturgeschichte*, 6th ed. (Göttingen, 1799), sec. 8, note **, p. 16.

ly to designate and distinguish a specific force (uniting in
itself the mechanical and teleological modalities) whose constant effect can be known from experience, but whose cause,
like the causes of all other natural forces, even those generally
acknowledged, will remain for us in this world a *qualitas
occulta* in the proper sense of the term.[35]

Actualising this architectonic project, the *Bildungstrieb* involves the
various functional powers that will later unfold in the operations
connected with the different organic structures; the concepts that
account for the *nisus* as subsuming causation under a *telos*, govern, on
this inferential account, our understanding of all physiological
phenomena.

There is no place here to compare Blumenbach's theses with the
analysis of physiological teleology proposed by Kant in his *Kritik der
Urteilskraft* (1790). But it is at least noteworthy that Kant stressed the
idea of functional integration as the fundamental ground for the
Blumenbachian type of physiological theory. This idea stems from a
reflective use of the understanding in the synthesis of empirical data
concerning vital phenomena. It means finally that a theory like
Blumenbach's anticipates a sufficient reason for the physiological
order beyond the necessary determination of concepts that would
form an objective synthesis of empirical data. Hence, one has to identify the concepts of functional forces in Blumenbach's physiology as
subjective (either metaphorically or transcendentally subjective) and
grant them either an invalid or a regulatory use in theorising. But it
should be granted that Blumenbach meant to subordinate the determination of forces to a 'rational conjecture', one that would account
for the integrative organic order. *Ueber den Bildungstrieb* initiates a
type of physiological theory in which speculation plays a major role,
that is a type of theory that takes leave from the epistemological
model directly inspired by Newton's physics (even though Blumenbach vouches at times that he proceeds on a strictly Newtonian
model). The resulting methodology may raise serious doubts and
objections (as it did in fact), but it focuses on a new concept, essential
for physiological theorising (that of functional integration), and he
tries to make regulatory use of it for directing analysis of physiological
phenomena. This concept has some content in Blumenbach's doctrine itself, but more important, Blumenbach suggests that it should
account for the multiplicity of empirical features corresponding to the
architectonic dispositions in the living body, and he gives it an
heuristic function in any attempt at building physiological theory.

35 Ibid., sec. 9, n. 2, p. 18.

III

The physiology of John Hunter (1728–93) is not without affinities with the methodological positions of Barthez and Blumenbach, but it could hardly be said to have formed in the same way or to fit the same epistemological requirements. In order to set acceptable terms of comparison, it will prove convenient to resketch the theoretical principles of Hunter's physiology on the basis of his *Lectures on the Principles of Surgery*, delivered in 1786–7. Other texts will complement this exposition, especially the posthumously collated notes of the *Observations on Natural History*.

Two aspects of Hunter's doctrine deserve to be considered: (1) his arguments for the irreducibility of physiological phenomena; (2) his theoretical constructs concerning the principle of life. The first aspect is more apparent, and I suspect that Hunter's vitalism can be easily misinterpreted if confined to it.

Hunter sets forth a distinction between common matter and animated matter (the latter comprising living vegetable and animal matter). Common matter is defined by general properties, namely solidity, fluidity, vapour (gaseous state), form and weight. To account for the fundamental requirement of cohesion, one should add the more abstract type of property that has gone by the name of 'attraction'. In particular, figure and magnitude, which represent form, depend upon an elective attraction of cohesion, and differences in attraction make for specific weights. Properties of common matter are known through sensation. Hunter seems to adopt some Condillacian type of derivation of ideas from sensation when he states that properties are identified by combining sensations of different senses, by analysing the cluster of impressions made by phenomenal bodies as a combination of representative sensations, and by using analogy from sensation to proceed to the unperceivable combinations of elementary properties, for instance in the case of hypothetical elements such as phlogiston.[36]

But general properties and derivable specific properties do not suffice to account for physical phenomena, which entail modes of action. Hunter's interpretation is that if properties make bodies into fit subjects for mechanics (and the derived sciences), some kind of life is needed to produce the interplay of properties and regulate bodily structures: 'Thus we find something like the life of mechanics, which is not matter, but a property belonging to it; what is simply mechan-

---

36 *Observations on Natural History*, in *Essays and Observations on natural history, anatomy, physiology, psychology, and geology, being Hunter's posthumous papers*, 2 vols. (London, 1861), I, p. 7.

ical, that is made of inert matter, must have, as it were, a soul to put and continue it in motion.'[37] The term 'soul' should not surprise in this instance. As Hunter explains in his *Observations on Natural History*, the modes of action of properties, even in the case of inanimate matter, remain essentially unknown; since they are regulative of phenomenal changes, they tend to be accounted for as properties embodying 'a species of intelligent quality'. Hunter's point is that they should not be conceived as presiding extraneously over material structures. They are strictly correlative of the phenomenal actions bodies are involved in, and animism as such is to be discarded.[38] Those dynamic properties foreshadow the status of physiological phenomena, but in this latter case we are dealing with drastic changes in bodily manifestations, so drastic that they shall be accounted for by heterogeneous dynamic properties. It is as if monstrosity had happened in the combination of matter.[39] The main aspect of this monstrosity is that the new-type bodies subsist through change by preparing within themselves matter similar to their own, which entails constancy in modes of action and in dispositions to act.

Hunter's description of vegetable and animal matter is built around the specific properties it manifests. These properties are taken to depend on a power superadded to common matter. When this power ceases to act, the living body returns to the condition of common matter, the phase of transition being characterised by special chemical reactions, namely, those of fermentation. We can consider animal and vegetable matter at three stages: as it manifests in the state of life the power of continuance and self-production; in its chemical composition, that is, in the inanimate state of death; and in its progressive degradation to the state of common matter after death. It is the contrast of stage 1 with both stages 2 and 3 that governs the characterisation of living matter.

Stage 2 shows the result of two processes, vegetalisation and animalisation, but at the same time it demonstrates that these two processes are not amenable to chemical analysis. Certainly one could

37 *Lectures on the Principles of Surgery*, in *The Works of John Hunter*, ed. James F. Palmer, 4 vols. (London, 1837), I, p. 213.
38 See *Essays and Observations*, I, pp. 7–8: 'Matter being endowed with properties which become the cause of our sensations, and the modes of action of those properties being hardly known these properties become the foundation of the idea of spirit, viz. a species of intelligent quality that presides over and directs the actions of matter. But, as causes and effects of matter seem to be entirely connected with matter itself, and to be a property inherent in and inseparable from it, and as these are becoming better known the "presiding spirits" are every day vanishing, and their authority becoming less.'
39 See *Works*, I, p. 214: '. . . seeming, as it were, a monstrosity in the combination of matter'.

proceed to such an analysis of organic matter rendered inert; one could start with 'products' of organic activity and try to reduce such products to a specific cluster of lower-level properties; what could not be accounted for this way are natural productive actions, such as digestion, blood formation and the manifold secretions. In other words, Hunter believes that no synthesis could be achieved through the regular modes of action connected with lower-level properties, so as to issue the various compositions of living matter.[40] Fermentation itself, as stage 3, is not amenable to common chemical processes, because it is spontaneous, meaning that it is unconstrained by external necessitating factors as in chemical reactions of common matter. But even if this proves tempting, it is not possible to generalise fermentation to make up for the synthetical processes of living matter. Degradation of living combinations does not afford an analytical means to account for such combinations, and the production of substances in the living organism is not to be assimilated to fermentation, except if one proceeds from very broad analogy and therefore on arbitrary ground. Indeed, it is tempting to judge Hunter's position as motivated by the fact that biochemical syntheses had not been achieved in his time and that they seemed properly unachievable. This interpretation would not, however, do full justice to the case. Indeed, some arguments play that way: For instance, Hunter states that the known processes cannot account for the material formation of vegetables and animals and that digestion achieves synthetical productions unparalleled by any fermentations. But the major arguments are of a different kind: They stress the specificity in *modes of action* and *powers* more than in properties. It is because the operations in living matter depend upon the exercise of determinate functions that the 'chemical' characteristics of organisms should be segregated from the common chemical properties. The misreading of his arguments elicited from Hunter the following reply:

> In my Lectures on Surgery I began with distinguishing the difference between vegetable matter and animal matter, and also the matter of the globe; saying, that common matter has

40   Ibid., I, p. 217: 'The production of many juices of plants, such as gums, acids, sugar, would seem to be of this kind; but all arise from natural action of the vegetable, and do not belong to chemistry. No chemist on earth can make out of the earth a piece of sugar, but a vegetable can do it. Digestion, the formation of the blood, and all the secretions of an animal, might at first appear to be of this sort; but that they really are not chemical products I am clearly convinced. If an ingenious man undertook to account for every change in matter by fermentation, there is no change in nature that might not be brought within his definition . . . for if you make a definition you may bring together under it a thousand things that have not the least connexion with it.'

undergone a very considerable change in producing the vegetable and the animal, in which was not to be found a particle
of any species of common matter, therefore an entire new
arrangement or combination of common matter; but they had
sprung from common matter, were supported by it, and
returned to it again. This was with a view to make our distinctions in the actions of the body more accurate; distinguishing with more precision between the actions of animals, the
decompositions and combinations of common matter which
are chemical, and the operation of combinations of common
matter on each other, which is mechanical. And also to show
that the vegetable and animal had powers and modes of
action totally different from those of common matter, either in
its chemical or mechanical operations, and which depended
upon their combination with the living principle.[41]

This last argument may be complemented by the statement that
components in vegetable matter, as well as in animal matter, do not
suffice to account for the formations taking place in organisms. The
principle of form in crystals may be attributed to the specific structure
of elementary components, but this does not seem to be the case with
organisms in which structures are produced and maintained by complex modes of endogenous activity. Chemical analysis would reveal a
few relatively amorphous components whose 'mechanical' combinations could not produce the equivalent of the functional activities
engendering living structures and taking place consequently within
the self-supporting organism. It is evident that by chemical analysis
Hunter means a decomposition into more elementary substances,
and not necessarily the analytical formulation of abstract laws of
structure and reaction for biochemical compounds. He has in mind
that knowing the properties of elements will not help us ascribe analogical properties to the organic and living bodies. For him, the only
way to go about this problem is to proceed to 'another mode of
investigation'.[42] It would consist in analysing physiological phenomena from their observable functional relations with one another,
and in admitting theoretical concepts about the modes of action involved consistent with the identified functions. With organisms, one
faces as initial data 'singular combinations of matter'.[43] Compared
with inanimate bodies framed from common matter, they appear as
machines with preternatural actions, resulting in self-production and

41 *Essays and Observations*, I, p. 13.
42 Ibid., I, p. 12.
43 *Works*, I, p. 219.

self-preservation. The methodological task is to find means for systematically analysing those actions. Hunter suggests significant approaches, for instance resorting to lower-order functional combinations (in more rudimentary organisms) to account for more complex ones, or correcting the aprioriness of any functional analysis by considering pathological or anomalous modalities of functions.[44] Hunter's idea seems to be that physiological, lawlike statements can only be obtained comparatively from the analysis of the functional modes of action themselves. The generally stated reason for this methodological move is that vegetalisation and animalisation of material compounds do not take place in direct relation with the available components, but are 'effected by the actions of the vegetable or animal'.[45] Any attempt at mechanical or chemical reductions reveals only that there is a *sui generis* circle of vital activities, which should be accounted for as such. 'Principle of life' is the concept used to identify this interconnectedness of vital phenomena in self-reiterating, as the following statement shows:

> In treating of any animal body I shall always consider its operations, or the causes of all its effects, as arising from the principle of life, and lay it down as a rule that no chemical or mechanical property can be the first cause of any of the effects in the machine . . . The living principle . . . in itself is not in the least mechanical, neither does it arise from, nor is it in the least connected with any mechanical principle.[46]

Hunter admits that once the organic structures have been produced, some effect might result that could be analysed as mechanical, if induced by external causes intervening on the geometrical characteristics of the living body; but such motions as happen then are subordinate to the form of the individual. In the same way, certain chemical reactions can take place involving the organic compound under constraint from external conditions, but these reactions are to be distinguished from the physiological syntheses operated by the self-supporting organism.

In line with these views, Hunter associates the living principle with form-building in organic body and distinguishes it both from the structures involved and the actions due to the mechanics of such structures. The principle of life is therefore initially defined as a

44 Ibid., I, p. 220: 'A monster is either from a deficiency of parts which can be produced from art (and often is from necessity, as in operations), or else from a modification caused by a wrong arrangement or construction of parts, which will produce an unnatural action, by which means the natural action may be known.'
45 Ibid., I, p. 218.
46 Ibid., I, p. 219.

power of self-formation, a kind of *Bildungstrieb*, which is conceived as
analogous with powers determining modes of action in machines, but
as issuing effects of a functional nature, even in a properly amorphous
matter. Hunter states:

> Organization and life do not depend in the least on each
> other; . . . organization may arise out of living parts, and
> produce action; but . . . life never can arise out of, or depend
> on, organization. An organ is a peculiar organization of mat-
> ter (let that matter be what it may), to answer some purpose,
> the operation of which is mechanical: but mere organization
> can do nothing even in mechanics: it must be something
> corresponding to a living principle, namely, some power. I
> had long suspected that the principle of life was not wholly
> confined to animals, or animal substances endowed with
> visible organization and spontaneous motion: I conceived that
> the same principle existed in animal substances devoid of
> apparent organization and motion, where there existed simply
> the power of preservation.[47]

Those statements concern the blood, as a structureless organic substance, endowed with fundamental vital power, which is architectonic in character. Indeed, the issuing organisation is capable of
mechanical operations. But the physiological operations in a complete
organism are not to be restricted to this kind, since functional phenomena are subsumed under the concept of architectonic activity.
This we shall examine later. To complete Hunter's theory of 'living
matter', we must now consider what differentiates animals and vegetables as organisms.

On this question, Hunter starts from the general thesis that animals
and vegetables partake in a 'power of action within themselves'[48]
whose main effects are production of the organic structure and maintenance of it for functional operation. It is most likely that vegetables
and animals differ in their chemical compositions and specific structures (considered when they are dying or dead); but in their operations and actions, they afford significant terms of comparison. They
differ in their systems of assimilation: In a complex animal, it is done
through digestion; in a vegetable, it seems to be done in the organs of
destination themselves. But one should distinguish between vegetalisation and animalisation on the one hand, and vivification on the
other. The first two refer to the formation of organic compounds

---

47 *A Treatise on the Blood, Inflammation, and Gun-shot Wounds* (1793), *Works*, III, p.
106.
48 *Works*, I, p. 214.

compatible with the living body; vivification refers to the fact that at a final stage compounds are assimilated to existing structures or transform into such structures and are correlatively endowed with the living principle. Vegetalisation operates either on common matter or on already vegetalised matter; animalisation generally requires previously vegetalised or animalised matter.[49] Hunter's view is that vegetalisation and animalisation are analogous processes; the only significant difference is their taking place in structures of distinct kinds. In particular, each part of the plant may act as an equivalent of a specialised 'stomach'; this generality of the assimilating structure in the vegetable goes along with a diversity of effects according to the action of the part. Parts tend to be functionally specialised in animals and so are generally unable to play other roles or to regenerate the whole structure, while engrafting is a constant proof of functional versatility of vegetal parts under the specific type involved:

> A vegetable is a perfect plant in every point, every point is capable of producing what the whole is capable of producing; but this is not the case with an animal. An animal is a compound of parts totally different in their sensations, stimuli, powers, and uses, from one another; each part doing one office and no more, and all obliged to one source for support and sensation.[50]

This explains the limits of regeneration in animal structures. Only when the part truly forms a compound of the whole can it restore a perfect animal; this is the case with some lower-order animals, for instance protozoa or hydrozoa. In more complex animals, the specialised functions of partial structures entail that there be systems for circulating animalised supplies and systems for communicating and co-ordinating powers of action: the vascular and nervous networks fill those needs.

The main distinction between vegetables and animals is that for animals the living principle achieves architectonic and other functional operations in a variety of specialised structures, whereas for

49 See ibid., I, p. 230: 'Animalization is the first; vivification the second. To prove this, I observed that an animal is increased and supported by many substances which previously had not the properties of animal matter, and of course not the principle called animal life, I observed, too, that it was also supported by substances which were of animal origin, but which had not then the living principle: in other words, an animal can be supported on dead vegetable and animal matter. In the next place it was remarked that these substances, before they can increase or support the animal, must all be converted into animal matter; and lastly, that the substances must be so prepared, or animalized, as to become part of the body, and of course to be endued with the living principle.'
50 *Essays and Observations*, I, p. 18.

vegetables the architectonic and functional activities seem to combine in parts that are essentially of common pattern and disposition. The ultimate consequence of Hunter's views on this matter is that physiological investigation should concentrate on the powers and modes of action rather than on the structural dispositions and that it should hypothesise patterns of organisation and architectonic analogies as theoretical concepts to account for the autonomous phenomena signified by the term principle of life.[51]

Theoretical constructs concerning the principle of life fit two objectives: They either serve to define the principle for the sake of building a research methodology or are used in fostering an explanation of physiological processes. Those two objectives are not treated separately by Hunter, except that one specific chapter, 'On the Vital Principle', in the *Lectures on the Principles of Surgery* has more to do with the first one, and the second one is illustrated by sets of arguments in the course of specific enquiries.

Though compounded in its effects by agency of complex phenomena, life 'is reducible to one simple property in every animal'.[52] This inference is based on the integrative nature of physiological phenomena, which seem to entail an architectonic idea to be achieved by various combinations of means. But such an abstract characterisation would not help investigate specific phenomena and therefore one needs a model for it.

In producing this model, one should not overstate the dependence of the property termed 'life' on highly organised structures. In a

51 This statement is in line with some of Stephen J. Cross's conclusions in 'John Hunter, the Animal Oeconomy, and Late Eighteenth-century Physiological Discourse', *Studies in the History of Biology*, V (1981), pp. 1–110. In that extensive study, Cross underlines the 'physiological' concepts governing J. Hunter's conception of comparative anatomy. And so, the first part of the paper offers views concurring with my own approach, except that my analysis is more concerned with the physiological theories and less with the doctrines of comparative anatomy illustrated by the Hunterian collections and forecasting Cuvier's reformulation of principles. The second part of the paper focuses on the main concepts expressing Hunter's idea of life: vital principle, power of action, susceptibility of impression, disposition to deviant action, internal oeconomy, system of 'sympathies' and so on. Though many considerations may be kept from Cross's analysis, it suffers from a major flaw because Cross wants to reduce those concepts to the epistemic strategy of a physiology based on specific properties (along the Hallerian paradigm). In my view, with the vitalists' generation represented by Barthez, Blumenbach and John Hunter, the Hallerian model is subjected to disruptive tensions. Instead of a structural repertoire of specific properties expressing Haller's ideal of *anatome animata*, the new physiology stresses the necessity of representing functional and architectonic sequences of phenomena by concepts that offer a *raison d'être* for the holistic and integrative features of functions.
52 *Works*, I, p. 221.

comparison of dead and living organic matter, structural dispositions are found to be quite similar; therefore, even if one presumes that the living principle emerges from specific structural modifications, it is to be considered as readily detachable from the specific structures involved. In the same way, it should appear as correlative of a wide diversity of structures and, consequently, relatively independent of the more complex structures the growing organism will produce. The conformation of organs as such will rather permit more mechanical activities than the fundamental action of life. It is a simpler arrangement that will prove required for the principle of life to operate, whether or not it emerges from this arrangement. Thus a first analytical concept for this principle will be afforded by defining it as a principle of preservation that maintains the structure, whether initial and rudimentary or complex and derived, in a state of relative immutability to changing external conditions that could prove disruptive. This concept is akin to Stahl's notion of an organism as opposed to a mechanism.

A further defining formula proposes that the living principle is a principle of action as well as of preservation. Such a principle is required because, as it seems, a living organism operates through endogenous, spontaneous activity. But the problem is to conceive how the living principle can determine materially that activity. Hunter's text is apparently ambiguous:

> It was not sufficient that animal matter should be endowed with . . . the principle of preservation, it was necessary that it should have action or motion within itself. This does not necessarily arise out of the arrangement for preservation; on the other hand, the arrangement for preservation, which is life, becomes the *principle* of action, not the *power* of action, for the power of action is one step further. The *power of action* must arise from a particular position of those living parts, for before *action* can take place the matter must be arranged with this view. This is generally effected by the union of two or more living parts, so united as to allow of motion on each other, which motion the principle of action is capable of effecting when so disposed.[53]

I infer from the text that the power of action that is required for physiological activities arises from the interrelationship between organic parts. This is not to say that such a power is strictly dependent upon the inert structure of any of those parts. Powers are prop-

53 Ibid., I, p. 222.

erties by themselves capable of stirring bodily structures into motion. It is clear that the power of action depends upon the principle of action, which itself depends upon the principle of preservation. The difference between power and principle rests, in my opinion, on the fact that principles are supposed to control or direct the motive processes in pursuance of given goals. In this instance, however, the conditions for physiological activity and more precisely the power of action emerge out of an architectonic process directly enacted by the principle of preservation. Principles therefore seem to be endowed with a twofold role, regulative and causal, whereas powers of action are derivatively causal. We are presented with an account of the 'special' mechanics of physiological processes based on theoretical presuppositions combining causation with teleology.

The principles of self-preservation and action represent the idea of life: They correspond to properties, but with the special features of autonomy and self-regulation expressed in our intellectual assessment of life. The link of such 'abstract' properties with the more mechanical properties, namely, the organic powers of motion, is conceived through a kind of monadological model, although Hunter never uses such an expression or seems to have had direct connection with monadologists. First, structural combinations arise from two or more 'simple acting parts'[54] uniting to allow special kinds of motion; the example of such elementary combinations is the muscular fibre with its characteristic motion of Hallerian irritability. But many more combinations are possible involving various kinds of animal matter, and various levels of complexity, higher ones corresponding to organs and combinations of organs. The 'powers of action' depend upon compounding arrangements of 'living particles',[55] and particles are living because animal matter is endowed with the principle of life in any of its least parts. Those minute living parts may possess enough of the principle to persist in existence regardless of the alterating conditions in the surrounding matter. Or they may be more active in fostering powers of motion in the combinations in which they partake. When more active, the principle of life in the organic particle stimulates the dynamical dispositions in the other particles conjoined with it, which act on their own. This monadic autonomy of motion is the ground for the 'self-equilibrating' character of the integrated motions: Action is harmonic instead of properly mechanical. The principle of life engendering moving powers endows them with

54 Ibid., I, p. 223.
55 Ibid.

functional dispositions in reciprocation; causal efficiency is thus confined to a special type, that of mutual stimulation of functional
dispositions.

> The principle of life has been compared to the spring of a
> watch, or the moving powers of other machinery; but this is
> not the case with an animal; animal matter has a principle of
> action in every part, independent of the others, and whenever
> the action of one part (which is always the effect of the living
> principle,) becomes the cause of an action in another, it is by
> stimulating the living principle of that other part, the action in
> the second part being as much the effect of the living princi-
> ple of that part as the action of the first was of the living
> principle in it. The living principle, then, is the immediate
> cause of action in every part; it is therefore essential to every
> part, and is as much the property of it as gravity is of every
> particle of matter composing the whole. Every individual
> particle of the animal matter, then, is possessed of life, and
> the least imaginable part which we can separate is as much
> alive as the whole.[56]

To complete his model for the concept of living principle, Hunter
stresses the fact that actions taking place in consequence of the principle may modify in return the internal conditions of life for the organism concerned. This kind of feedback process can be represented as
taking place between the action and the principle of action, which is
kept either stimulated or preserved by those self-regulating motions.
The feedback process is also required to adjust the activity of the
whole according to the species of action intervening in various parts.
Action is a stimulus for further action of a more harmonious kind; it is
through retroactive stimuli that the dispositions of the elementary
parts are set in regulative operation.[57] Interestingly enough, Hunter
happens to use the metaphor of consciousness to express the teleological connection between more or less active parts when they partake in the same co-ordinate processes. For instance, in absorption,

56   Ibid.
57   See ibid., I, p. 224: 'It would appear, then, that life is not *action*, but it is
continued or supported by it when it takes place. Action creates a necessity of
support, and furnishes it. It is not necessary that *action* should continue in all parts;
in some it is only necessary that the principle and power of action should be
continued, but in others it is necessary that *action* should take place even for the
preservation of the principle of action. Action is necessary for the various purposes
for which the animal is intended, and if one species of action takes place, it brings
the whole into action, as all the parts and actions of an animal body are dependent
upon one another.'

there must be some kind of harmony in the internal dispositions of the absorbed and absorbing living parts in the organic compound to operate jointly a functional activity.[58] Notwithstanding the metaphorical phrasing, such expressions as 'consciousness in the parts' are used as equivalents of the common self-programming dispositions theoretically required to account for physiological phenomena, even if no direct empirical justification is available. Hunter explains:

> I have used the word consciousness, because we have no
> language existing answerable to all my views of the animal
> oeconomy, and to coin words would not answer the purpose,
> because then I must have a dictionary of my own. I have not
> a word for expressing the cause of those actions which take
> place in the body, as if it was conscious that such and such
> things were going to take place. There are actions in the body
> which come the nearest to consciousness of the mind of
> anything that I can conceive, and therefore I make use of this
> word; but it is commonly applied by philosophers only to the
> mind.[59]

In the same way, a given susceptibility to stimuli is a theoretical construct justified for the sake of interpreting the functional phenomena involved in simple life, applying this expression to the case of elementary organic structure. The powers of action in specific parts are roused into operation by impressions of various kinds, but this does not suffice to describe the 'monadological' activity that implies a kind of reflective disposition to react as well as an ability to coordinate with the same reflective dispositions in other parts: 'Animal matter having internal actions, these actions are producing impressions which are forming dispositions to action in the parts impressed . . . : the impressions will be according to the nature of the impressions and part impressed conjoined'.[60]

Having developed his concept of living principle into this kind of

---

58　See ibid., I, p. 255: 'The remote cause of absorption of whole and living parts implies the existence of two conditions, the first of which is a consciousness, in the part to be absorbed, of the unfitness or impossibility of remaining under such circumstances, whatever they be, and therefore they become ready for removal, and submit to it with ease. The second is a consciousness of the absorbents of such a state of the parts. Both these concurring, they have nothing to do but to fall to the work. Now the part that is to be absorbed is alive, it must feel its own inefficacy and admit of absorption. The vessels must have the stimulus of imperfection of this part, as if they were sensible that this part were unfit; therefore take it up. There must be a sensation in both parts. When the part to be absorbed is a dead part, as nourishment and extraneous matter of all kinds, then the whole disposition is in the absorbents.'

59　Ibid., I, p. 236.
60　Ibid., I, p. 267.

methodological model, Hunter applies it in interpreting physiological functions. We shall take only a few instances of such applications. A very interesting case is that of the functions of the blood. The centrality of this topic in Hunter's physiology is evident from his *Treatise on the Blood, Inflammation, and Gun-shot Wounds* (1793), but for our interpretation we shall rely essentially on the more theoretical approach in the *Lectures on the Principles of Surgery*.

Hunter draws a significative distinction between organisation of animal matter and the self-supporting conditions for the living principle in very rudimentary forms of material structures. He thus has no problem attributing vitality to organic fluids, and especially to blood. Provided it has undergone change in the lungs, blood appears to transmit life to the bodily structures; these produce specific actions (e.g., sensitive action in the nervous network), but are themselves unable to produce the substantive condition for the living principle to operate. Blood or equivalent organic fluids in bloodless organisms seems to foster the expansion and regeneration of the principle. The fluidity of blood is itself dependent upon vital principle in both the fluid and the vessels. Coagulation of extravasated blood is the normal outcome of the vital processes taking place in blood itself, since a tendency for the parts of blood to separate and solidify manifests itself in cases of inflammation: The functional disturbance in the solid parts determines a functional reaction in the blood flowing by.[61] Inflammation expresses a meaningful 'harmony' of blood with the solids. One significant interpretation of coagulation is to suppose that fluidity depends upon a kind of 'consciousness of the use of motion', which is superseded when functional requirements shift to other purposes in the normal repair and growth of organic parts, or which is lost in some devitalising extravasations. In any event, coagulation is defined as a kind of attraction between some component parts of blood; this attraction results from stimuli inducing an irritation. Hunter considers that it is by a sort of coagulation from blood or its equivalent that solid parts are either generated or repaired. In this operation, the materials contained in the fluid conjoin with the living principle, whatever the mode of this combination. The result is some part fit for living action, which will adjust itself to the type of sur-

---

61 See ibid., I, p. 235: 'If the blood does become inflamed in passing through an inflamed part, we must suppose that it immediately loses that disposition when it meets with parts in perfect health. These properties, namely, increased disposition to separate, and a disposition to become a firmer solid, always show increased disposition for action in the living principle, and also, most probably, increased power. It is one of the signs of strength of the living powers although the materials for action are weak.'

292   *François Duchesneau*

rounding parts and perform organic functions accordingly. The
powers of action in blood are those of simple life, but by entering
complex organic structures the extravasated blood compounds will
combine elementary powers of action so as to produce higher-level
functional activity.

Speaking of organisation in a living body, Hunter stresses that
complex structures should be understood as originating in combining
powers of action amongst more elementary parts, in contrast with the
notion of a mechanic put into motion by the exercise of an isolated
power: 'An [animal] must have power in every part, so that his
powers are diffused through the whole animal, which is almost composed of powers.'[62] At the same time, Hunter distinguishes between
two kinds of physiological operations: (1) actions common to every
part and depending upon the intrinsic principle in these parts
('growth, alteration, building up, taking down [absorption], etc.'); (2)
'those actions which are of whole parts, and which vary according to
their composition or construction, being employed chiefly respecting
other matters, not for the immediate use of themselves, as in those
above mentioned, but still absolutely necessary for the first'.[63] In the
latter case, Hunter mentions stomach, heart, organs of respiration,
organs of sensation, mind and will. The idea is that such complex
organic systems with their high level of functional activity are on the
one hand built from combining powers of elementary parts and, on
the other, instrumental to the pursuance of the more fundamental
operations of life: mainly generation, growth, reproduction. This
view is quite original in the context of eighteenth-century physiology;
it is somewhat similar to one of Caspar Friedrich Wolff's theses, but
very foreign to the views of most physiological theorists. Notwithstanding, it represents probably the specific feature of Hunter's system of 'vitalist' physiology. Hunter mentions that

> [specialized complex organs] may be called labourers, being
> subservient to the first [individual elementary parts], which,
> as being engaged in laying down and taking up parts, may be
> called the bricklayers. It is the first which compose the move-
> ments of the true animal, being those which are immediately
> employed about itself. It is the operations of these which
> properly constitute the animal oeconomy respecting itself.[64]

I would tend to reinterpret such a statement as indicative of what I
call a monadological model for theoretical constructs in an account of

62 Ibid., I, p. 242.
63 Ibid., I, p. 243.
64 Ibid.

physiological phenomena. The vital powers and principles embodied in elementary structures afford sufficient reason for more complex structures and functional activities. But this is only conceivable if one admits that powers and principles comprise an architectonic disposition to be displayed at successive levels of complexity in the form of integrative actions.[65] This qualification points to the restricted meaning of vitalism when applied to Hunter's physiological system.

It may readily be concluded from the survey of such physiological systems as Barthez's, Blumenbach's and John Hunter's that they have some basic assumptions in common. These basic assumptions form the argument for identifying a special brand of vitalism. On the other hand, there are significant disparities between these systems and they point to a second area of theoretical presuppositions that suggest divergent approaches to the methods and concepts of physiological theory. Both subsets of propositions played a role in fostering research methodologies in the early nineteenth century, and as such they might deserve further consideration, beyond the limits of this essay.

Barthez, Blumenbach and John Hunter share the opinion that analysis of physiological phenomena cannot be operated fully by locating determining conditions in microstructural dispositions of a mechanical or chemical type. Haller, for instance, tried to combine phenomenal analysis with theoretical constructs about micromechanical dispositions and resulting properties. The new trend is towards emphasising the teleological aspects of phenomena in adequate constructs, which should account for the fact that organic activity is integrative and represents a special kind of architectonic disposition in nature. Hence, we get concepts of *principe vital*, *Bildungstrieb* and *living principle*, which in each case have to be detailed in a series of methodological models, for instance about synergies and sympathies, about derivative forces and properties in complex organic structures (contractility, irritability, proper life, sensitivity), about modalities of the principle in self-preservation or action and in specific powers of action. The architecture of principles and derived concepts is called upon to play a twofold role: determining a system of *raisons d'être* to

---

65 For instance, it seems relevant to interpret Hunter's contribution to pathology as incorporating a specific research interest on tissues conceived as fundamental organic elements at a level of complexity allowing for functional activity. This aspect of Hunter's doctrine has been specially examined by Othmar Keel in 'La pathologie tissulaire de John Hunter', *Gesnerus*, 37 (1980), pp. 47–61; and 'Les conditions de la décomposition "analytique" de l'organisme: Haller, Hunter, Bichat', *Les études philosophiques* (1982), pp. 37–62.

classify and organise the physiological data, and to represent at the theoretical level the architectonic competence of nature in framing and operating the organic structures. This second and more dynamic function becomes the leading one and determines the transition beyond iatromechanism, and animism, even beyond Haller's analytical system of vital properties, and beyond most solidist systems that had attempted to integrate specific physiological forces in imitation of Newtonian forces. Obviously this is not to say that the new trend has freed itself from arbitrary speculative constructs. In a way, the theories involved had been speculative to the point of integrating teleological concepts of a metaphorical or reflective nature, concepts that appealed to design for interpreting the production of functional effects. But they would have used them for analytical purposes and mainly as heuristic devices.

Once that generic characterisation has been achieved, it is impossible to avoid acknowledging the specifics of each system. Barthez treats complex functional activities on an analytical scheme, and he aims at formulating lawlike statements about the correlations of physiological phenomena; his explanatory principles relate to general systematic properties underlined by analysis of functional effects considered apart from structural conditions. His models are at once abstract and epiphenomenal. General sensitivity and nervous sympathies afford him his privileged object of enquiry. Blumenbach aims at combining Hallerian type of analysis for the complex structures and derivative forces with epigenetic presupposition about the initial stages of organic formulation and regeneration. His concept of *Bildungstrieb* inserts the architectonic disposition within a special force otherwise analogous to Newtonian properties and principles. But the initial architectonic disposition is used to complete the analysis of subordinate and derived phenomena by combining the teleological aspect of self-regulatory functions with the determining structural aspects. John Hunter displays his original manner in resorting to a kind of 'monadology' of the living principle broken down into the elementary organic compounds. He avoids, however, falling back on a doctrine of organic molecules *à la* Buffon or even *à la* Needham. The intrinsic architectonic of these elementary powers of vital action may result in the complex organic activities of specialised physiological systems. The phenomena of generation and growth remain the fundamentals of physiological activity, the more complex functions such as nervous sensitivity being only instrumental to what I would call, using a more modern language, metabolic processes. And Hunter has in view that metabolic and plastic processes are but two differential aspects of the power of living matter and that living matter needs to be analysed into regulatory dispositional 'elements', elements inevitably of a conceptual nature that would form the proper meaning of physiological phenomena, as well as into chemical compounds or microstructural devices of a mechanical kind.

10

William and John Hunter: breaking the Great Chain of Being

W. D. IAN ROLFE

Introduction

William Hunter (1718–83) acquired from his mentor, James Douglas, not only many of his books and papers but also the introduction to, and inspiration for, the subsequent interests of his life.[1] One of these abiding interests was natural history, exemplified by Douglas's 1718 description of the flamingo, anatomy of the armadillo (1716) and demonstration of the development of the frog (1712).

William published only three papers on natural history: on the mastodon (1768), on fossil mammals from Gibraltar (1770) and on the nylgau antelope (1771).[2] He wrote one other paper, on moose and Irish 'elk', which has recently been published.[3] When compared with his twenty-eight medical and human anatomical works, these four papers constitute only a small fraction of his writings.[4] In contrast,

1 C. H. Brock, 'James Douglas (1675–1742), Botanist', *Journal of the Society for the Bibliography of Natural History*, 9 (1979), 137–45; C. H. Brock, 'Dr. William Hunter's Museum, Glasgow University', *Journal of the Society for the Bibliography of Natural History*, 9 (1980), 403–4; K. B. Thomas, *James Douglas of the Pouch, and his Pupil William Hunter* (London, 1964), p. 76; J. L. Thornton, *Jan Van Rymsdyk* (Cambridge, 1982), p. 23; J. Young and P. H. Aitken, *A Catalogue of the Manuscripts in the Library of the Hunterian Museum in the University of Glasgow* (Glasgow, 1908), nn. 522–4.
2 W. Hunter, 'Observations on the Bones, Commonly Supposed To Be Elephants' Bones, Which Have Been Found Near the River Ohio in America', *Philosophical Transactions of the Royal Society of London*, 58 (1768), 34–45; W. Hunter, 'An account of the Nyl-ghau an Indian Animal Not Hitherto Described', *Philosophical Transactions of the Royal Society of London*, 61 (1770), 170–81; W. Hunter, 'Account of Some Bones Found in the Rock of Gibraltar', *Philosophical Transactions of the Royal Society of London*, 60 (1771), 414–16.
3 W. D. I. Rolfe, 'William Hunter (1718–1783) on Irish "elk" and Stubbs's *Moose*', *Archives of Natural History*, 11 (1983), 263–90; W. D. I. Rolfe, 'A Stubbs Drawing Recognised', *Burlington Magazine*, 125 (1983), 738–41.
4 In the MS catalogues of William Hunter's papers prepared by Dr C. Helen Brock, there are 142 lots of medical and human anatomical manuscripts, but only 52 natural history manuscripts; 230 sets of illustrations of medical and human anatomical subjects, but only 14 of animal subjects.

John Hunter wrote thirty natural history (including comparative anatomical) works but only twenty on human anatomy and medicine.[5]

Nevertheless, it was William who gave John his introduction to
comparative anatomy, during the ten years that John spent working
as anatomical assistant to William in London, after 1748.[6] William
Hunter promoted John Hunter's, as well as Hewson's and Cruikshank's, researches into the comparative anatomy of various organs
and made original contributions to mammalian embryology, not only
through his own work, but also by sponsoring that of Cruikshank.[7]
'He cultivated all branches of natural history.'[8]

William Hunter had relatively 'few preparations in comparative
anatomy, having always objected strongly to them',[9] but he published his own approval of John's comparative anatomical work[10] and
turned to him in connection with his own mastodon work. It was
John who 'at first sight told me that the grinder was certainly not an
elephant's'.[11]

The extent of such collaboration between William and John Hunter,
in collecting as well as research, has yet to be fully explored: Both
William's and John's publications contain many references to the assistance John rendered William. That their interests were close is
shown not only by their collections, but also by the frequent misiden-
tification of the one for the other, even in contemporaneous literature. As Broussonet wrote to Sir Joseph Banks in 1783: 'William
Hunter's place would have been filled by his brother, if he had not
been confused with him.'[12]

It is in their museums that the subsequent divergence of interests
between the two brothers can best be discerned. John's museum, 'his
great unwritten book', was explicit: the exposition of his new approach to the Animal Oeconomy, showing the interdependence of
structure and function.[13] As such, it has been much documented

5 J. Dobson, John Hunter (Edinburgh and London, 1969), pp. vii–xi.
6 C. H. Brock, ed., 'William Hunter: A Reassessment,' In S. F. Simmons and J.
Hunter, An Account of the Life and Writings of the Late William Hunter (1783) (Glasgow,
1983), pp. 45, 62.
7 Ibid., p. 63.
8 Vicq d'Azyr, 'Éloge historique: Hunter', in Oeuvres, 5 vols. (Paris, 1805), II, p.
382.
9 Brock, ed., William Hunter, p. 25, but see also S. J. Cross, 'John Hunter, the
Animal Oeconomy, and Late Eighteenth-Century Physiological Discourse', Studies in
the History of Biology, 5 (1981), n. 30.
10 Dobson, John Hunter, p. 36.
11 W. Hunter, 'Elephants' Bones', p. 37; Brock, ed., William Hunter, p. 19.
12 W. R. Dawson, ed., The Banks Letters (London, 1958), p. 155. Dr Helen Brock
tells me this refers to the place as foreign associate in the Académie Royale des
Sciences, made vacant by William Hunter's death. Brock, ed., William Hunter, pp.
xiii, 20.
13 Cross, 'Animal Oeconomy', pp. 1, 13. Dobson, John Hunter, p. 190.

since, so that his museum's original form and function are relatively well known.[14] William's museum, the outstanding collection of human anatomy and pathology, was largely extraordinary in its variety and extent.[15] It was brought to life as a teaching museum of anatomy, and it was through his school of anatomy, even more than through his writings, that William Hunter's great influence made itself felt.[16] The museum required his presence to bring it alive: 'At once simple and profound . . . subjects which were uninteresting in themselves were rendered interesting by the liveliness of his descriptions.'[17] When the collections were removed to Glasgow in 1807 they were inevitably disturbed, and the first subsequently produced catalogue of the museum was by an outsider unacquainted with Hunter's purposes.[18] Later catalogues[19] confirm the importance of the human anatomical series but give little indication of the original arrangement of the whole museum. Detailed analysis of the contemporary and Trustees MS catalogues of the museum has yet to be made, but Vicq d'Azyr's *Éloge*[20] gives hints of its comparative anatomical arrangement, in series of functions.

It is by these collections that William Hunter's interest in natural history is revealed, although the contemporary relevance of much of his material has still to be evaluated. Brock summarises the collections, which included material from the Cook voyages – insects arranged and first described by Fabricius, shells and other specimens collected by Banks's artist Parkinson and rocks in the form of tools or implements made by the natives.[21] With his purchase of Fothergill's collection, Hunter acquired a shell collection second only to that of

14 References in Cross, 'Animal Oeconomy', n. 31.
15 Brock, ed., *William Hunter*, p. 67.
16 J. H. Teacher, *Catalogue of the Anatomical and Pathological Preparations of Dr. William Hunter* (Glasgow, 1900), p. xxii.
17 Brodie in Teacher, *Catalogue*, p. lxvii. Vicq d'Azyr's 1805 eulogy records that by that date the museum 'had lost the great part of its merit. The precious and rare fragments that one admired there have not been arranged to meet the eye. Under the hand of William Hunter each was a centre of instruction and illumination. Surrounded by his museum, Hunter was more expert, and his collection itself took on a new aspect and inspired a new interest. Now, the chain of all these truths is broken; all is mute in this vast building [the Windmill Street house, museum, lecture theatre and dissecting room], where everything declares the loss of a great man' (Translation of Vicq d'Azyr, 'Éloge', p. 387).
18 J. Laskey, *A General Account of the Hunterian Museum, Glasgow* (Glasgow, 1813), devotes seventy-seven pages to listing the natural history collections or displays, twenty-three pages to human anatomy and only eighteen to other fields, showing the predominance of the subject from his point of view. Although post-Hunter additions had been made to the collections, they had occurred to most sections of the museum.
19 Cross, 'Animal Oeconomy', n. 30.
20 Vicq d'Azyr, 'Éloge', pp. 382–3.
21 C. H. Brock, 'Dr Hunter's South Seas Curiosities', *Scottish Art Review*, 14, no. 2 (1973), 6–9, 37–8; Brock, 'Hunter's Museum'; Brock, ed., *William Hunter*, pp. 24, 67–8.

the duchess of Portland and a coral collection that was 'the foremost in Europe'.[22] It also included the only currently recognisable shell from Tradescant's collection, as well as the second known specimen of a living crinoid.[23] Queen Charlotte gave Hunter specimens from her menagerie, including the corpse of the first nylgau seen in Britain, which had been depicted by Stubbs. A fuller account of the possible significance of some of his 'geological' collections is given by Durant and Rolfe.[24] Minerals formed a large part of his natural history collections, but he started collecting these only in about 1765. 'Before this he held such collections in contempt and was always out of humor with his Brother who had begun a collection of ores.'[25] Part of his interest lay in medical mineralogy, perhaps inculcated by his teacher Cullen. Most of his minerals were obtained by purchase from the leading European dealers of the day, notably Jacob Forster and Peter Woulfe. Far from being a collection of mere curios, his collections and library were sought out by contemporary scholars. Although the specimens were valuable, he encouraged analysis of them, as by Fordyce in studying the chemical composition of minerals, and by Bedford in classifying iron ores. Many of these collections recognisably reflect current issues of the day, such as the volcanist debate. His fossil collection was relatively small but significant, (as will be seen in the section entitled 'Mastodon, Moose and Extinction'). Almost nothing is known of his herbarium of thousands of plants.

The Great Chain of Being

In the following account a selection of William Hunter's collections will be used to illustrate links in the Chain of Being. According to this concept a continuous chain extended from inert matter and stones, through laminated stones and plants via zoophytes eventually to Quadrupeds, Man and through the Realms of Angels to God (Figs. 10.1, 10.2).[26]

The idea has its roots in Aristotle's notion of continuity and gradation between adjacent kinds of being when hierarchically arranged, and in Plato's principle of plenitude – that all the possible kinds of things exist. 'It gained particular biological significance in the eighteenth century through its endorsement in the writings of Leibniz,

22 J. C. Lettsom, *Memoirs of J. Fothergill*, 4th ed. (London, 1786), p. 55.
23 J. Ellis, 'An account of an Encrinus &c', *Philosophical Transactions of the Royal Society of London*, 52 (1762), 357–62.
24 G. P. Durant and W. D. I. Rolfe, 'William Hunter (1718–1783) as Natural Historian: His "Geological" Interests', *Earth Sciences History* 3 (1984), 9–24.
25 Brock, ed., *William Hunter*, p. 24.
26 A. O. Lovejoy, *The Great Chain of Being* (Cambridge, Mass., 1936); P. C. Ritterbush, *Overtures to Biology* (New Haven, Conn., and London, 1964), p. 71.

IDEA OF A SCALE OF NATURAL BEINGS.

BY M. BONNET.

Man.

Orang-outang
Monkey

Quadrupeds.

Flying fquirrel
Bat
Oftrich

Birds.

Aquatic bird
Amphibious bird
Flying fifh

Fifh.

Creeping fifh
Eel
Water-ferpents

Reptiles.

Slug
Snail

Snails (with fhells)

Pipe-worms
Moth

Infects.

Gall-infects
Tape-worm
Polypus
Sea-nettle
Senfitive plant

Plants.

Lichens
Mouldinefs
Mufhrooms
Truffles
Coral
Lithophytes
Amianthes
Talcs, Gypfums, Selenites
Slate

Stones

Figured ftones
Chryftallized ftones

Salts.

Vitriols

Metals.

Semi-metals

Brimftone.

Bitumens

Earths.

Pure Earth

Water.

Air.

Fire.

More Subtile Matter

Fig. 10.1. Bonnet's Ladder of Being (1764), as translated by White. In White's 1799 original, the right hand-column continued below that on the left. In Bonnet's 1779 version, the words occupy spaces between the rungs of a typographical ladder.

Buffon and Bonnet.'[27] Bonnet's version of the Chain[28] is shown in Figure 10.1.

To view some of Hunter's natural history collections from the standpoint of the Great Chain of Being is not to imply that William Hunter necessarily regarded his own collections in this light. The Chain does, however, form a convenient framework by which to order this account. Nevertheless, with his interest in earlier views of medicine, evinced so well by his library,[29] Hunter would probably have known of traditional notions of the 'graduating' of medicine,[30] which are in turn related to the *Scala natura* or the Chain of Being. The medieval belief in the value of contemplation of the 'Scale of Nature as a vehicle whereon . . . we may ascend to God' (Fig. 10.2)[31] was abandoned only in the early eighteenth century. The principle of plenitude suggested 'man's duty was to keep *his* place, and not to seek to transcend it'.[32]

Although allegiance to the Chain continued throughout the eighteenth century, new progressivist thinking inspired scientists to "temporalise" the Chain and view it as a ladder that organisms might climb rather than a rigid ranking of immutable entities. This new view of nature penetrated everywhere (Fig. 10.3).[33] As Condorcet wrote in

27 P. Sloan, 'Chain of Being', in W. F. Bynum and R. S. Porter (eds.), *Dictionary of the History of Science* (London, 1981), p. 63. Full details of the Great Chain concept and its implications are set out in Lovejoy's *The Great Chain of Being*. Supplementary accounts to this work are given by E. M. W. Tillyard, *The Elizabethan World Picture* (London, 1943); Ritterbush, *Overtures*; W. F. Bynum, 'The Great Chain of Being after Forty Years: An Appraisal', *History of Science*, 13 (1975), 1–28; S. J. Gould, *Ontogeny and Phylogeny* (Cambridge, Mass., 1977), pp. 23–8, 34, 36; 'Bound by the Great Chain' and 'Chimp on the Chain', *Natural History*, 92, no. 11 (Nov. 1983), 20–4 and no. 12 (Dec. 1983), 18–27; and E. Mayr, *The Growth of Biological Thought* (Cambridge, Mass., 1982), pp. 18, 201–2, 326–7. See also Cross, 'Animal Oeconomy', n. 64.
28 C. White, *An Account of the Regular Gradation in Man, and in Different Animals and Vegetables; and from the Former to the Latter* (London, 1799), pp. 17, 18.
29 J. Baldwin, *William Hunter 1718–1783 Book Collector* (exhibition catalogue) (Glasgow, 1983); M. Ferguson, *The Printed Books in the Library of the Hunterian Museum in the University of Glasgow: A Catalogue* (Glasgow, 1930); N. R. Ker, *William Hunter as a Collector of Medieval Manuscripts* (Glasgow, 1983); Young and Aitken, *Catalogue of Manuscripts*.
30 F. A. Yates, 'The Art of Ramon Lull', *Journal of the Warburg & Courtauld Institutes*, 17 (1954), 144; and in *Lull & Bruno, Collected Essays* (London, Boston and Henley, 1982), p. 42.
31 Illustration: Yates, 'Ramon Lull', plate 14a; F. A. Yates, *The Art of Memory* (London, 1966), fig. 4; Yates, *Lull & Bruno*, plate 7a. Statement in caption: Lovejoy, *Great Chain of Being*, p. 92.
32 Lovejoy, *Great Chain of Being*, p. 200.
33 D. V. Erdman, J. E. Grant, E. J. Rose and M. J. Tolley, *William Blake's Designs for Edward Young's 'Night Thoughts', A Complete Edition*, 2 vols. (Oxford, 1980), II, colour plate NT258; Lovejoy, *Great Chain of Being*, p. 80; M. D. Paley, 'Blake's "Night Thoughts", An Exploration of the Fallen World', in A. H. Rosenfeld (ed.), *William Blake Essays for S. Foster Damon* (Providence, R.I., 1969), p. 148.

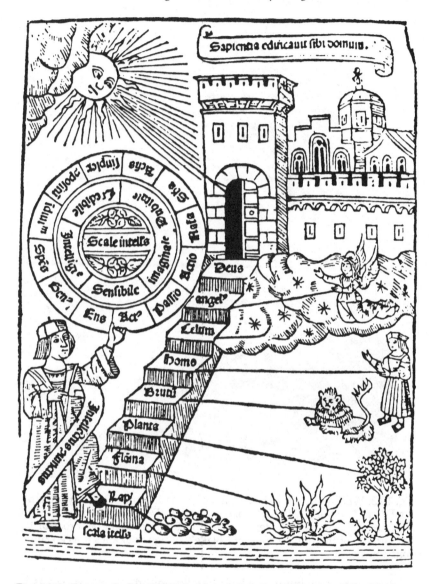

Fig. 10.2. Ramon Lull's (1305) *Ladder of Ascent and Descent of the Mind,* as depicted in the first printed edition of 1512. Although it incorporates an abbreviated Chain of Being, such a ladder was intended to lead contemplation upwards to the One, not to preoccupation with the Many, steps of created things.

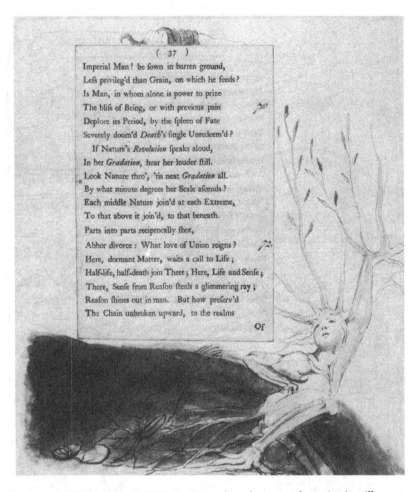

(37)

Imperial Man ! be fown in barren ground,
Lefs privileg'd than Grain, on which he feeds ?
Is Man, in whom alone is power to prize
The blifs of Being, or with previous pain
Deplore its Period, by the fpleen of Fate
Severely doom'd *Death*'s fingle Unredeem'd ?
     If Nature's *Revolution* fpeaks aloud,
In her *Gradation*, hear her louder ftill.
Look Nature thro', 'tis neat *Gradation* all.
By what minute degrees her Scale afcends ?
Each middle Nature join'd at each Extreme,
To that above it join'd, to that beneath.
Parts into parts reciprocally fhot,
     Abhor divorce : What love of Union reigns ?
Here, dormant Matter, waits a call to Life ;
Half-life, half-death join There ; Here, Life and Senfe ;
There, Senfe from Reafon fteals a glimmering ray ;
Reafon fhines out in man. But how preferv'd
The Chain unbroken upward, to the realms
                                                      Of

Fig. 10.3. William Blake's 1795–7 vision of gradation and continuity, illustrating Edward Young's 1745 *Night Thoughts on Life, Death and Immortality* (Night VI, lines 707–25). Young's text praises the Chain of Being as proof of the immortality of the human soul, but Blake's design embodies it as a state of consciousness.

1793:' The perfectability of Man is really boundless; the progress of this perfectability, henceforth independent of any power that would arrest it, has no other limit than the duration of the globe where nature has set us.'[34]

> When minds ascend,
> Progress, in part, depends upon themselves . . .

34   Gould, *Ontogeny*, p. 34.

O be a man! and thou shalt be a god!
And half self-made! Ambition how divine![35]

Calculi

Calculi are often inert, laminated stones forming concretions in the body that must have seemed to connect lower regions of the Chain with higher regions. Over many years – dated drawings indicate at least from 1764 to 1778 – Hunter was amassing records for an account of bodily concretions or calculi. His brother John experimented with the formation of calculi and communicated the results to William, who taught them to his pupils in 1761.[36] Unfortunately, William Hunter's manuscript on this topic seems to have been lost, perhaps during the period of Baillie's use of the museum, 1783–1807.[37] Baillie's interest in this topic is shown by his providing Wollaston[38] with a calculus for his work. Many of William Hunter's calculi still exist in the Hunterian Museum's pathological collections at Glasgow's Royal Infirmary.[39] The three volumes of superb drawings of calculi, many of them by Jan van Rymsdyk,[40] together with proofs of the twenty-one etched plates and most of the plates themselves, are preserved in the Hunterian Library (T.3.7–9). One of these hitherto unpublished plates is included here (Fig. 10.4).[41] It shows the high quality of William Hunter's work, which was not to be equalled until the production of the 1845 *Catalogue of Calculi* in his brother's museum at the Royal College of Surgeons, London. The pre-eminence of the latter collection was recognised by the transfer to it, early in the nineteenth century, of the British Museum's calculi, including Sir Hans Sloane's own material.

Undoubtedly, Hunter's prime interest in such concretions was medical – calculi were a widespread cause of illness at the time, because of dietary deficiencies, particularly of vitamin A. As a contemporary writer put it:

No malady entail'd upon human creatures, more frequently
occurs; no disease carries along with it more excrutiating

35 Young (1745), *Night* IX, lines 1993–8, see Lovejoy *Great Chain of Being*, p. 263.
36 J. F. Palmer, ed., *The Works of John Hunter, F.R.S.*, 4 vols. (London, 1835), II, p. 42.
37 Brock, ed., *William Hunter*, pp. 22, 39–40.
38 W. H. Wollaston, 'On Gouty and Urinary Concretions', *Philosophical Transactions of the Royal Society of London*, 87 (1797), 395.
39 Teacher, *Catalogue*, pp. lxi, 858–937.
40 Cf. Thornton, *Rymsdyk*.
41 Teacher, *Catalogue*, p. 908 (no. 53.53) and p. 929 (no. 53.137) respectively; Young and Aitken, *Catalogue of Manuscripts*, p. 450.

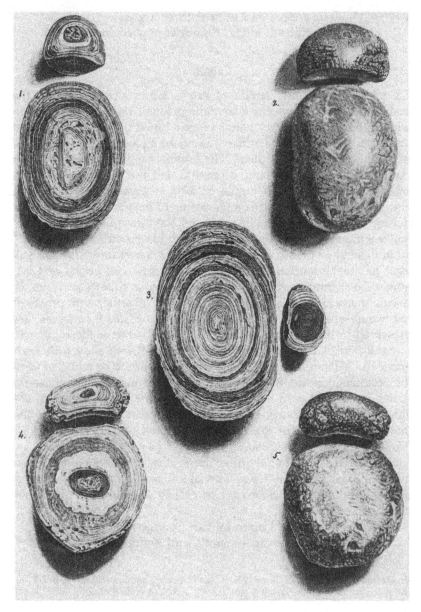

Fig. 10.4 Urinary calculi, printer's proof of plate 12 from William Hunter's unpublished work on calculi. 1, 2, uric acid bladder calculi; 4, 5, mixed-phosphate bladder calculi – the 'fusible calculus' of Wollaston. Glasgow University Hunterian Library T.3.9.

torture, nor a more formidable train of symptoms; neither is any cure attended in more barbarous circumstances, than that of freeing persons from the attack of stony, petrify'd substances found in the cavity of human bladders, by the only effectual means hitherto known; to wit, the operation of Lythotomy.[42]

It was another of the topics in which Hunter inherited his interest, as well as much literature, from his mentor, James Douglas.[43] The possible connection of this subject with views on the formation of fossils – a connection that John Hunter maintained in comparing the fossilisation of wood with the formation of calculi[44],– requires exploration. Rudwick has drawn attention to the pervasiveness in the sixteenth century of the 'stoniness' problem and the important analogy of the growth of stones in the body with fossils in the ground: microcosm and macrocosm.[45] Lhwyd expressed a similar view in the late seventeenth century and linked it with monstrosities.[46] The latter were to be utilised in Diderot's 1749 theory of nature's self-creative dynamism: 'All matter quick and bursting into birth'.[47] Diderot proposed, and reiterated in his 1769 *d'Alembert's Dream*, 'a more or less continu-

42   Anon., *A Dissertation on the Stone in the Bladder* (London, 1738), p. 8. Hunter had a good library on mineral waters, part of which was relevant to the search for a calculus solvent; T. Short, *A General Treatise on the Different Sorts of Cold-Mineral Waters in England . . . to Which is Added an Account of Several Experiments Made in Search After a Solvent of the Human Calculus . . .* (London, 1766); Durant and Rolfe, 'William Hunter . . . His Geological Interests'. Shortly after having learned the technique at Monro's lectures, William Hunter gave soap as a lithontriptic; J. Parsons, *A Description of the Human Urinary Bladder* (London, 1742). See also A. J. Viseltear, 'Joanna Stephens and the Eighteenth Century Lithontriptics', *Bulletin of the History of Medicine*, 42 (1968), 199–220. 'The great Hunter' is also recorded as bathing, something that caused his contemporaries to view the activity as more than a simple luxury (A. Leitzmann and C. Schuddekopf, eds., *Briefe – G. C. Lichtenberg*, 3 vols. [Hildesheim, 1966], III, p. 100), a view that Tobias Smollett (*An Essay on the External Use of Water* [London, 1752]) would have shared.
43   Thornton, *Rymsdyk*, p. 23; Young and Aitken, *Catalogue of Manuscripts*, nn. 522–4. Douglas devised a widely adopted operation for the stone, and it is worth noting that at least one of Hunter's pupils, Charles White, became a noted lithotomist (*Dictionary of National Biography*).
44   J. Hunter, *Observations and Reflections on Geology* (London, 1859), p. xl. Amongst the few extraneous fossils in the trustees' 1790s catalogue of William Hunter's minerals is a collection of fossil woods. This included Lough Neagh wood, purchased at Richard Mead's sale in 1754, which was the subject of much contemporary discussion of the fossilisation question; see J. Hill, *Natural History of Fossils* (London, 1748), p. 639.
45   M. J. S. Rudwick, *The Meaning of Fossils* (London and New York, 1972), pp. 24–5.
46   J. Raven, *John Ray, Naturalist* (Cambridge, 1942), pp. 436–7.
47   L. G. Crocker, 'Diderot and Eighteenth Century French Transformism', in B. Glass, O. Temkin and W. L. Straus (eds.), *Forerunners of Darwin 1745–1859* (Baltimore, 1959), p. 120; A. Pope, *Essay on Man* (London, 1733), line 234.

ous form of generation that could produce complex organic structures directly from matter at almost any time'.[48] It is in this context then that Hunter's own collection of monsters is to be viewed, together with his comment on them:

> Even monsters, and all uncommon, and all diseased animal productions, are useful in anatomical enquiries; as the mechanism, or texture, which is concealed in the ordinary fashion of parts, may be obvious in a preternatural composition. And it may be said, that nature, in thus varying and multiplying her productions, has hung out a train of lights that guide us through her labyrinth.[49]

In Hunter's day, Maupertuis believed life resided in the simplest forms of matter[50] and that fossils and metals lay 'in that uncertain frontier region where one does not know whether one ought to speak of life or not'.[51] The history of science of calculi has yet to be written, but Hunter's work pre-dates that which led to the important work of geologist Wollaston[52] and the discovery of uric acid in calculi by Scheele in 1776.

Corals

Corals seemed to provide a key link in the Chain of Being, between the inert and living worlds.[53] They literally played a constructive role in Whitehurst's 1778 *Theory of the Earth*.[54] Some years earlier, however, Ellis (1755) had been the first to show that corals and zoophytes were true animals,[55] and it was this significant collection that Hunter obtained from Dr John Fothergill after the latter's death in 1780.[56] As 'rock which grew', corals reiterated the 'stoniness' problem and, significantly, had been compared with calculi.[57] A special room was

48 P. J. Bowler, 'Evolutionism in the Enlightenment', *Journal of the History of Ideas*, 12 (1974), 163.
49 W. Hunter, *Two Introductory Lectures Delivered by Dr. William Hunter to his Last Course of Anatomical Lectures at his Theatre in Windmill Street* (London, 1784), p. 4.
50 Cross, 'Animal Oeconomy', p. 39, n. 126.
51 M. Foucault, *The Order of Things* (London, 1970), pp. 161–2, 232.
52 Wollaston, 'Gouty Concretions', pp. 386–400.
53 Crocker, 'Diderot', pp. 116, 117, 134; Ritterbush, *Overtures*, pp. 113, 127–34.
54 B. Smith, *European Vision and the South Pacific 1768–1850* (Oxford, 1960), p. 74; Durant and Rolfe, 'William Hunter . . . His Geological Interests'.
55 J. Ellis, *An Essay towards the Natural History of the Corallines* (London, 1755).
56 In 1768, Fothergill had written to Hunter advising him how to clean and mount these specimens, promising him that 'some are reserved for Dr Hunter's museum when it is ready to receive them'; B. C. Corner and C. C. Booth, *Chain of Friendship* (Cambridge, Mass., 1971), p. 282.
57 R. Porter, *The Making of Geology* (Cambridge, 1977), pp. 49–50.; L. Clendening, *Source Book of Medical History* (New York, 1960), pp. 247–50.

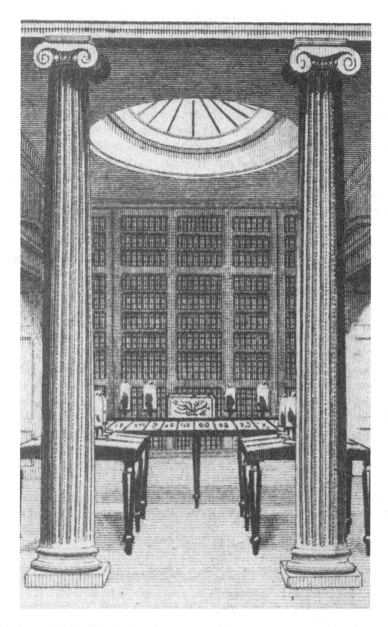

Fig. 10.5. Detail of early nineteenth-century bookplate for the Hunterian Library, showing a fan-coral from Fothergill's collection occupying pride of place in the library of the 1807 Hunterian Museum at Glasgow University. Other corals can be seen 'placed up and down the museum, covered with glass bells', as recommended to Hunter by Fothergill in 1768. Here also was displayed the second known specimen of a living crinoid.

planned in 1804 to house them in Glasgow University's purpose-built Hunterian Museum (Fig. 10.5).[58]

Mastodon, moose and extinction

For centuries, the principle of plenitude, one of the unit ideas in the Chain of Being, made the possibility of extinction unthinkable. Hooke claimed in the seventeenth century that ammonites were extinct organisms, but argued that this maintained the theory of plenitude, rather than destroying it. This did not convince his contemporaries, however: Both Lister and Ray argued against his view.[59] Furthermore, those organisms were a long way down the *Scala naturae*. Strong, large, powerful and useful creatures like the elephant and horse were high in the Chain of Being.[60]

Buffon's 1761 suggestion that the fossil elephant from the Ohio River was extinct,[61] was therefore of great importance. However, almost immediately, in 1762 Daubenton tried to disprove the suggestion by showing that the tusks and femora of the fossils were like those of the one living elephant species then recognised. The isolated, aberrant teeth were explained away as being admixed hippopotamus teeth, and by 1764 Buffon had accepted Daubenton's view that the fossils were the same as living elephants.[62] Voltaire also attacked the concept of the Chain of Being:[63] 'Continuity is nowhere evidenced in nature. Let the proof of that be that there are extinct species in both animal and vegetable kingdoms'.[64] He also accepted that species might be exterminated by man: 'If the rest of the world imitated the English, there would be no more wolves on Earth.'[65] But despite such an attack, as well as that by Dr Johnson in 1757, the concept continued to operate powerfully. It was against this background that William Hunter wrote his *Ohio incognitum* (mastodon) paper in 1767. He differed from Daubenton, showing the femora of the fossil and living elephants to be quite different. Furthermore, he

---

58 Laskey, *Hunterian Museum*, pp. 86–7, 106–8.
59 Rudwick, *Meaning of Fossils*, p. 65.
60 W. Lynskey, 'Goldsmith and the Chain of Being', *Journal of the History of Ideas*, 6 (1945), 363–74.
61 A point picked up by Goldsmith in his introduction to Brooke's 1763 *Natural History* (A. Friedman, *Collected Works of Oliver Goldsmith*, 5 vols. [Oxford, 1966], V, p. 238).
62 Buffon, G.-L. Leclerc, Comte de, *Histoire naturelle, générale et particulière*, vol. 13 (Paris, 1764); J. C. Greene, *The Death of Adam* (Ames, Iowa, 1959), pp. 100–1.
63 Lovejoy, *Great Chain of Being*, p. 252.
64 L. Formigari, 'Chain of Being', in *Dictionary of the History of Ideas*, 5 vols. (New York, 1968), I, pp. 329–30.
65 Lovejoy, *Great Chain of Being*, p. 252.

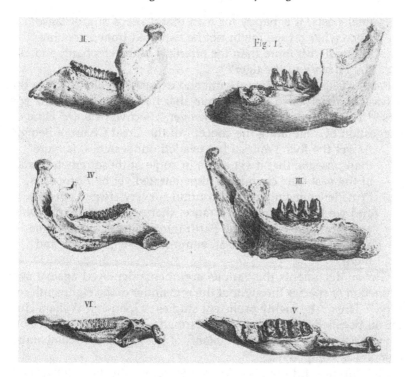

Fig. 10.6. William Hunter's 1768 illustration of a fossil mastodon jaw with the teeth *in situ* (I, III, V), for comparison with a recent elephant's jaw from John Hunter's collection (II, IV, VI). The engravings are reversed from Rymsdyk's original drawings, which are preserved in the Hunterian Library (Glasgow University HF 92).

found one of the supposed hippopotamus teeth *in situ* in an *Ohio incognitum* jaw in the British Museum. By publishing a drawing of the fossil jaw alongside that of a living elephant, Hunter made the difference in the *Ohio incognitum* inescapable (Fig. 10.6).[66] He therefore concluded that 'though we may as philosophers regret it, as men we cannot but thank Heaven that its whole generation is probably extinct'.[67]

Goldsmith rewrote this in his own inimitable way:

It is the opinion of Doctor Hunter that the [fossil teeth] must have belonged to a larger animal than the elephant; and differing from it, in being carnivorous. But as yet this formidable creature has evaded our search; and if, indeed, such an an-

66 Durant and Rolfe, 'William Hunter . . . His Geological Interests', fig. 1.
67 W. Hunter, 'Elephants' Bones', p. 45.

imal exists, it is happy for man that it keeps at a distance;
since what ravage might not be expected from a creature,
endued with more than the strength of the elephant, and all
the rapacity of the tiger![68]

Raspe visited Hunter's museum and expressed Voltaire's idea that
it was the destructive hand of man that had exterminated the species.[69] The influential Pennant, however, effectively denied Hunter's
suggestion by reiterating the concept of the Great Chain of Being:[70]

As yet the living animal has evaded our search; it is more
than possible that it yet exists in some of those remote parts
of the vast new continent, unpenetrated yet by Europeans.
Providence maintains and continues every created species;
and we have as much assurance, that no race of animals will
any more cease while the Earth remaineth, than seed time
and harvest, cold and heat, summer and winter, day and
night.[71]

Greene documents the various arguments deployed against such
extinction of species throughout the remainder of the eighteenth century.[72] Thus, 'the highly proficient studies of John and William Hunter on petrified mammalian remains made little impact for lack of a
community with the requisite blend of geological and comparative
anatomical competences'.[73]

That Hunter did not abandon the topic of extinction, however, is
shown by a paper he wrote between 1770 and 1773, intended for the
Royal Society, on moose and Irish 'elk'.[74] The paper also explains
why, in 1770, Hunter commissioned the artist George Stubbs to depict the first bull moose to enter England. It had always been thought
that William Hunter, like his brother John, was interested in such
novelties for their own sake, as exemplified by his 1771 nylgau de-

68   O. Goldsmith, *A History of the Earth and Animated Nature*, 8 vols. (London, 1774),
IV, pp. 283–4. On predation and the Great Chain, see P. Fuller, 'Variations on a
Theme', *New Society*, 70(1140) (1984), 139–40.
69   R. E. Raspe, 'Dissertatio epistolaris de ossibus et dentibus elephantum, aliarum-
que Belluarum in America Septentrionali', *Philosophical Transactions of the Royal Society
of London*, 59 (1769), 126–37; Raspe, *An Account of Some German Volcanos, and Their
Productions with a New Hypothesis of the Prismatical Basaltes: Established upon Facts*
(London, 1776).
70   T. Pennant, *Synopsis of Quadrupeds* (Chester, 1771), p. 192.
71   This possibility of survival in remote regions is, inevitably, a hardy perennial. It
has recently been exhumed to suggest the existence of mammoths in the northern
USSR; H. Bowser, 'When Elephants Roamed the Ranges', *Science Digest*, 19, no. 6
(June 1983), 66.
72   Greene, *Death of Adam*, pp. 106–33. See also L. B. Miller, 'Charles Willson Peale
as History Painter: *The Exhumation of the Mastodon*', *American Art Journal*, 13 (Winter
1981), 47–68.
73   Porter, *Making of Geology*, p. 167.
74   Rolfe, 'Stubbs's Moose'; Rolfe, 'A Stubbs Drawing'.

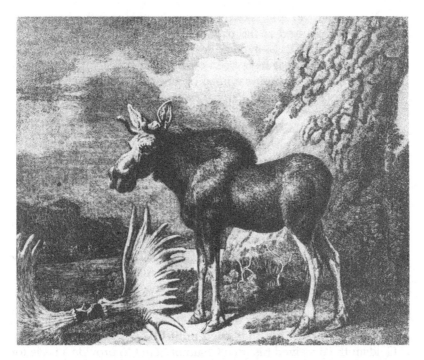

Fig. 10.7. Mazell's 1783 etching of Stubbs's 1770 painting, commissioned by William Hunter, of the first bull moose to enter Britain. The adult moose antlers in the foreground were provided to show their difference from the fossil Irish 'elk' antlers depicted by Molyneux in 1697.

scription, but it is now obvious that his interest in the moose lay much deeper.

Since 1697, opinion had favoured Molyneux's view 'concerning the large horns frequently found under ground in Ireland, concluding from them that the great American deer called a Moose, was formerly common in that island'. The moose, like the European elk, was poorly known in eighteenth-century England, and Hunter found it impossible to decide whether they were different animals. He was highly critical of the illustrations published by the French Academicians in 1671, and of those published by Buffon in 1764. Stubbs's picture was thus the first accurate portrayal of a moose. In the foreground of the picture the artist depicted a pair of adult moose antlers (Fig. 10.7).[75] As Hunter put it:

75 From T. Pennant, *Arctic Zoology*, 2 vols. (London, 1785), I, plate viii. Molyneux's illustration is reproduced in S. J. Gould, *Ever Since Darwin, Reflections in Natural History* (New York, 1978), p. 80; Rolfe, 'Stubbs's *Moose*', fig. 10.

Now, whoever will take the trouble to compare the horns
upon the ground of the picture with the figure of the Irish
horns which Dr. Molyneux has published will see that the
two animals must have been of different species . . . The Irish
Deer then was a noble animal of an unknown species, which
like the American elephant or *incognitum* is still now probably
extinct.[76]

Hunter never published his paper, however, because he could not
be certain that Irish 'elk' were not still living in the depths of western
Canada, in the form of an animal called the 'waskesser' as Pennant
had suggested in 1771. Although he drew up a questionnaire that
might have produced the answers to settle the matter, it is unclear
whether this was ever circulated. Hunter permitted Pennant to have
an etching made of Stubbs's painting of the moose for him to use in
his 1785 *Arctic Zoology*. Ironically, Pennant was the first to accept that
the Irish 'elk' was no longer living in Canada: The myth was probably
based on the largest living subspecies – the Alaskan moose *Alces alces
gigas* Miller. Hunter's prophecy of the Irish elk's extinction was therefore correct, but a morphological account comparable in detail to that
prepared by Hunter, *proving* the uniqueness of the giant Irish deer, as
it is now called, was not published until 1812, by Cuvier.

Goldsmith conceived his own Chain of Being to provide a basis for
the organisation of his *Animated Nature* (1774),[77] a work that is basically rewritten extracts, mainly from Buffon, Brookes, Pennant, Willughby and Pluche.[78] At the head of his chain was either the horse,
judged according to its usefulness to man, or the elephant, based on
its size and sagacity. Indeed, the elephant was 'the most sagacious
animal next to man . . . in every respect the noblest quadrupede in
nature'. Elk (i.e., moose) is listed with deer, fourth down Goldsmith's

76 Rolfe, 'Stubbs's *Moose*', p. 276.
77 Goldsmith, a great promoter of the Chain concept in his popular writings of
1763 and 1774 (Friedman, *Goldsmith*), was Professor of Ancient History at the Royal
Academy from 1770 to 1774, whilst William Hunter was Professor of Anatomy (J. M.
Oppenheimer, 'John and William Hunter and some Contemporaries in Literature
and Art', *Bulletin of the History of Medicine* 23 [1949], 27; S. C. Hutchison, *The History
of the Royal Academy 1768–1968* [London, 1968], p. 236). Tobias Smollett, an even
closer friend of William Hunter (J. M. Oppenheimer, 'A Note on William Hunter
and Tobias Smollett', *Journal of the History of Medicine*, 2 [1947], 481–6), is reputed to
have written the lengthy footnote dismissing the Chain concept, in his translation of
Voltaire's 1757 poem *The Lisbon Earthquake* (B. R. Redman, ed., *The Portable Voltaire*
[Harmondsworth, 1977], pp. 560–2). In fact, that footnote is by Voltaire and I have
been unable to trace the poem, or his *Philosophical Dictionary* entry on 'Chain of
Created Beings', in Smollett's *Works of Mr. Voltaire* 1761–5. It is therefore uncertain if
Smollett would have known of it, or discussed its implications with Hunter.
78 W. Lynskey, 'The Scientific Sources of Goldsmith's *Animated Nature*', *Studies in
Philology*, 40 (1943), 33–57; Lynskey, 'Goldsmith and the Chain'.

scale headed by the horse, and it may be significant that he mentions 'the Elk; the size of which, from current testimony, appears to be equal to that of the elephant itself'.[79]

Breaking the Great Chain

With these demonstrations of extinction, one published and one in manuscript, Hunter thus broke the Great Chain of Being twice – and at the high level of quadrupeds.[80] In both papers, he prefaced his use of 'extinct' by 'probably', a wise precaution should the animals indeed be found in unexplored regions. He had good reason to be circumspect on this crucial point since he knew of the living crinoid described only shortly after the first such specimen had been found.[81] This discovery vindicated Ray's opinion in the seventeenth century that such animals, known hitherto only from fossils, 'may be lodged so deep in the seas . . . that they may never come in sight' – a possibility reiterated in 1809 by Lamarck.[82] Hunter eventually acquired the specimen described by Ellis, as part of Fothergill's collection, in 1780. It was understood that Hunter would acquire Fothergill's collection long before then, however, as a letter of 1768 indicates.[83]

Hunter's proof of extinction broke the Chain in all three of its unit ideas: plenitude, continuity and gradation. The philosophical repercussions of this were profound, as Pope had foreseen in his *Essay on Man*:[84]

> Vast chain of being! which from God began,
> Natures ethereal, human, angel, man,
> Beast, bird, fish, insect, what no eye can see,
> No glass can reach; from infinite to thee,
> From thee to nothing. – On superior powers
> Were we to press, inferior might on ours;
> Or in the full creation leave a void,
> Where, one step broken, the great scale's destroy'd:
> From Nature's chain whatever link you strike,
> Tenth, or tenth thousandth, breaks the chain alike.

79 Goldsmith, *Animated Nature*, IV, pp. 252–3; II, p. 303, III, p. 140.
80 It may be significant that Hunter chose to work on two such large animals – moose, the largest terrestrial mammal of North America and Europe, and mastodon. Buffon's 'greatest fact', his theory of degeneration, was being actively discussed at that time (Rolfe, 'Stubbs's *Moose*', n. 54).
81 Ellis, 'Account of an Encrinus'.
82 Greene, *Death of Adam*, p. 97. Rudwick, *Meaning of Fossils*, pp. 63, 89. Mayr, *Growth of Biological Thought*, p. 348.
83 Corner and Booth, *Chain of Friendship*, pp. 281–3.
84 Lovejoy, *Great Chain of Being*, p. 60.

This is not to imply that William Hunter consciously set out to break the chain, or that he entertained religious doubts as a result of his discovery. Many quotations in Hunter's writings testify to his continued belief in God: 'Astronomy and Anatomy, as Fontenelle observes, offer a most striking view of two of the greatest attributes of the Supreme Being. The first gives an idea of his immensity, the last astonishes with his intelligence and art, in the variety and delicacy of animal mechanism.'[85]

I know of no explicit mention of the Chain in William Hunter's writings. John Hunter, however, 'had a keen awareness of the scale of beings'. He had a self-consciously new approach to comparative anatomy, based on graded series of organs that emphasised physiological *functions*, as a key factor in the life of animals and plants.[86] John was a keen exponent of gradation, one of the three key concepts in the Chain of Being, and this is epitomised by the series of skulls in the background to his portrait by Reynolds[87] (Fig. 10.8).[88] Although

85 W. Hunter, *Introductory Lectures*, p. 63.
86 Cross, 'Animal Oeconomy', pp. 10, 13, 66.
87 The series of skulls from human to crocodile in Reynolds's 1786 portrait (Cross, 'Animal Oeconomy', n. 51) is essentially the same as that chosen in 1799 by Charles White (*Gradation in Man*) to show the Chain of Being. White (ibid., p. 144, n. 7) refers to an engraving of this portrait as indicating John Hunter's ideas of gradation. This and Camper's 1791 *Dissertation* were the inspiration for White's own depiction (recently reproduced: Gould 'Bound by the Great Chain', p. 20; Ritterbush, *Overtures*, plate 7) with its emphasis on Camper's facial angle. White was led to his own views from having heard 'Mr. John Hunter's remarks on the gradation of skulls, as he stated in the introduction to the course of lectures on midwifery, which he delivered last winter at the Lying-in hospital in Manchester' (White, *Gradation in Man*, p. iii). This cannot therefore be brother John, who died in 1793 (see Cross, 'Animal Oeconomy', n. 64); it is the Dr John Hunter who lived *c.* 1730–1809 (T. Bendysshe, *The Anthropological Treatises of Johann Friedrich Blumenbach* [London, 1865], p. 359; *Dictionary of National Biography*. Cf. A. Keith, 'A Discourse on the Portraits and Personality of John Hunter', *British Medical Journal* 1 [1928], 207). White, however, was a friend of our John Hunter and was a fellow student with him under William Hunter in 1748–9. His notes of those lectures have been published: N. Dowd, *Hunter's Lectures of Anatomy* (Amsterdam, London, New York, 1972).
   Although John Hunter's manuscript on gradation was destroyed by Home (J. Hunter, *Essays and Observations on Natural History, Anatomy, Physiology and Geology*, 2 vols. [London, 1861], II, p. 495), Clift's transcripts survive to give an idea of Hunter's views. In his section 'On the origin of species,' Hunter wrote: 'Does not the natural gradation of animals, from one to another, lead to the original species? And does not that mode of investigation gradually lead to the knowledge of that species? Are we not led on to the wolf by the gradual affinity of the different varieties in the dog?' (J. Hunter, *Essays*, I, p. 37). This should not be read in a later, fully evolutionary sense, but as an attempt to discover the original species from which existing species had been derived (Cross, 'Animal Oeconomy', nn. 51, 57). It is perhaps an early expression of the new form of essentialism that was to flourish in the idealistic morphology and *Urbilden* of the *Naturphilosophen* (Mayr, *Growth of Biological Thought*, pp. 38, 457–8; Ritterbush, *Overtures*, pp. 208–9).
88 For caption up to last sentence: J. Hunter, *Essays*, I, p. 37. For last sentence of caption: Palmer, *Works of John Hunter*, IV, pp. 236, 237, 239, 245.

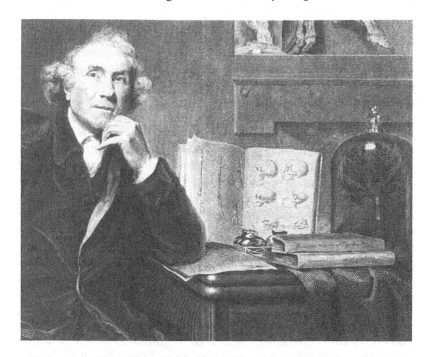

Fig. 10.8. John Hunter's view of gradation, epitomised by 'hands' and skulls: a detail from William Sharp's 1788 engraving of Reynolds's 1786 portrait of John Hunter (Hunterian Art Gallery). According to Keith the skull series runs from European human and Australian aboriginal (top) through chimpanzee and macaque monkey (middle) to dog and crocodile (bottom). The 'hands' run horse, ox, pig (top) and dog, monkey, man (bottom). The two juxtaposed sequences may illustrate Hunter's point that 'the declension of animals from the Human to the brute, or more distant brute, is faster in the head . . . than in the four extremities'. Furthermore, although 'the declension of animals from the most perfect to the most imperfect is in regular order or progression . . . it is far from being an equal one'. The reversal of the two sequences on the facing pages may be significant, although Hunter stated that the 'more perfect animals have compounded joints' and actions, as in the human hand.

John used the linear chain for sequences of *organs*, he rejected its applicability to a chain of *beings*.[89] He found that the sense of progression derived from any one organ system, and traced from one major animal group to another, could be reversed if another organ system was selected.[90] William would have known intimately of this work, which occupied much of John's life and which started early on in his

89 Cross, 'Animal Oeconomy', pp. 19, 26; Ritterbush, *Overtures*, pp. 194–5.
90 Vicq d'Azyr made a similar point in 1774 and White's (1799) linear chain was made possible only by a series of evasions (Gould, 'Bound by the Great Chain', p. 23).

318   W. D. Ian Rolfe

own dissecting rooms.[91] John, therefore, also played a part in falsifying the concept of the Chain.[92]

J. F. Blumenbach was acquainted with the Hunters' work and shared many of their views.[93] He accepted two periods of extinction and had explicitly discarded the Chain of Being and its social implications by the late eighteenth century.[94] Cuvier brought together and enlarged the examples of extinction in fossil vertebrates[95] and put an end to the debate about the reality of extinction. In 1809, Lamarck suggested an evolutionary solution to the problem: 'that the fossils in question belonged to species still existing, but which have changed since that time, and have been converted into the similar species that we now actually find'.[96] Nevertheless, it was well into the nineteenth century before the Chain was abandoned as an intellectual framework. Even then, its influence can be discerned in Owen, Agassiz and Darwin,[97] and perhaps a vestige survives to this day in Lyell's expression 'missing link'.

Both John and William Hunter can thus be seen to have played their separate parts in changing the climate of opinion in that 'period of transformation in the most basic fabric of the knowledge of living beings'. A detailed study of William's work, like Cross's structuralist study of John's discourse, would be required to reveal whether William also showed 'a mode of knowing and speaking of life fundamentally discontinuous with later developments'.[98]

Acknowledgements

I am indebted to C. Helen Brock, S. Clark, G. P. Durant, J. Egerton, A. Fletcher, N. Fogg, M. Hopkinson, R. P. S. Jefferies, E. M. Rayer

91 Dobson, *John Hunter*, p. 36.
92 Ritterbush, *Overtures*, p. 194; cf. p. 197.
93 Blumenbach's views on irritability and sensitivity, for example, were similar to those of John Hunter, deriving from Glisson and Haller (M. Neuburger, 'British Medicine and the Göttingen Medical School in the Eighteenth Century', *Bulletin of the History of Medicine*, 14 [1943], 462). British physicians were much quoted in Göttingen, where Blumenbach was appointed professor in 1776. He visited John Hunter's museum (Palmer, *Works of John Hunter*, p. xxxviii), and made use of Banks's library and museum in 1792 (Bendysshe, *Blumenbach*, p. 149). Soemmering, a devotee of Blumenbach, spent much time with John Hunter in 1778. Blumenbach's views were the basis for Stubbs's *Comparative Anatomical Exposition* (J. Egerton, *George Stubbs, Anatomist and Animal Painter* [London, 1976], pp. 15, 34).
94 Mayr, *Growth of Biological Thought*, p. 347; Bynum, 'The Great Chain . . . : An Appraisal', pp. 21–2.
95 G. Cuvier, *Recherches sur les ossemens fossiles*, vol. 4 (Paris, 1812); Rudwick, *Meaning of Fossils*; Bynum, 'The Great Chain . . . : An Appraisal', p. 8.
96 Mayr, *Growth of Biological Thought*, p. 349.
97 Bynum, 'The Great Chain . . . : An Appraisal', p. 22.
98 Cross, 'Animal Oeconomy', p. 73.

and H. S. Torrens for assistance in preparing this essay. Figure 10.3 is reproduced by courtesy of the Trustees of the British Museum and Oxford University Press; Figures 10.4 and 10.5, with the permission of the Librarian and Keeper of the Hunterian Books and Manuscripts, Glasgow University.

PART IV. OBSTETRICS

11

The pleasures of procreation: traditional and biomedical theories of conception

ANGUS McLAREN

A recent chronicler of eighteenth-century childbearing has argued that so great were the dangers and diseases that inevitably accompanied parturition that women in past times must have loathed and feared sexual intercourse.[1] But cultural anthropologists tell us that every aspect of social life is culturally conditioned.[2] The ways in which people perceive their experiences are as important as the experiences themselves. Fertility is, according to such researchers, never found to be 'natural'; conception, pregnancy, childbirth and nursing are all socially determined. In this essay I will attempt to follow up on these insights of the cultural anthropologists' in order to understand how British people in the past viewed the process of procreation and how such views began to change in the course of the eighteenth century.

In 1776 John Hunter supervised the first successful attempt at artificial insemination. He instructed a linen draper who suffered from hypospadias how he could use a warm syringe to impregnate his wife. The operation worked and pregnancy ensued, but because of Hunter's fear of the criticisms of moralists it was reported only posthumously, twenty-three years later in the *Philosophical Transactions* of the Royal Society.[3] It is surprising that Hunter's success has received so little attention from historians, because no other act so dramatically demonstrated the separation of the principles of sexual

1 Edward Shorter, *A History of Women's Bodies* (New York, 1982), 16.
2 See, e.g., Clifford Geertz, *The Interpretation of Cultures* (New York, 1973).
3 Everard Home, 'An Account of the Dissection of an Hermaphrodite Dog', *Philosophical Transactions of the Royal Society* (1799), 162 and see also F. N. L. Poynter, 'Hunter, Spallanzani, and the History of Artificial Insemination', in L. G. Stevenson and R. P. Multhauf, eds., *Medicine, Science and Culture: Historical Essays in Honor of Oswei Temkin* (Baltimore, 1968).

pleasure and procreation that, they tell us, occurred as the 'modern mind' emerged.

How did early modern British men and women perceive sexuality? Was it pleasurable? Was it a similar experience for both sexes? According to the historians who have most recently plotted the rise of the modern family, it was only in the eighteenth century that the enjoyment of sexuality became, for women, at least a possibility. Lawrence Stone, Edward Shorter and Randolph Trumbach all advance what is in the main a Whig interpretation of the history of the family according to which only recently did love, affection and a concurrent concern for the sexual gratification of one's mate emerge.[4] They attribute the possibility of women's enjoyment of sexuality to the growth of a new individualism linked to market capitalism and to the freedom from pregnancies offered by the expansion of contraceptive knowledge. There is much of value in such arguments concerning the eighteenth century but they fail to explain why in the nineteenth century the double standard continued to hold sway. Far from enjoining women to anticipate sexual pleasure, the majority of early Victorian writers who broached the subject counselled stoicism and passivity. The historians of the family also fail to explain why – if the 'pleasure principle' were to appear only in the eighteenth century – the sixteenth and seventeenth centuries were marked by an earthy attitude towards sexuality strikingly absent in the sentimental late 1700s and the prudish early 1800s.

Hunter's work does, I believe, provide a useful benchmark against which such shifts in both popular and scientific attitudes towards procreation can be plotted. In what follows the literature devoted to the issues of sexual pleasure and procreation prior to Hunter's activities will be reviewed with the intent of casting a fresh light on the history of British attitudes towards sexuality. It will be argued that from the sixteenth to the eighteenth centuries it was commonly assumed that women not only found pleasure in sexual intercourse but they positively had to if the union were to be a fruitful one. It was only in the 1700s that a new scientific appreciation of the process of procreation began to spread, which held that pleasure and procreation were not necessarily linked. As a consequence, by the beginning

4 Randolph Trumbach, *The Rise of the Egalitarian Family: Aristocratic Kinship and Domestic Relations in Eighteenth-Century England* (New York, 1978); Lawrence Stone, *The Family, Sex, and Marriage in England, 1500–1800* (New York, 1977); Edward Shorter, *The Making of the Modern Family* (New York, 1976). For a more complex view of the eighteenth century see Roy Porter, 'Mixed Feelings: The Enlightenment and Sexuality in Eighteenth Century Britain', in P. G. Boucé, ed., *Sexuality in Eighteenth Century England* (Manchester, 1982), 1–27.

of the nineteenth century, one could speak of two sexual cultures: a 'low' culture of traditional beliefs in which women's sexuality was accepted, and a 'high' culture of scientific understanding in which women's sexuality had little place.[5] We shall be asking the sorts of questions that anthropologists, sensitive to the issue of sexual tensions, have posed: Who takes the initiative in sexual encounters? Who is supposed to gain more pleasure? Who controls fertility? We shall seek to understand why the answers made to such questions in the seventeenth century differed from those of the nineteenth century.

The evidence most often advanced to support the argument that sixteenth- and seventeenth-century sexual attitudes towards sexuality were not 'puritanical' is ironically enough drawn primarily from Puritan sources. From Edmund Morgan to Edmund Leites the assertion has been made that Puritans in both England and New England recognised the importance of love, friendship and sexuality in marriage.[6] Traditional Christianity portrayed women as the daughters of Eve and accordingly as lacking in rational control and sexually voracious. Woman's innate interest in sex was a matter not so much of her sensibly seeking pleasure as giving in to self-destructive urges. With the rise of the ideal of the 'spiritualised household' in both humanist and Puritan thought in the sixteenth century, however, there came a new legitimation of marital sexuality, a stress on the virtues of family life, and an acceptance of female sexual needs as natural. Women's libidinal drives were now taken by Protestants as a good thing inasmuch as they helped hold together the family, whereas conservative Catholics, so the argument runs, would continue to prize celibacy and view female sexuality with distaste. So we find William Gouge in *Of Domesticall Duties* (1622) claiming spouses owed each other 'due benevolence'. 'To deny this duty being justly required, is to deny a due debt, and to give Satan a great advantage.' This Puritan pamphleteer went on to assert that sexual relations should continue even after a woman became pregnant. 'Conception is not the only

5 On the notions of high and low cultures see Natalie Davis, *Society and Culture in Sixteenth Century France* (Stanford, Calif., 1975); Peter Burke, *Popular Culture in Early Modern Europe* (London, 1978); Christopher Hill, *The World Turned Upside Down: Radical Ideas During the English Revolution* (London, 1972).
6 See Edmund S. Morgan, 'The Puritans and Sex', *New England Quarterly*, 15 (1942), 591–607; Edmund Leites, 'The Duty to Desire: Love, Friendship, and Sexuality in Some Puritan Theories of Marriage', *Journal of Social History*, 15 (1982), 383–408; W. and M. Haller, 'The Puritan Art of Love', *Huntingdon Library Quarterly*, 5 (1941–2), 235–72; M. Todd, 'Humanists, Puritans, and the Spiritualized Household', *Church History*, 49 (1980), 18–34.

end of this duty: for it is to be rendered to such as are barren.'[7] Similarly, Thomas Gataker in *A Good Wife, God's Gift* (1623) claimed, 'In the first place cometh the Wife, as the first and principall blessing, and the Children in the next . . . If Children bee a Blessing, then the root whence they spring ought much more to bee so esteemed.'[8] In short, such writers shifted the focus on the ends of marriage from procreation to companionship.

Such interpretations are useful, but a reliance on religious tracts has led historians to overlook far more obvious sources relating to sexuality, the traditional medical texts.[9] In this large corpus of works devoted to the questions of conception and gestation, sexuality necessarily figured centrally. How one moved from non-being to being was from the time of the Greeks a key philosophical and scientific conundrum. It gave rise to an extended discussion over the centuries on embryological development. It was a discussion that until the new medical experimentation of the sixteenth century was highly speculative, one in which laymen, doctors and priests all participated and accepted as given the linking of pleasure and procreation.

Early modern Europeans looked back to Aristotle, Hippocrates and Galen for explanations of how life was created. For Aristotle, who was ignorant of the functions of the ovaries and testicles, both male and female produced 'sperma' from their blood – seed for the male and menstrual fluid for the female. The woman, because of her natural coldness, could not concoct real seed, and as proof Aristotle noted: 'A sign that the female does not emit the kind of seed that the male emits, and that generation is not due to the mixing of both as some hold, is that often the female conceives without experiencing the pleasure that occurs in intercourse.'[10] The male fluid had to be, given Aristotle's preconceptions regarding male dominance, qualitatively superior; he asserted that it provided the elements of form and movement for the new being, while the female fluid was characterised as providing matter and passivity. Aristotle suggested that, as in the making of cheese the inert milk was activated by rennet, so too in procreation the active semen produced life from the passive menstrual fluid. He went so far, some have argued, as to deprive women not only of pleasure, but even of maternity and presented them as being little more than incubators. Beyond this, he claimed that semen

7 William Gouge, *Of Domesticall Duties: Eight Treatises* (London, 1622), 223.
8 Gataker cited in James T. Johnson, 'English Puritan Thought on the Ends of Marriage', *Church History*, 38 (1969), 430.
9 On French views of sexuality see Pierre Darmon, *Le Mythe de la procréation à l'âge baroque* (Paris, 1977).
10 Aristotle, *De Partibus Animalium I and De Generatione Animalium I*, trans. D. M. Balme (Oxford, 1972), 48.

tried to produce the highest form of life, that is the male; should it fail, the result was an imperfect product, the female.[11]

More popular in the long run than Aristotle's views were those of Hippocrates, who on the whole tended towards an egalitarian model of procreation. He argued that because of the 'intensity of the pleasure involved', the seminal fluids were distillations drawn from all parts of both spouses' bodies, and accordingly hereditary traits of either could appear.[12] The two fluids or 'semence' were similar in nature and their mixing produced life. This Hippocratic line was taken up in the second century A.D. by Galen, who attempted to synthesize it with Aristotelian medicine.[13] This compilation of medical theories was to dominate Western thought for the next fifteen hundred years. For the purposes of this study, what is of interest is that in contrast to Aristotle's male-oriented explanation of procreation the Galenic was 'feminist' inasmuch as both sexes were presented as contributing equally in conception and accordingly both had to experience pleasure. The female seed was said to move like the male and the fact that a woman could not bear children if her ovaries were removed was advanced as proof that she was more than the mere 'nest' Aristotle suggested. Anatomically, the two sexes were presented in Galenic accounts as complementary, the difference being that the man's genitalia were on the outside and the woman's on the inside. The clitoris was likened to the penis and the ovaries considered 'testicles' or 'stones' that produced seed. The male seed was, it is true, depicted by Galenists as superior in having 'spiritual' qualities lacking in the female, but Galen's reproductive schema was nevertheless far more egalitarian than Aristotle's.

The semence or two-seed theory was to have a long life in Western culture.[14] Thomas Raynald asserted that the woman's seed differed from the man's but was no less perfect and her sensual appetites no less demanding: 'For if that the God of nature had not instincted and

11 Anthony Preus, 'Science and Philosophy in Aristotle's Generation of Animals', *Journal of the History of Biology*, 3 (1970), 1–52.
12 Cited in Howard B. Adelman, *Marcello Malpighi and the Evolution of Embryology* 5 vols. (Ithaca, N.Y., 1966), II, 737.
13 Anthony Preus, 'Galen's Criticisms of Aristotle's Conception Theory', *Journal of the History of Biology*, 10 (1977), 65–85. On hostility to the Galenic view that women produced seed see M. Anthony Hewson, *Giles of Rome and the Medieval Theory of Conception* (London, 1975).
14 On the semence theory in the Middle Ages see Helen R. Lemay, 'Human Sexuality in Twelfth Through Fifteenth Century Scientific Writings', in Vern Bullough and James Brundage, eds., *Sexual Practices and the Medieval Church* (Buffalo, N.Y., 1982), 187–203; for the Renaissance see Ian Maclean, *The Renaissance Notion of Woman* (Cambridge, 1980), 28–33; for sixteenth-century England see Levine Lemnie, *The Touchstone of Complexions*, trans. Thomas Newton (London, 1581), 108; Thomas Cogan, *The Haven of Health* (London, 1584), 245.

inset in the body of man and woman such a vehement and ardent appetite and lust, the one lawfully to company with the other, neyther man nor woman would ever have been so attentive to the works of generation and increasement of posterity.'[15] Why, asked Nathaniel Highmore, would women have 'testicles' if not for the purpose of producing seed? 'When also in coition ye shall observe the same delight and concussion as in Males; why should we suppose Nature, beyond her custome, should abound in superfluities and uselesse partes?'[16] Sir Thomas Browne advanced the same views when combating the report that a woman could be passively impregnated by bathing in a tub in which a man had left semen. ' 'Tis a new and unseconded way in history to fornicate at a distance, and much offendeth the rules of physic, which say, there is no generation without joint emission, nor only a virtual, but corporal and carnal contraction.'[17] William Harvey provided a useful summing-up of early seventeenth-century views:

> Conception, according to the opinion of medical men, takes place in the following way: during intercourse the male and the female dissolve in one voluptuous sensation, and inject their seminal fluids [*geniturae*] into the cavity of the uterus, where that which each contributes is mingled with that which the other supplies, the mixture having from both equally the faculty of action and the force of matter; and according to the predominance of this or that geniture does the progeny turn out male or female.[18]

Although the microscope was to permit in the late seventeenth century the beginnings of a more precise definition of the different contributions of the two sexes in procreation, one still found in the popular literature of the late eighteenth century the assumption that the seed of the two were similar. Nicolas Venette spoke of two seeds in *Conjugal Love Reveal'd* (1720); John Maubray in *The Female Physician* (1724) declared that both sexes contributed 'seminal matter'; and the best known of the popular sex manuals, *Aristotle's Masterpiece*, held (until the 1755 edition) to the semence view.[19]

15 Thomas Raynald, *The Birth of Man-Kinde* (London, 1634), 41; see also Helkiah Crooke, *A Description of the Body of Man* (London, 1618), 202, 216, 261, 295.
16 Nathaniel Highmore, *The History of Generation* (London, 1651), 85.
17 *Sir Thomas Browne's Works*, ed. S. Wilkins, 4 vols. (London, 1835), III, 345.
18 *The Works of William Harvey*, trans. Robert Willis (London, 1865), 294.
19 A Physician [Nicolas Venette], *Conjugal Love Reveal'd* (London, 1720), 37; John Maubray, *The Female Physician* (London, 1724), 20; and see also Henry Bracken, *The Midwife's Companion* (London, 1737), 12. On the changing presentation of conception compare *Aristotle's Masterpiece* (London, 1690), 10, to *The Works of Aristotle* (Derby, 1840?), 15. On the semence view in France see the French equivalent of *Aristotle's Masterpiece*, the anonymous *Les admirables secrets d'Albert le Grand* (Cologne, 1722), 2.

What was the importance of the continuation of the belief that both sexes produced seed? In reviewing the literature in 1755 Michel Procope-Couteau noted that to hold such a view implied that both sexes had to experience pleasure in order to procreate.[20] Indeed, in the popular literature, what was most striking was the maintenance of basically Galenic theories of equal responsibility and pleasure in sexual activity.[21] Such texts continued to ask the traditional sorts of questions about conception and gestation: Do women experience pleasure? How does conception occur? How can it be prevented or encouraged? Can one predetermine the sex of offspring? The new, scientific literature of the late seventeenth century shelved these old questions – at least overtly – and explored the narrower issues of the organisation and development of the embryo. Whether or not the scientific approach was free of sexual bias we will attempt to discover at the end of this essay, but it is first necessary to provide an account of procreation as described in the traditional texts.

The best example of the popular works on sexuality was *Aristotle's Masterpiece*, the anonymously authored compendium of information that drew from Nicholas Culpeper, Albertus Magnus and common folklore.[22] The first editions appeared in the late seventeenth century, and there were more editions of it in the eighteenth century than of any other medical text. Over time it was viewed by the respectable as being in increasingly bad taste. In fact, it changed very little and, if anything, became more modest in its anatomical descriptions. It would come to appear vulgar, however, because it crystallised and maintained what were in effect late seventeenth-century beliefs about sexuality.[23] By drawing on *Aristotle's Masterpiece* and other pre-scientific accounts, we can piece together a picture of early modern sexual beliefs.

The first point made in such manuals is that women experience pleasure in the sexual act. According to *Aristotle's Masterpiece*, at age

20 M*** [Michel Procope-Couteau], *L'Art de faire garcons ou nouveau tableau de l'amour conjugal* (Montpellier, 1760 [1st ed., 1755]), 25.
21 For one woman's acknowledgement of her and her husband's 'inordinate love, and the great delectation they each had in using the other' see the fourteenth-century work, *The Book of Margery Kemp* (New York, 1944), 6; see also on the earlier period Edith Whitehurst Williams, 'What's So New About the Sexual Revolution?' *Texas Quarterly*, 18 (1975), 46–55.
22 But for the argument that Venette best captured the late seventeenth-century portrayal of sexuality see the stimulating introduction by Roy Porter, ed., Nicholas Venette, *The Mysteries of Conjugal Love Revealed* (London, in press).
23 See Otho T. Beall, '*Aristotle's Masterpiece* in America: A Landmark in the Folklore of Medicine', *William and Mary Quarterly*, 20 (1963), 207–22; Vern Bullough, 'An Early American Sex Manual: or Aristotle Who?' *Early American Literature*, 7 (1973), 236–46; Janet Blackman, 'Popular Theories of Generation', in John Woodward and David Richards, eds., *Health Care and Popular Medicine in Nineteenth Century England* (London, 1977).

fourteen or fifteen the menses 'incite' the body and mind of the girl. If the young woman is deprived of sex she ultimately becomes a 'green and weasel coloured' old maid. For the married deprived of companionship by the death of a spouse, there is the additional problem of stilling a delicious habit. Such women were described as the 'brisk' widows whose passions were difficult to calm.[24]

Sexual pleasure was, according to the popular texts, not simply vaginal. Great attention was paid to the importance of the clitoris. According to the *Masterpiece* it was clitoral stimulation that gave 'delights' and such knowledge was essential, 'for without this, the fair sex neither desire mutual Embraces nor have pleasure in 'em, nor conceive by 'em'.[25] Henry Bracken in *The Midwife's Companion* (1737) likewise stated that the clitoris 'by its fullness of nerves and exquisite sense affords unspeakable Delight'.[26] Sibly wrote in 1794 that both sexes necessarily experienced 'voluptuous gratification'.[27] Indeed, the suggestion was made in works like Venette and *Aristotle's Masterpiece* that women might experience more pleasure than men; that they would be 'more recreated and delighted in the Venerial Act' because they both gave and received seed while the man only gave.[28]

The second point made in the texts was that women not only experienced pleasure, they were actively seeking it in sexual embraces. These were certainly not the passive Victorians lying back and thinking of the empire. Lazarus Riverius in *The Practice of Physick* (1658) poetically imagined that the woman's womb,

> skipping as it were for joy, may meet her Husband's Sperm, graciously and freely receive the same, and draw it into its innermost Cavity or Closet, and withal bedew and sprinkle it with her own Sperm, and powered forth in that pang of Pleasure, that so by the commixture of both, Conception may arise.[29]

24 *Aristotle's Masterpiece* (1690), 2. Similarly, Johannes Johnstonus warned in *An History of the Wonderful Things of Nature* (London, 1657), 326–27, that the unexpended 'seed' of widows and virgins caused melancholy.
25 *Aristotle's Masterpiece* (1690), 98; see also *Aristotle's Compleat Masterpiece* (London, 1749), 16.
26 Bracken, *Midwife's Companion*, 10.
27 E. Sibly, *The Medical Mirror or Treatise on the Impregnation of the Human Female* (London, 1794), 23.
28 Venette, *Conjugal Love*, 161; *Aristotle's Masterpiece* (1690), 23–4; Johnstonus, *History*, 330. On the Continent Agrippa of Nettesheim went so far as to twist Galen's theory to assert that children were products of the female seed alone. 'It is the seed of woman alone, as Galen and Avicenna say, that is the matter and nutriment of the fetus, least of all the man's which enters into the woman as an accident into the substance.' Cited in Arlene Miller Guinsburg, 'The Counterthrust to Sixteenth Century Misogyny: The Work of Agrippa and Paracelsus', *Historical Reflections/Réflexions historiques*, 8 (1981), 3–28.
29 Lazarus Riverius et al., *The Practice of Physick* (London, 1658), 503.

James McMath presented the same scene while describing in *The Expert Midwife* (1694) the causes of infertility.

Sterility happens likewise, from the Womans Disgust, and Satiety of the Venereal Embrace; or her dullness and insensibility therein: When the Orifice bids shut against the *Yard*: Which else (while eager upon it, strenuously and naturally *Tickled* and *Roused* therein) applyes to it, delightfully opens, and ravenously attracts the mans *Seed* (which is then sufficiently darted into the Recesses of the *Womb*) emits also her own: Whence *Conception*.[30]

Bracken and Sibly described the womb 'embracing' the penis,[31] while Guillemeau declared that 'in some Women the wombe is so greedy, and lickerish that it doth even come down to meet nature, sucking, and (as it were) snatching the same, though it remaine only about the mouth and entrance of the outward orifice thereof'.[32] There could, it was recognised, be problems arising from women's sexual desires. Jane Sharp argued that 'the most frequent cause of Barrenness in young lusty women . . . is . . . their great desire of copulation'.[33]

The third point made in the texts was that the woman's pleasure was necessary to ensure conception. Venereal delights opened the cervix so admitting the man's seed and precipitating the woman's. Philip Barrough asserted in 1658, 'Also unwilling carnall copulation for the most part is vaine and barren: for love causeth conception, and therefore loving women do conceave often.'[34] Riverius held that it was enjoyment that led the woman to give 'down sufficient quantity of Spirits wherewith her Genitals ought to swel at the instant of Generation'.[35] Nicholas Culpeper stated in *A Directory for Midwives* (1660): 'Want of Love between man and wife, is another cause of Barrenness. That there is an Essential Vital Spirit in the Seed of both sexes, is without all question.'[36] John Sadler agreed:

Aetuis and Sylvius ascribe one maine cause of barrennesse to compel'd copulation, as when parents enforce their daughters

30 James McMath, *The Expert Midwife* (Edinburgh, 1694), 3.
31 Bracken, *Midwife's Companion*, 10; Sibly, *Medical Mirror*, 17.
32 James Guillemeau cited in Audrey Eccles, *Obstetrics and Gynaecology in Tudor and Stuart England* (London, 1982), 29. See also Robert H. Michel, 'English Attitudes Towards Women, 1640–1700', *Canadian Journal of History*, 13 (1978), 43–4.
33 Jane Sharp, *The Compleat Midwife's Companion: or the Art of Midwifery Improved* (London, 1725 [1st ed., 1671]), 109; and see also the comments of a recent historian of seventeenth-century chapbooks: 'Certainly, the whole tenor of the merry books conveys that seventeenth-century women enjoyed their own sexuality and were expected to enjoy it.' Margaret Spufford, *Small Books and Pleasant Histories: Popular Fiction and Its Readership in Seventeenth Century England* (London, 1981), 63.
34 P. Barrough, *The Method of Physicke* (London, 1583), 157.
35 Riverius, *Physick*, 503.
36 Nicholas Culpeper, *A Directory for Midwives* (London, 1660), 70.

to have husbands contrary to their liking, therein marrying
their bodies but not their hearts and where there is want of
love, there for the most part is no conception; as appears in
women which are deflowered against their own will.[37]
Indeed so widespread was the belief that affection was necessary for
conception that it was held that rapes were necessarily sterile. Should
a woman who was assaulted bear a child, it could be advanced as
proof of her complicity. Samuel Farr in *Elements of Medical Jurisprudence* asserted, 'For without the enjoyment of pleasure in the venereal
act no conception can probably take place.'[38]

Any physical problem that rendered the pleasure of the woman
difficult to achieve was also believed to hamper procreation. John
Pechey referred, for example, to 'some distemper in the Vessels dedicated to generation, and then the woman perceives very little or no
pleasure in the act of copulation'.[39] John Bulwer warned, 'circumci-
sion detracts somewhat from the delight of women by lessening their
titillation'.[40] Jane Sharp directed particular attention to the clitoris in
The Compleat Midwife's Companion (1725). It was the clitoris, in her
words, that 'makes Women lustful and take delight in Copulation;
and were it not for this they would have no desire nor delight, nor
would they ever conceive'.[41]

The variety of sources one can draw on to illustrate the continued
vitality of Galenic ideas provides support for one of the main conten-
tions of this study, namely that until the seventeenth century there
existed in England a common culture of procreational knowledge in
which woman's sexual pleasure was seen by both laymen and doctors
as necessary for fecundity. In the seventeenth century this common
culture was undermined. What one finds happening is that a new
'high' culture of scientific embryology emerged that severed the traditional linking of pleasure and procreation. What had been the common culture became the 'low' culture. As indicated by the reprintings
of traditional works such as *Aristotle's Masterpiece*, the older interpretations did not disappear, but they were increasingly viewed by
the educated and respectable as aspects of the mind-set of the lewd
and vulgar.

37 John Sadler, *The Sick Woman's Private Looking Glass* (Norwood, N.J., 1977 [1st
ed., 1636]), 108–9.
38 Samuel Farr, *Elements of Medical Jurisprudence* (London, 1815 [1st ed., 1788]), 46;
for similar views see *Aristotle's Last Legacy* (London, 1789), 363, and *Aristotle's
Compleat and Experienced Midwife* (London, 1700), 132.
39 John Pechey, *The Compleat Midwife's Practice Enlarged* (London, 1694), 243.
40 John Bulwer, *Anthropometamorphosis: Man Transform'd; or the Artificial Changeling*
(London, 1650), 213.
41 Sharp, *Compleat Midwife's Companion*, 36.

From the late sixteenth century onward, medical scientists who adopted the experimental method were faced with the problem of reconciling their new observations with the models of procreation set out by Aristotle, Hippocrates and Galen. The first discoveries were incorporated in the old model, but as enough contradictory evidence was accumulated it became necessary to construct a new paradigm.[42] The dominant view of embryological development up until the sixteenth century has been called epigenetic. That is, the idea was that all parts of the new creation developed sequentially. The weakness of the theory was that it did not satisfactorily explain how such a complicated process as the creation of life took place. A rival theory to that of epigenesis was that of preformation. Some early writers like Plato and Aeschylus argued that a miniature embryonic life was already in place within the parent – like an egg – and embryological development consisted only of growth, not creation.[43] Such an argument allowed one to avoid the issue of how life was created, but the problem with it was that no human egg had been discovered. William Harvey has been hailed by some as the founder of modern embryology for his 1651 work, *De generatione animalium*, but in fact he did not find an egg and he also failed to find semen in the uterus and so fell back on a contagion theory to explain conception. He followed an epigenetic line of reasoning and held that the egg was the *product*, not the cause of conception.[44]

The real changes in embryological thought came with the emergence of preformation theories in the late seventeenth and early eighteenth centuries. On the Continent, Malpighi's important work on the embryological development of the chick provided the basis for a more sophisticated view of conception.

> By its very nature the uterus is a field for growing the seeds, that is to say the ova, sown upon it. Here the eggs are fostered, and here the parts of the living [foetus], when they have further unfolded, become manifest and are made strong. Yet although it has been cast off by the mother and sown, the egg is weak and powerless and so requires the energy of the semen of the male to initiate growth.[45]

In England, Henry Power and William Croone have been credited with advancing similar preformation theories in the 1660s, but the breakthrough came when Regnier de Graaf, without the aid of the

42 See Eccles, *Obstetrics and Gynaecology*, and Jacques Roger, *Les sciences de la vie dans la pensée française du XVIIIᵉ siècle* (Paris, 1963).
43 Adelman, *Malpighi*, II, 733–77.
44 Harvey, *Works*, 362.
45 Adelman, *Malpighi*, II, 861.

microscope, discovered what were to be known as the Graafian follicles, which contained the mammalian egg.[46] De Graaf's work was available in England by 1672. In fact, the actual mammalian egg was not to be found until 1827 by von Baer, but the view that the woman, like the chicken, held within her miniature offspring gained rapid popularity in the scientific community.[47] Thus in John Case's *The Angelical Guide* (1697) we find references to the human egg being shaken by the sperm into the Fallopian tubes; Joseph Blondel went so far as to refer to semen as mere manure for the ovum; Alexander Hamilton in 1781 declared that the child existed in the ovaries and the act of generation was 'only the means intended by providence to supply it with life'; and William Cullen's edition of Albrecht von Haller, although reviewing conflicting theories on generation, held that the foetus was excited into life only by the 'seminal worms'.[48]

In the preformationist school the ovists – those who held that the miniature being already existed in the mother's egg – formed one group. The animalculists – those who argued that a tiny being existed in the spermatozoa – formed the other. The strength of the ovist argument was based on the analogy with egg-laying animals; the animalculists, however, could point to the discovery in semen of microscopic beings by Leeuwenhoek in 1677. The animalculists either denied the existence of the egg or argued that it existed only to provide nourishment for the tiny beings within the drop of semen. As in Aristotle's original formulation the woman was again perceived as little more than a nest or *nidus*.

Whatever the preferred line of attack, preformation theories budded in the 1670s and blossomed in the first half of the eighteenth century.[49] They presented an image of a mono-parental embryo in

46 For overviews see Elizabeth B. Gasking, *Investigations into Generation 1651–1828* (Baltimore, 1967); Charles W. Bodemer, 'Embryological Thought in Seventeenth Century England', in A. G. Debus, ed., *Medicine in Seventeenth Century England* (Los Angeles, 1968), 1–25; Joseph Needham, *A History of Embryology* (New York, 1959), 115–230.

47 Helen Brock informs me that a claim can be made that W. Cruikshank discovered the egg as early as 1778 and reported it in the *Philosophical Transactions* in 1797. See also Needham, *History of Embryology*, 217.

48 John Case, *The Angelical Guide* (London, 1697), 53; Joseph Blondel, *The Strength of Imagination in Pregnant Women Examin'd* (London, 1727), 42; Alexander Hamilton, *A Treatise on Midwifery* (London, 1781), 40; William Cullen, ed., *First Lines of Physiology by the Celebrated baron Albertus Haller* (Edinburgh, 1786), II, 206–8; and see also 'A Physician', *A Rational Account of the Natural Weaknesses of Women* (London, 1727), 62.

49 Although it is not especially important for the purposes of this study, it should be noted that strictly speaking 'preformation' theory held that the formation of each new being took place through the activities of the soul or spirit in the parents' body whereas only 'pre-existence' theory or *emboîtement* held that all organisms were created at one ime in the past. See Peter Bowler, 'Preformation and Pre-existence in the Seventeenth Century', *Journal of the History of Biology*, 4 (1971), 221–44.

which conception implied simply an enlargement of what was already there.[50] There was no 'creation' *per se*. The power of this new theory was based in part on microscopic findings. Indeed the microscope in revealing a miniature hidden world fired men's imaginations with the idea of worlds even tinier. The theory was also supported by ideological concerns. It nicely countered the radically rationalist view of Cartesians that the law of motion had in the beginning created life, which in turn supported the concept of abiogenesis or spontaneous generation. The idea of pre-existence or *emboîtement* also complemented seventeenth-century Calvinist and Jansenist ideas of predestination. Science could be seen as confirming the religious idea that all human beings had been created by God at one point in time.[51] Swammerdam, for example, noted that in embryology, 'even the foundation of original sin itself would already have been discovered, since the whole of mankind would have been concealed in the loins of Adam and Eve, and to this could be added as a necessary consequence that when these eggs have been exhausted the end of mankind will be at hand'.[52] John Wilkins agreed that the microscope proved the existence of some 'wise intelligent being', and William Paley exulted in the fact that the scientific investigation of reproduction made it more, rather than less, mysterious: 'He [the parent] is in total ignorance why that which is produced took its present form rather than any other. It is for him only to be astonished by the effect.'[53] Science could thus be turned to defend Christianity against mechanical, rationalist arguments.

The pre-existence and preformation theories were not without their weaknesses. How did one explain hereditary traits that might vary

50 George Garden, 'A Discourse Concerning the Modern Theory of Generation', *Philosophical Transactions of the Royal Society*, 196 (1691), 474–8.
51 In addition to the ovists and animalculists there was a third and even more bizarre school of thought – that of the 'panspermists', who argued that all beings were created by God at one moment in time, that such tiny beings were suspended in the atmosphere and that they passed from the air into the man and then into the woman and then were born. For example William Wollaston wrote that all souls were created in the beginning but that the material forms of beings were effected later. 'If then the *semina* out of which animals are produced, are (as I doubt not) *animalcula* already formed; which, being dispersed about, especially in some opportune places, are *taken in* with aliment, or perhaps the very air; being separated in the bodies of the *males* by strainers proper to every kind, and then lodged in *their* seminal vessels, do *there* receive some kind of addition and influence; and being thence transferred into the wombs of the females, are *there* nourished more plentifully, and grow, till they become too big, to be longer confined' (N. N. [William Wollaston], *The Religion of Nature Delineated* [London, 1722], 65). Microscopic studies were thus turned to the purpose of Christian apology.
52 Swammerdam cited in Adelman, *Malpighi*, II, 908.
53 John Wilkins, *Of the Principles and Duties of Natural Religion* (London, 1673), 83; William Paley, *Natural Theology* (London, 1802), and see also John Ray, *The Wisdom of God Manifested in the Works of Creation* (London, 1691).

from child to child? How did one explain the polyp's ability (discovered in the 1740s) to regenerate itself? And on a commonsense
level, was one really to believe that Adam and Eve contained within
them every generation of mankind ever to live?[54] Clearly this was a
theory that easily lent itself to spoofing, a temptation given in to by
writers like Sterne.[55] Moreover the defenders of the animalculist theory had the particular problem of explaining why, if each sperm was a
potential man, God permitted such a wholesale slaughter of millions
of beings in every sexual act.

For our purposes what is most interesting is how the theories related to the role of the sexes. One finds that the animalculists presented
women as being little more than passive recipients of the male gift
and returned them to their Aristotelian role of breeding machines.
The ovist line of argument would appear at first glance to have been
more 'feminist' inasmuch as it credited the mother with carrying
preformed beings. In fact the ovists also portrayed the woman as
playing a far more passive role than that attributed to her by the
defenders of the old semence or two-seed theory. Previously it had
been argued that the woman had to be aroused and delighted for
conception to occur. Now it was stated that her active involvement
was minimal. The sperm was active and the egg almost inert. The egg
was presented by scientists as 'shaken' into life by the sperm or
allowed by its intervention to 'escape' into the Fallopian tube. William Smellie, for example, wrote: 'The *Ovum* being impregnated, is
squeezed from its *Nidus* or husk into the tube by the contraction of the
Fimbria, and thus disengaged from its attachments to the *Ovarium*, is
endowed with a circulating force by the *Animalculum*, which has a *vis
vitae* in itself.'[56]

In the latter half of the eighteenth century there was a shift away
from preformation theory and back to epigenetic views in large part
because of unhappiness with the weaknesses of the former model.
But there was no return to the theory of the double semence of two
homogeneous fluids; rather one saw the elaboration of the idea of two
distinct sorts of building blocks for the new creation.[57] For the pur-

54 Michael H. Hoffheimer, 'Maupertuis and the Eighteenth-Century Critique of
Preexistence', *Journal of the History of Biology*, 15 (1982), 119–44.
55 Louis A. Landa, 'The Shandean Homunculus: The Background of Sterne's
"Little Gentleman" ', in Carol Camden, ed., *Restoration and Eighteenth Century
Literature* (Chicago, 1963), 49–68.
56 W. Smellie, *A Treatise on the Theory and Practice of Midwifery* (London, 1752), 115;
see also Hamilton, *Treatise on Midwifery*, 40.
57 On doctors' appreciation of the embryological debate at the end of the eighteenth century see, e.g., John Aitken, *Principles of Midwifery* (Edinburgh, 1785), 42–4,
and Charles Severn, *First Lines on the Practice of Midwifery* (London, 1831), 31. On the
scientific level see Shirley A. Roe, *Matter, Life and Generation: Eighteenth Century
Embryology and the Haller-Wolff Debate* (Cambridge, 1981).

poses of this study what is important to note is that in stressing the idea of different male and female sex roles both preformation theories and the later more sophisticated epigenetic theories undercut the older notion of the necessity of both men and women experiencing sexual pleasure.

The common argument advanced in histories of science is that between the sixteenth and nineteenth centuries scholasticism slowly but surely gave way to empiricism.[58] In analysing progress in embryological thought, however, we find that although a science emerged that was more accurate than Galen's in particulars – for example in demonstrating the differentiation of functions in male and female sexual organs – it did not give rise to a general explanation of procreation any more satisfying than that sketched out two thousand years before. Indeed the new explanation appeared in many ways impoverished inasmuch as it said less and less about the social and cultural aspects of sexuality that ordinary men and women assumed were of utmost importance.

Women's pleasure in sexuality had been traditionally justified on the grounds that their sexual organs were very much like men's. Men had to be aroused to ejaculate and it followed logically enough that women also had to experience pleasure if they were to produce seed. Modern science revealed that this was not so, that men and women were anatomically different, that the ovaries were not 'testicles' producing seed. It was thanks to such new knowledge that John Hunter was able to direct the first successful attempt at artificial insemination. Theoretically there was no reason why such more accurate and detailed accounts of physiological fact should have led to a denigration of women's right to pleasure, but in fact they did.[59]

The new embryological knowledge of the sperm and the egg – the one active and the other purportedly passive – led to new expectations, or was employed to rationalise new expectations, of differing male and female sexual experiences. William Harvey began this reappraisal of sexual performance innocently enough when he observed that not all females presented an 'effusion of fluid' during intercourse.

> But passing over the fact that the females of all the lower animals, and all women do not experience any such emission of

58 See, e.g., Roger's work cited in footnote 42.
59 Hilda Smith anachronistically attacks seventeenth-century writers such as Culpeper for not adopting a 'straight forward informational approach' in their discussion of gynaecology and so implies that in a scientifically based medicine social and sexual preoccupations would not intrude. This chapter argues that such an overlap always occurs. See Hilda Smith, 'Gynecology and Ideology in Seventeenth Century England', in Berenice A. Caroll, ed., *Liberating Women's History* (Urbana, Ill., 1976), 97–115.

fluid, and that conception is nowise impossible in cases where
it does not take place, for I have known several, who without
anything of the kind were sufficiently prolific, and even some
who after experiencing such an emission and having had
great enjoyment, nevertheless appeared to have lost somewhat of their wonted fecundity; and then an infinite number
of instances might be quoted of women, who, although they
have great satisfaction in intercourse, still emit nothing, and
yet conceive.[60]

But those who followed Harvey chose to stress the notion that the
pleasure of women was not only unnecessary for procreation but was
likely not even attainable. Thus we find la Vauguion saying, 'We see
every day, that some women are impregnated without emission of
Seed, or receiving the least Pleasure.'[61] Procope-Couteau asked in
1755 if it were not true that many women never felt pleasure in the
sexual act.[62] An anonymous author writing in 1789 asserted that pleasure was felt by few women but was in any event not necessary.[63]
Fodéré informed his female patients that in place of passion, 'com-
plaisance, tranquility, silence, and secrecy are necessary for a prolific
coition'.[64] By the mid-nineteenth century Dr Acton was declaring:

There can be no doubt that sexual feelings in the female is in
the majority of cases in abeyance . . . and even if raised (which
in many instances it never can be) is very moderate compared
with that of the male . . . As a general rule, a modest woman
seldom desires any sexual gratification for herself. She submits
to her husband, but only to please him and, but for the desire
of maternity, would far rather be relieved from his attentions.[65]

But patients apparently did not abandon old theories as quickly as did
their doctors. In the 1860s Sims complained that it was still,

. . . the vulgar opinion, and the opinion of many savants that,
to ensure conception, sexual intercourse should be performed
with a certain degree of completeness, that would give an
exhaustive satisfaction to both parties at the same moment.
How often do we hear husbands complain of coldness on the

---

60 Harvey, *Works*, 298–9.
61 M. de la Vauguion, *A Compleat Body of Chirgurical Operations* (1699), cited in
Eccles, *Obstetrics and Gynaecology*, 35.
62 [Procope-Couteau], *L'Art*, 25.
63 'A Physician', *Speculations on the Mode and Appearances of Impregnation in the
Human Female* (Edinburgh, 1789), 43.
64 Fodéré cited in Michael Ryan, *The Philosophy of Marriage* (London, 1837), 331.
65 Dr William Acton, *The Functions and Disorders of the Reproductive Organs* (London,
1857), 213, and see also John S. and Robin M. Haller, *The Physician and Sexuality in
Victorian America* (Urbana, Ill., 1974), 96–101.

part of the wives; and attribute to this the failure to procreate. And sometimes wives are disposed to think, though they never complain, that the fault lies with the hasty ejaculation of the husband.[66]

The new view of women – which held that as far as conception was concerned it was of no importance how indifferent or indeed hostile they might be to the sexual act – did result in one unexpected reform. In cases of rape nineteenth-century courts would no longer assume that the pregnancy of the victim implied her acquiescence. 'It was formerly supposed', wrote E. H. East in 1803, 'that if a woman conceived it was no rape, because that showed her consent; but it is now admitted on all hands that such an opinion has no foundation either in reason or law.'[67]

Thus in the medical literature one moved from the picture of the sexually active woman of the seventeenth century to the passionless creature of the nineteenth. Some have suggested that the rise of evangelical religion was responsible for the new stress on women's chastity, decorum and purity.[68] Others have argued that doctors rather than priests played a key role in counselling moderation – that purity and suspicion of sexuality were exploited by physicians in order to enhance their positions as counsellors and confessors.[69] Still others have suggested that the emergence of a new economic view of the world that lauded thrift, prudence and self-control necessarily negatively influenced sensual enjoyments.[70] And finally some have argued that 'passionlessness' was in part a strategy seized upon by women to protect themselves from male sexual demands, in particular in order to limit pregnancies but more generally as a way of allowing women at least a negative control over sexuality.[71] The purpose of this essay has been to examine the role played in this evolution by medical scientists who were influenced by, but who also obviously influenced, the other participants in the debate over sexuality. The

66 James Marion Sims, *Clinical Notes on Uterine Surgery* (London, 1866), 369.
67 E. H. East, *A Treatise of the Pleas of the Crown*, 2 vols. (London, 1803), I, 445, and see also Susan S. M. Edwards, *Female Sexuality and the Law* (Oxford, 1981), 123–4.
68 M. Quinlan, *Victorian Prelude* (New York, 1941); Peter Fryer, *Mrs. Grundy: Studies in English Prudery* (London, 1963).
69 Stephen Nissenbaum, *Sex, Diet, and Debility in Jacksonian America: Sylvester Graham and Health Reform* (Westport, Conn., 1980), 28; Charles E. Rosenberg, 'Sexuality, Class, and Race in Nineteenth Century America', *American Quarterly*, 25 (1973), 131–53.
70 Peter Cominos, 'Innocent Femina Sensualis in Unconscious Conflict', in Martha Vicinus, ed., *Suffer and Be Still: Women in the Victorian Age* (Bloomington, Ind., 1972), 158–62.
71 Nancy F. Cott, 'Passionlessness: An Interpretation of Victorian Sexual Ideology, 1790–1850', *Signs*, 4 (1978), 219–36.

main argument of this work is that the rights of women to sexual pleasure were not enhanced, but eroded as an unexpected consequence of the elaboration of more sophisticated models of reproduction.[72]

Why did doctors participate in the rejection of the old image of the lusty female and in the new portrayal of the solemnity and sacredness of procreation that required female submissiveness? Margaret Jacob, surprised to find that so many eighteenth-century scientists were religious and turned their ideas to support a natural theology, concluded that to understand the Newtonians one had to appreciate the extent to which they tailored their philosophy of nature to serve the social and political purposes of liberal, Protestant interests.[73] In a remarkably similar fashion medical scientists appear to have turned the later eighteenth-century discussion of procreation to the purposes of bolstering a new, middle-class image of the respectable, asexual female.[74] The notion of aggressive female sexuality did not disappear but would henceforth be associated by medical men only with working-class women. Doctors in this way contributed to the effort made on a variety of fronts by the middle classes to elaborate new social and sexual roles to differentiate their enlightened lives from the unthinking, hedonistic existences of both the upper and lower orders.

It follows from my conclusions that we have to question seriously the assertion of Stone, Shorter and Trumbach that the eighteenth century saw the dawning of a new era of sensual enjoyment. But although I take issue with the idea that the sexual pleasure of women was unknown in early modern Britain, I do not want to be taken as saying that in contrast to the constrained Victorian world there once existed a Merrie Englande of 'uncontrolled' sexuality. What we find upon examination is that in every century women's roles are prescribed and given elaborate medical and biological justifications. For reasons we cannot go into here it appeared subversive to argue in the early nineteenth century that spouses had the same sexual needs, but

72 Carolyn Merchant has some interesting things to say about the rise of the 'machine metaphor' in late seventeenth-century medical discussions of women's sexual passivity, but in presenting male chauvinism as unchanging from Aristotle to Harvey to Darwin she fails to produce a believable explanation of shifts in attitudes towards procreation. See *The Death of Nature: Women, Ecology, and the Scientific Movement* (San Francisco, 1980).

73 Margaret Jacob, *The Newtonians and the English Revolution, 1689–1720* (Ithaca, N.Y., 1976) and on eighteenth-century Enlightenment thought and women see also Jacob's *The Radical Enlightenment: Pantheists, Freemasons, and Republicans* (London, 1981), 208.

74 Marlene Legates, 'The Cult of Womanhood in Eighteenth Century Thought', *Eighteenth Century Studies*, 10 (1976), 21–40; A. D. Harvey, '*Clarissa* and the Puritan Tradition', *Essays in Criticism*, 28 (1978), 38–51.

from the sixteenth century to the eighteenth a commonplace assumption was that the bed was one place in which men and women were more or less equal.[75] The view was fairly egalitarian but not entirely so given that male physical and psychological needs were taken as the norm against which women's acts and feelings were measured. According to much of the popular literature all women were lascivious and amorous, and it must be recalled that in examining such texts we are gaining insights into what were often mere male fantasies about female sexuality. Nevertheless a review of this literature suggests that it is a gross over-simplification to argue that love, affection and sexual enjoyment were unknown in the 'World We Have Lost'.

Acknowledgement

This essay first appeared in *Reproductive Rituals: The Perception of Fertility in England from the Sixteenth Century to the Nineteenth Century* (London: Methuen, 1984). I would like to thank Methuen for its permission to reprint this material.

75 Carl Degler has attacked the notion that Victorian doctors denied women's sexuality and has asserted that 'it was recognized that the sex drive was so strong in a woman that to deny it might well compromise her health'. But to make his case Degler has to rely on works written in the 1870s and later; the early nineteenth-century material, which would undermine his argument, is ignored. See Carl N. Degler, 'What Ought to Be and What Was: Women's Sexuality in the Nineteenth Century', *American Historical Review*, 79 (1974), 1467–90; *At Odds: Women and the Family in America From the Revolution to the Present* (New York, 1980). That sexual repression percolated down to the working classes is indicated by the inability of nineteenth-century artisan autobiographers to discuss their sex lives. See David Vincent, 'Love and Death and the Nineteenth Century Working Class', *Social History*, 5 (1980), 223–48.

12

William Hunter and
the varieties of man-midwifery

ADRIAN WILSON

Introduction

Historians tell us that the eighteenth century witnessed a 'revolution in obstetrics': From the 1730s there was a sudden increase in male attendance in childbirth, and the 'men-midwives' who thus came into being rapidly displaced the traditional midwife, instituted classes in midwifery, brought about an explosion of technical knowledge and further promoted their new activities by means of lying-in hospitals, wards and charities. The *causes* of this change (it is said) were the forceps and fashion. The design of the forceps was published in 1733; the instrument was taken up at once by male practitioners, for whom it served as 'the key to the lying-in room'. Fashion promoted the new man-midwifery, which began at the top of the social scale and spread inexorably downwards as each social rank aped its betters.[1]

William Hunter was himself a leading 'man-midwife' in mid-eighteenth-century London. Yet in trying to connect Hunter's practice with the wider 'revolution in obstetrics', we encounter an obstacle: Hunter's strenuous *opposition* to the midwifery forceps, made famous through remarks reproduced by Spencer in his *History of British Midwifery*. 'Where they save one, they murder twenty', Hunter said, adding that it was 'a thousand pities they were ever invented'. Can the forceps then have been the 'key to the lying-in room'? If not, how can the rise of man-midwifery be explained? And why did Hunter take this particular view – unlike such fellow men-midwives as William Smellie?[2]

---

1 The quoted phrases are from J. H. Aveling, *English Midwives: Their History and Prospects* (London, 1872), p. 86, and Walter Radcliffe, *Milestones in Midwifery* (Bristol, 1967), p. 30. See also Jean Donnison, *Midwives and Medical Men* (London, 1977), pp. 21–41; Audrey Eccles, *Obstetrics and Gynaecology in Tudor and Stuart England* (London, 1982), p. 124.
2 Herbert R. Spencer, *The History of British Midwifery from 1650 to 1800* (London, 1927), pp. 72–3.

The approach I shall take to these questions involves a focus on male obstetric practice rather than precept; a widening of view, to embrace the seventeenth century as well as the eighteenth; and, so far as is practicable, a shift of attention from 'obstetrics' or 'midwifery' to *childbirth*. To begin with, I shall outline certain features of childbirth itself that provide a necessary context for approaching the nature of male obstetric practice. The central section of the essay will be concerned with the different forms that man-midwifery could take; I shall then suggest provisional answers to the initial questions and conclude with some historiographical reflections.

The critical features of childbirth, in any society, are the social arrangements made for its routine management, the biological forms it can take and the technical means available for intervention. As to the social arrangements, childbirth in mid-eighteenth-century England was routinely managed not by male practitioners but by midwives, and it was usual for the birth to be attended by several other women – 'gossips', who were variously the friends, relatives and neighbours of the childbearing mother. Of the biology of childbirth the most important thing to be said is that most births, then as now, were normal and spontaneous, needing no assistance at all for a safe delivery. If difficulty arose, or was perceived to have arisen, there were three main techniques available: podalic version, craniotomy and forceps extraction.

The biological and technical dimensions deserve some amplification. From both modern and historical sources, we can derive the following picture of the incidence of different types of birth:

1. About 96 per cent of births were normal and spontaneous. Most of these (93 percent) came by the head, the remainder (about 3 per cent) by the breech.
2. The remaining 4 per cent of births involved serious obstruction and could not be delivered without intervention. Most of these cases of obstruction (around 3 per cent of all births) came by the head, just as did most of the spontaneous deliveries. The other 1 per cent of all births comprised roughly equal numbers of obstructed breech births (particularly footling breech, the rarest of the breech varieties but also the most dangerous) and cases of arm or shoulder presentation (all of which became obstructed, save only those few where the child was premature and thus very small).
3. Some births were subject to complications, either major or minor. The minor complications included fainting, vomiting and tearing of the perineum. The major complications, which were of much greater moment as they threatened the mother's life, were haem-

orrhage (flooding) and convulsions (what is now called eclampsia). The incidence of such minor complications is very difficult to assess, but a working guess of 1 per cent may not be too wide of the mark.

Complications were more likely in association with obstruction, and thus we cannot simply add the two together to assess the incidence of serious difficulty. Rickets, leading to a distorted female pelvis and thus to a greater likelihood of obstruction, seems to have been quite rare and thus not to have increased the likelihood of difficulty as much as might be expected. Thus, although there is some indeterminacy about this, we can say with confidence that serious difficulty (whether due to obstruction or to complications) was of the order of 4 per cent in frequency; that obstructed labour was the commonest source of difficulty; and that obstruction by the head was the most frequent form this took.

The different surgical techniques were designed for specific forms of obstruction, though they also had other applications. Both craniotomy and forceps extraction were used for obstructed births by the head; each in its different way permitted traction on the head (aiding the mechanical force of the uterus) and reduced the size of the head (permitting an easier passage through a fixed bony channel). Craniotomy could be used only on a dead child; it opened the skull. The midwifery forceps could be used if the child was alive or dead, for they grasped the head externally. The other chief technique, podalic version, was designed for malpresentations, notably for births presenting by the arm or shoulder; this method consisted literally in 'turning the birth to the feet' and it succeeded (in the hands of a skilled practitioner) because the feet of the child were both small (permitting an adult hand to pass) and easily grasped – in both respects unlike the head of the child, which was large, smooth and slippery. Thus, in theory, podalic version would have been used only for malpresentations, craniotomy only for delivering a dead child coming by the head, and the forceps for a child (living or dead) coming by the head. This was, on the whole, true, but in practice there were qualifications. For one thing, podalic version could be used for births by the head; for another there was the alternative technique of cephalic version (turning to the head) in malpresentations, though this was difficult to use and was seldom effectual; and third, it has to be added that craniotomy instruments were sometimes used on a living child, in the hope of saving the mother's life. (In very rare cases, with great luck and skill, a practitioner could even draw a living child with a craniotomy device.)

It is appropriate here to mention very briefly the well-known histo-

ry of the midwifery forceps.[3] The instrument was invented, in the
early seventeenth century, by one of the Chamberlens, a family of
Huguenot refugees who had settled in England in the late sixteenth
century. Practising in London throughout the seventeenth century,
the Chamberlens kept the forceps a secret until about 1700 – after
which date the design leaked out to a series of individual practitioners. By the 1720s the instrument had been demonstrated in Paris
(though in a different form), and was being used by at least two
London practitioners outside the Chamberlen family (and probably
by many more than this). In the early 1730s the former secret burst
into print, in the writings of Butter (1733), Chapman (1735) and
Giffard (edited posthumously by Hody, 1734). Thereupon the forceps
was widely available, and it was indeed taken up by large numbers of
young surgeons. One such individual was William Smellie, who in
the next decade settled in London and offered classes in midwifery at
which the use of the forceps was taught. From this point on, man-
midwifery and the forceps were widespread and also controversial.

The dramatic effects of the publication of the forceps design create
the impression that man-midwifery was novel in the eighteenth
century and that it was indeed the forceps that promoted man-
midwifery. Yet the forceps story itself, beginning as it does a century
earlier, qualifies this picture; and in fact there is abundant evidence of
male obstetric practice in seventeenth-century England, *outside* the
Chamberlen family. In the case of Percival Willughby of Derby, it is
thanks to the lucky accident that he wrote a midwifery treatise which
survived in manuscript that we know he had an extensive obstetric
practice in the Midlands in the mid-seventeenth century. From other
sources we learn of Willughby's counterparts, in the late seventeenth
and early eighteenth centuries, in other county towns and also in
large market towns. These seventeenth-century practitioners were
not usually *called* men-midwives; rather, they were described by the
routine practitioner-labels of the time, that is as physicians, surgeons,
apothecaries.

Nonetheless, although male obstetric practice before the publication of the forceps was more common than has been thought, it was
indeed unusual. The norm in childbirth was delivery by a midwife,
and this remained true at least up to the middle of the eighteenth
century, even in such centres of man-midwifery as London and Edinburgh. And it is this that sets for us the central question here: By what
routes did male practitioners enter the lying-in chamber at all? What

3 See J. H. Aveling, *The Chamberlens and the Midwifery Forceps* (London, 1882);
Kedarnath Das, *Obstetric Forceps* (Calcutta, 1929); Walter Radcliffe, *The Secret Instrument* (London, 1947).

were the *paths to childbirth* of men like Willughby in the seventeenth century, and Hunter in the eighteenth?

Eight paths to childbirth

The materials that most easily enable us to answer this question are the midwifery treatises written by these men, especially where such treatises include illustrative case histories. Such case histories are not necessarily representative of the practices from which they are drawn; yet for the present purpose this need not matter unduly, since we are concerned in the main with the 'range' of the phenomena, and rather less with their 'central tendency'. It is a reasonable assumption that male treatises will include at least some examples of all the major 'paths to childbirth' experienced by their authors. What follows is a descriptive account, based on that assumption. For this purpose I have used three treatises and one set of lecture notes. The treatises are those of Willughby, Giffard and Smellie; the lecture notes are from a student of Hunter's, and they are used in default of an actual treatise by Hunter himself.

A brief word is in order about these sources and their authors.[4] Percival Willughby (1596–1685) practised in Derby from about 1630 to at least 1672; he wrote his 'Observations in Midwifery' between 1660 and 1672, and it contains cases variously written down from recall (as far back as 1630 or earlier) and recorded as soon as they occurred (particularly from the 1660s). The treatise remained unpublished during Willughby's lifetime, but found its way into print in 1754, 1863 and 1972. It contains over a hundred deliveries performed by Willughby and introduced into the text to support his didactic arguments. The *Observations* was a polemic for non-intervention in normal births, and for podalic version in cases of obstruction. It claimed repeatedly that midwives, particularly young midwives in the countryside, were ignorant and injudicious practitioners.

William Giffard (fl. 1720s) was a London surgeon about whom little is known. He acquired an obstetric forceps during the 1720s, and

---

4 Percival Willughby, *Observations in Midwifery*, ed. Henry Blenkinsop (Warwick, 1863; reprinted with introduction by John L. Thornton, Wakefield, 1972). The 1754 edition was in Dutch; see Thornton's introduction. A slightly earlier, manuscript version of this treatise is in the British Library, Sloane MS 529, fols. 1–19, paginated 1–35. William Giffard, *Cases in Midwifery . . . Revis'd and publish'd by Edward Hody* (London, 1734). William Smellie, *A Treatise on the Theory and Practice of Midwifery*, 3 vols. (London, 1752, 1754, 1764; vols. 2–3 entitled *A Collection of Cases in Midwifery*). Reprinted (London, 1876–8), edited with annotations by Alfred H. McClintock. William Hunter: Royal College of Surgeons, London, MS 42.d.25, Lecture notes on midwifery taken from Hunter's lectures, n.d. (?1760s).

from that point (if not before) made a record of many of his obstetric cases, over 200 in all. After his death, these cases were edited and published by Edward Hody, FRS, as one of his first communications in print about the forceps.

William Smellie (1697–1763) was trained as an apothecary in Lanark, was acquainted with William Cullen, and practised obstetric surgery as part of a general rural practice in the 1720s and early 1730s. On learning of the forceps, he took steps to educate himself in their use, travelling first to London and then to Paris in a search for instruction. From Grégoire in Paris he gained the idea of using phantoms for teaching purposes, and he returned to London where he set up both as a practitioner and as a teacher. During the 1740s he had some 900 male pupils, who enrolled in courses of varying lengths for a sliding scale of fees; and he also taught some midwives, though it is not known how many. Subsequently, he wrote his *Treatise* for the further education of his former pupils. He retired from practice in 1759, and then produced two supplementary volumes of case histories – mostly his own, but a substantial number taken from other treatises (including Giffard's) and from his own ex-pupils' correspondence with him. There are over 500 cases in the treatise.

William Hunter needs no introduction in the present context, but two features of his career deserve mention. First, he began his medico-surgical education in the late 1730s, that is after the design of the forceps had been published. Second, he spent a year of training under Smellie, from late 1740 to late 1741. This was when Smellie's classes were just beginning, but it is safe to assume that his main ideas and practices were well settled by this time; Hunter, by contrast, was still learning. Hunter went on to become surgeon, physician, man-midwife and anatomist, and the lecture notes of his students show that he gave courses on all these topics with the possible exception of physic.

I shall also be referring briefly to two other male practitioners, both of the early eighteenth century.[5] Hugh Chamberlen was the last of the forceps family dynasty; something of his practice is known from aristocratic family papers investigated by Randolph Trumbach, and it is in this connection that I shall be mentioning him. James Houstoun attempted to become a man-midwife, but did not succeed; I shall

5 Randolph Trumbach, 'The Aristocratic Family in England, 1690–1780. Studies in Childhood and Kinship' (PhD thesis, Johns Hopkins University, 1972), p. 31. James Houstoun, *Memoirs of the Life and Travels of James Houstoun, M.D., Collected and Written by His Own Hand* (London, 1747), pp. 73–4.

consider his training in obstetrics, which he recounted in his autobiography.

When I began preparing this essay, it was my belief that men came to childbirth by just three distinct routes or 'paths'. As I worked through the material, however, it emerged that my theme was better chosen than I had actually imagined, for I found that the paths to childbirth numbered not three but eight. I wanted to contend that man-midwifery was complex, but the historical evidence surpassed my contention: The distinctions between different paths require to be drawn in three different dimensions. These dimensions concern the timing of the call for male attendance; whether or not the call had been anticipated; and finally, the presence or absence of a midwife in addition to the male practitioner.

The first dimension to consider – that of the timing – enables us to distinguish between three types of call, which I shall term advance calls, onset calls and emergency calls. In an *advance* call, the practitioner was summoned by the mother to come and reside in her house at some point during her pregnancy, to advise her on her diet and course of life, to remain until the birth itself, to be in attendance during the birth, and to continue for some time afterwards to supervise her post-partum recovery. An *onset* call summoned the practitioner to the delivery as soon as labour commenced; an *emergency* call sent for him only after some serious difficulty had arisen.

In the second dimension (anticipation), we have to distinguish between *booked* and *unbooked* calls. The male practitioner could be 'engaged'(as Willughby put it) or 'bespoke' (Smellie's term) for attendance, and this constituted a booked call; if there had been no such prior arrangement, the call was unbooked. All advance calls were by definition booked; onset and emergency calls, by contrast, could be either booked or unbooked. The booking amounted to an engagement to attend on the due summons; that summons could itself be of the onset or emergency type. This may seem strange in the case of an emergency call, yet it did indeed happen, at least in Willughby's practice. The effect of such an engagement was probably that he had to refuse all other calls, except emergencies close to hand.

Our third dimension concerns the presence or absence of a midwife. In both advance and onset calls, the male practitioner could be called either *in addition to* a midwife, or *in lieu of* a midwife; his own role differed radically in these two distinct situations. If a midwife was involved, the man's place was to be on hand in case difficulty arose; thus a further, subsidiary 'call' was required to bring him into the delivery room itself. If, by contrast, there was no midwife, then the man's task was to effect the actual delivery. As for emergency calls, we may assume for the sake of initial simplicity that these always involved the prior attendance of a midwife, though we shall later see that this requires qualification.

Our sources by no means make it explicit in every case-description just which of these eight possible paths had been followed; the main difficulty lies in identifying onset calls and in specifying the particular variety within that broad category. Nonetheless, there is every indication that each of these eight distinct routes did in fact occur historically. The eight paths are summarised in Figure 12.1, and an illustration of each, drawn from the treatises of Willughby and Smellie, is given in the Appendix.

It is obvious that these calls will have been made to different extents amongst different social classes, and that they must have commanded different fees. *Advance* calls, in particular, could be made only by mothers of the gentry or merchant classes, since these women alone would have had the large houses required for entertaining the male practitioner as a living-in guest. Again, advance calls must have earned very large fees, since they tied the practitioner down; in theory, he was not permitted to accept any other engagement, although leave might be granted to answer an emergency call or to attend from its onset the delivery of a regular patient.[6] On the evidence of Willughby's cases, it would seem that *onset* calls came from a slightly wider circle of patients (the 'semi-gentry' or wives of clergymen and professionals as well as the gentry) and that *emergency* calls took him to mothers of all social classes; a preliminary examination of Giffard's and Smellie's cases suggests a similar picture for these two later practitioners. The size of the fees depended greatly upon the reputation and achievements of the individual practitioner, as well as on the wealth of the patient and on the type of call. It is impossible to be precise on this score, but it seems certain that there was a great difference in fees between advance calls, onset calls and emergency calls; and it is likely that advance calls commanded tens of pounds, onset calls one or a few pounds or guineas, and emergency calls perhaps a pound or less. On some occasions, particularly emergency calls, a practitioner might give his services free of charge.

Why were male practitioners called at all? On the evidence of Willughby's and Smellie's cases, it seems that both advance and onset calls were usually made because the mother (or someone else) ex-

6 See Willughby, *Observations*, p. 141, for an example of this.

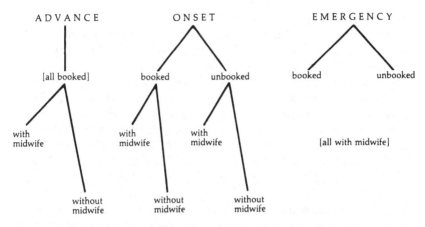

Fig. 12.1. Classification of paths to childbirth

pected that the birth would be difficult. This might be because of difficulty in previous births, through fear of the first birth or because there had been some problem in pregnancy such as a fever or discharge. Emergency calls, by definition, arose because of difficulty. Thus male practice, at least in its origins, was very largely connected with abnormal birth or with the expectation of such abnormality.

What I have presented so far is a framework of classification, designed to capture the 'varieties of man-midwifery' and at the same time to facilitate comparisons between different practitioners. But this framework leaves out the important question of *who made* the different types of call. Here I can only offer an impressionistic account, surveying the main features of the problem – together with the observation that this is a crucial question on which much more work is needed. First, it seems that whenever 'booking' was involved, it was done either by the mother herself or by her husband. Second, and similarly, it was again the mother or husband who made 'advance' and 'onset' calls *without a midwife*. Third, there is a further dimension in those 'advance' and 'onset' calls that were made *with* a midwife. For, as we have seen, in these cases the original task expected of the male practitioner was merely to stand by in case of difficulty; and so the question arises as to who decided that 'difficulty' had indeed occurred, and thus that the male practitioner standing by should be asked to lend his active services. In practice, it seems (though this is a preliminary conclusion) that it was usually *the midwife* who made this decision. Thus in these two of our eight 'varieties', the 'calling' of a male practitioner actually took place in two stages, and was undertaken by different parties: first, the original booking, which was made by the mother or her husband; and second, the further summons to the delivery room, which might or might not occur, but which if it were made was made by the midwife.

This leaves just one of our eight varieties, namely *unbooked emergencies*. In practice, these were the commonest kinds of calls in all our sources – and it is here that the act of calling was at its most complex. There were several possible 'calling agents': the mother, her husband, the midwife, the various women attending the birth, and finally people outside the delivery room who knew the mother and were associated with the given male practitioner. In Willughby's cases we find all of these different possible agents named as having initiated the call. There are some cases where *combinations* of calling agents are mentioned, such as the mother and midwife or 'all the women'; there are also a few instances of conflict, where one party wanted Willughby to be called but another was opposed to this. Further, there appears to have been a difference between Willughby's practice in Derby (where he spent most of his working life) and London (where he lived for some four years, practising 'among the meaner sort of women'). In Derby, few of the emergency calls came from midwives, and there are examples of midwives being opposed to his being called. In London, it was the midwives themselves who usually called him, and we also find that Willughby was much more kindly disposed towards London midwives than towards their Midlands counterparts. Interestingly, we find that Giffard's and Smellie's cases – occurring in London some seventy to ninety years later – also show many emergency calls by midwives. Thus there seems to have been a tradition in London of better relations between midwives and surgeons than obtained in the provinces.

There is a further issue, pertaining especially to emergency calls, and just as important as the question of who made the call: namely *when and why* the call was made. So far, I have been writing as if the definition of an 'emergency' was unproblematical; but in fact, as the sources make abundantly clear, this definition was itself a social act. An emergency could consist in flooding – but how much flooding? In obstructed labour – but obstructed for how long? In danger to the mother's life – but how was this danger assessed? It was the participants in the birth who answered these questions, following their own beliefs about the nature of childbirth and the role of the male practitioner. A man-midwife might be called to deliver a living child, or a dead one; after twelve hours, or after ten days; in hope, or in fear. An obstetric emergency was, in short, *defined by* the participants in the birth: It was not a biological 'given', even though it was (so to speak) socially constructed out of biological raw materials. And the social 'definition' of an emergency was in fact highly complex, involving as it did a number of separate people in distinctive social roles.

A final set of complexities has to be mentioned in connection with emergency calls, particularly of the unbooked variety. So far, I have been assuming for the sake of simplicity that in such cases, the primary management of the birth had been in the hands of a midwife; but of course, emergencies could and did occur with a male practitioner in charge. Further, I have been assuming that in the event of an emergency, the first recourse was to a male practitioner; but in fact, a midwife could be called in this role. Indeed, certain midwives seem to have specialised in such emergency work, or at least enjoyed reputations for being able to deliver difficult births: Three such midwives are mentioned in Willughby's treatise. Sometimes a chain of practitioners was called: Willughby occasionally found three or more midwives present at a difficult birth, and Smellie records cases where he was the second or third male practitioner to have been summoned. Hunter described in his lectures a case that went from the midwife to a male practitioner to a second male practitioner and then back to the original midwife. This would appear to be unusual: So far as a pattern can be detected, this would seem to be for the delivery to pass from midwives to male practitioners, but not the other way around.

Further variants arose as by-products of man-midwifery itself, through lying-in hospitals on the one hand and through the teaching practice of William Smellie on the other. We can presumably regard delivery in a lying-in hospital as a special case of the onset call, but a definitive classification of such births must await research into the admission and management policies of the lying-in hospitals. Smellie devised for teaching purposes an ingenious arrangement: He induced poor women to permit him and his pupils to deliver them. The advantage for the mother was that the delivery was free (and indeed, Smellie arranged a maintenance fund for these women during their lying-in by subscriptions from his pupils). The advantage for Smellie and the pupils was a stock of natural labours for their instruction. These arrangements represented onset calls (presumably of the booked variety); often Smellie himself was left in the role of emergency consultant; and he kept a midwife employed to attend such labours if they proved normal but lingering.

Profiles of practice

Any individual practice can be conceived as having a specific *profile*, consisting of the relative and absolute frequencies of these different

354   *Adrian Wilson*

Table 12.1. *Profiles of practice: types of calls known to have been accepted by various practitioners (Willughby in Derby, all others in London)*

	Willughby (1660s)	Chamberlen (c. 1720)	Giffard[a] (1726–8)	Smellie (1740s)	Hunter (1740s–60s)
Advance	+	+	·	·	+
Onset	+	+	+	+	+
Emergency	+	?	+	+	+

Key: + = known to have occurred
     · = known not to have occurred
    ? = occurrence uncertain
[a]Cases 1–37 only.
Sources: See footnotes 4 and 5.

types of calls. In considering this question, I shall simplify the matter considerably by attending only to the distinction between advance, onset and emergency calls (i.e., suppressing the issues of booking and midwife presence). Table 12.1 shows, for five practitioners, which of these types of calls they are known to have attended. Here Giffard and Smellie stand out as not, apparently, having enjoyed the lucrative advance calls; all the five practitioners in question, however, received onset and (probably) emergency calls. For three of these practitioners (Willughby, Giffard and Smellie) a quantitative estimate can be made, provided we may assume that the cases in their treatises are representative of those in their practices. Table 12.2 displays this information, giving for Giffard and Smellie only provisional estimates based on small samples of their cases, whereas for Willughby's recorded cases the picture is complete.

We cannot, of course, assume that the cases in any individual's treatise are representative of those in his practice. On the contrary, we would expect the cases to be recorded selectively; and such selection might well distort the picture in the very dimension that concerns us. For instance, male practitioners might be expected to record more cases involving serious difficulty, to the relative neglect of normal births, which would have the effect of exaggerating the proportion of emergency cases. This problem can be resolved only by detailed work on each particular treatise, reconstructing the composition of the text, the distribution over time of different types of case, the purposes of the author, and so far as possible the socio-geographical catchment area of his practice. I have carried this out only for Willughby's treatise, but the results are very encouraging. Table 12.3 displays three tests that

Table 12.2. *Relative frequencies of advance, onset
and emergency calls in selected/sampled cases
of Willughby, Giffard and Smellie*

	Willughby	Giffard	Smellie
Numbers of cases			
Advance	11	—	—
Onset	6	4	9[a]
Emergency	47	28	22
Unknown	—	3	3
Total	64	35	34
Percentages			
Advance + onset	27	11–20	26–35
Emergency	73	80–9	65–74

Note: Cases used: Willughby – all his childbirth cases from
1660–1672, i.e., those occurring during the writing of his
treatise; Giffard – the first 35 childbirth cases (coming from
cases 1–37) of his treatise; Smellie – a stratified random
sample (1 case in 10) of all the cases in his treatise (vols. ii
and iii), replacing non-childbirth/non-Smellie cases with
Smellie childbirth cases where possible.
[a]Includes one case received by his pupils at onset of labour,
but which they referred to Smellie because an emergency
arose.

can be made of the representativeness of the cases included in the
previous table; if there was some particular bias (such as a bias in
favour of emergency cases), it would almost certainly be reflected in
one or more of these tests. In fact these measures show no such
distortion; what seems to have happened is that the variety of
Willughby's arguments had the accidental effect of making him record
different types of calls to roughly equal extents. We cannot, of course,
naïvely extend this finding to Giffard and Smellie, yet it is possible
prima facie that their case series, too, are approximately representative.

Thus encouraged, we may return to Table 12.2, from which two
main features stand out. First, Willughby was distinctive amongst
these three practitioners in receiving 'advance' calls at all. It may be
that the other cases in Giffard's treatise show a few such calls, but
even so the sample suggests that the incidence of these in Giffard's
practice must have been much lower than in Willughby's. As for
Smellie, I can confirm from a sifting of the cases that he records no

Table 12.3. *Reliability of the cases in Willughby's treatise*
as a source for his practice: numbers of cases in various categories

Similarity of two phases of the case series:[a]	1660–6	1667–72
Advance	5	6
Onset	3	3
Emergency	24	23
Totals	32	32
Types of case recording:	Primary[b]	Secondary[b]
Advance + onset	14 (27%)	3 (23%)
Emergency	37 (73%)	10 (77%)
Comparison with catchment area:	Observed	Expected[c] (with $N = 64$)
Advance + onset	17	9–28
Emergency	47	36–55

[a]These can be regarded as distinct 'phases', because Willughby's topics of concern changed in 1667.

[b]Primary cases are those involving the delivery of a mother whom Willughby had not delivered before; secondary cases are follow-up deliveries, i.e., further deliveries of mothers he had already delivered. It is likely that Willughby recorded all secondary cases (hence these are probably representative); it is certain that he recorded only a small fraction, about ⅕, of his "primary" cases (hence these are very probably unrepresentative).

[c]Basis of 'expected': Emergency practice estimated by various routes at 25–30 per year. Advance and onset cases estimated at 5–20 per year, on the assumption that amongst the eligible social classes and within Willughby's catchment area, the incidence of such calls could have been as low as 5 per cent or as high as 20 per cent. The figures given represent the extremes from these assumptions.

explicitly 'advance' cases at all. There may be some under the 'unknowns', but it is unlikely that this would have been a significant component of Smellie's practice without the fact ever being explicitly acknowledged; and of course Smellie was so busy with his teaching, and with his onset and emergency calls, that he lacked the incentive to accept advance calls. As we have seen, the advance calls were lucrative – but so was Smellie's teaching, which stood handsomely in place of an advance-call practice.

The second point that emerges from Table 12.2 is the overwhelming predominance of emergency calls in all three sets of cases. Around three-quarters of the cases – more amongst Giffard's, less amongst Smellie's – were of this type. If we compare the three sets in this respect (that is, ignoring the distinction between 'advance' and 'onset' cases that is relevant only in Willughby's practice) then their *similarity* is the striking finding. This serves to extend and underline a point I have made already, namely that 'man-midwifery' tended to be concentrated upon difficult births. Normal births were brought into male practice only via advance and onset calls, and even these calls were usually made because difficulty was *expected*. But the main component of male practice – at least, that of Willughby, Giffard and Smellie – was emergency work, and here of course difficulty had *already occurred*.

Finally, a 'profile of practice' should also include some assessment of the overall *rate* of practice, that is of how many births the given man-midwife attended in a typical year. For Willughby, some of this has already emerged (in Table 12.3): He saw in all perhaps thirty-five to forty births per year, and this is consonant with his socio-geographical catchment area. Notice that we have here a strong constraint on provincial obstetric practice by men: Willughby had a big local reputation, was seated in a county town, and practised over a ten-mile radius, yet given the distribution of population and the general restriction of his practice to emergency work, he could not have expected to attend as many as fifty births per year. The likely rate of practice for men-midwives in market towns must therefore have been still lower. In sharp contrast were the prospects in London, which had fifteen times as many births in the metropolitan area as occurred within Willughby's ten-mile radius of practice. Thus it is not surprising to find that Giffard seems to have attended something of the order of 50 to 100 births a year.[7] The rate of Smellie's London practice awaits investigation, but it seems overwhelmingly likely that this was at least as high as Giffard's.

Practice and precept

The 'profile of practice' of any given man-midwife dictated the actual experience of childbirth he accumulated. A practice dominated by emergencies would lead to much experience of malpresentations, obstructed labours and major complications; a practice involving

---

7 There are long gaps in Giffard's case series (as in Willughby's). If we look only at those cases without such long gaps between them, then from the first 37 cases in Giffard's treatise we find an average of a case every eight days, just under 50 per year. But there was a heavy concentration of cases in August, 1728 (cases 27–36, i.e., ten cases in all), including six uses of the forceps; this month may well have been more representative, and it would suggest over 100 cases per year. The true rate probably lay somewhere between these estimates.

more advance and onset cases might give far more opportunities to see the mechanism of normal labour, yet this could also depend on whether these cases involved a midwife as well as the male practitioner. This influence of the type of practice on the experiences of the practitioner can be brought out dramatically by contrasting two specific individuals: Percival Willughby and James Houstoun. We have already seen the broad contours of Willughby's practice: a delivery every ten days or so, mostly emergencies, but about once a month an advance or onset case – usually delivered, however, not by Willughby but by the midwife.

Houstoun's brief experience in man-midwifery was gained at the Paris Hôtel-Dieu. There, in the position of house surgeon, which he gained after arduous lobbying, he delivered in four months about 300 births – for which he was personally responsible, even though he was working in tandem with some fellow-trainee female midwives. It is therefore likely that he gained more experience of *normal birth* than Willughby acquired in a decade of practice, perhaps even in a lifetime. Yet precisely the opposite is true of *difficult* cases. If we take the florid example of arm/shoulder presentation, Houstoun probably saw only one such delivery; he may have seen none, or two, or just possibly as many as three, but it is highly unlikely that he delivered more than this.[8] Willughby, by contrast, delivered about six such cases every year; he became so adept at them that he could effect the delivery by podalic version in just seven minutes, and in the course of his practice he devised his own method of turning, improving on Paré's technique, which was the one he had learned initially. Moreover, there were qualitative differences between Willughby's experience and Houstoun's. In difficult births, Willughby was the practitioner of last resort; Houstoun, by contrast, 'called in the master-surgeon of the Hospital's assistance'. In normal births, Willughby usually played a subordinate role to the midwife; Houstoun's position was complex, since on the one hand he performed the delivery himself, while on the other hand 'we assisted one another, and had a mistress midwife who directed the whole'.

The actual experiences of the practitioner, together with his previous education, are what we should expect to have conditioned the attitudes he developed. Willughby provides a clear case in point, for his *Observations* record how he arrived at his strenuous belief in non-

---

8 Assuming that cases of arm/shoulder presentation occurred at a rate of 1 in 200 deliveries, in 300 births the odds are 14 to 1 against more than three such cases, using binomial probabilities.

intervention. His training had been confined to the use of the crotchet for craniotomies, and consequently, in advance and onset cases he 'gave way to the midwife' to do whatever she pleased. But different midwives managed deliveries in different ways: Some placed the mother on a midwife's stool, others in bed, still others kneeling on a bolster on the floor; some stretched the labiae with their hands and pulled the child, while others left the delivery to proceed naturally; some wanted to hurry labour, others to defer it. All this meant that Willughby had a rich pool of experience from which to learn – if he so desired. And he did indeed wish to learn, for he was horrified both at the sufferings of women in childbed and at the grisly work of craniotomy he might be called on to perform. Thus propelled to observe, Willughby 'took this observation': 'That those women were easiest or soonest delivered, that kept themselves warm and quiet, in or on their beds or pallets, deferring their labours to the very last, and patiently suffering nature to bedew with humours those places, and so to mellow and open by degrees their bodies, without midwives' enforcements.' The preconditions for this piece of learning were first, the different practices of different midwives, and second, Willughby's position on the sidelines in advance and onset cases – the fact that he usually did not have responsibility for conducting the delivery.

Smellie, Hunter and the revolution in obstetrics

In this light, I suggest, we can better understand the questions with which we began, concerning William Hunter's role in the eighteenth-century 'revolution in obstetrics'. Again, this is best brought out by a contrast – in this case, the contrast between Hunter and his teacher, rival and fellow-*émigré* from Lanarkshire, William Smellie.

Smellie's introduction to obstetric practice came in Lanark itself in the 1720s; he was then unacquainted with the forceps but could perform podalic version, and he seems to have had an emergency practice much akin to Willughby's. This means that the routine obstetric work Smellie was performing, as part of a general practice, consisted mainly of craniotomies. Now, compared to craniotomy, the forceps was a far more humane instrument – which is why Smellie, on reading about the forceps, acquired it and went about learning how to use it. As we have seen, his subsequent London practice included a significant proportion of normal births, yet numerically these were far outweighed by emergency cases. As Smellie tended to entrust onset calls to his pupils, and to give himself a consultant role, this pattern would have been enhanced. Given this pattern of experience, Smellie was likely to be a relative enthusiast for the forceps and for surgical intervention (whether manual or instrumental) in general.

William Hunter's development as a man-midwife, very different from Smellie's, can be summarised in terms of four stages. First, he came to medical practice (in 1737) after the design of the forceps had been published: He was not a man of the craniotomy era. Second, his initial training in midwifery came from Smellie himself, that is from the leading forceps practitioner of the day. Third, he left Smellie's household to live with James Douglas and thereby gained access (as Helen Brock has shown) not only to a vast wealth of anatomical techniques, ideas and preparations, but also to the polite, aristocratic practice of man-midwifery. Finally, from 1748 at the Middlesex Hospital, and then from 1749 at the newly founded Lying-in Hospital, Hunter had a position as a consultant man-midwife. We shall now see that the obstetric attitudes displayed in Hunter's lectures are intelligible as the product of these experiences.[9]

A striking feature of the lectures is the frequency with which Hunter referred to Smellie – and, no less so, the complexity of his attitude to Smellie. From the lecture notes, Smellie emerges not only as the foil against whom Hunter develops his own anti-interventionist stance, but also in the role of the great man. In the introductory, historical lecture Hunter referred to some thirteen authorities, Hippocrates being the first and Smellie (mentioned three times) the last; in the substantive part of the course, Smellie towered over all the rest, with twenty-seven citations as against eighteen for all other authors combined (La Motte with four citations being his nearest rival). Strikingly, Hunter made no mention at all of Ould, Exton or Burton, whereas he did refer to Chamberlen, Mauriceau and Daventer – proof enough that such references were highly selective. The thrust of the references to Smellie is much more evenly balanced than might have been expected: fourteen references are critical, ten are favourable and the remaining six are ambiguous or neutral. The criticisms are almost invariably in the direction of describing Smellie as too officious, too interventionist, and to this extent the received view is correct; but the presence of great praise alongside the blame, together

---

9 The lecture notes, cited in fn. 4, are paginated 1–176, followed by a few pages on the management of children. The themes I discuss are found on the following pages: references to Smellie, pp. 7, 8, 10, 25, 28, 32, 34, 35, 39 (twice), 47, 51, 59, 73f, 90, 92, 97, 101, 102, 104 (twice), 111, 115, 119, 122, 131, 134, 139, 147, 173. Forceps, pp. 102–16. Placenta, pp. 95 (from which I quote), 99f. Reputation and 'delicacy', pp. 39, 43, 44, 50, 51, 52, 53, 55, 58, 70, 79, 82f, 87f, 94, 95, 134, 150, 153, 168, 172–6 (my final quotation is from p. 176).

with the sheer weight of the references to Smellie, suggests something more: that in the sphere of midwifery, Smellie was something of a father-figure for Hunter.

What strengthens this picture is the fact that Hunter's own anti-interventionism was by no means as total or as doctrinaire as has sometimes been supposed. On the forceps, the lecture notes reveal that the classic quotation reproduced by Spencer has to be heavily qualified: Although inveighing several times against their injudicious and over-hasty use, Hunter devoted much time (some fifteen pages in the manuscript notes) to detailed instructions on how to apply the forceps. Similarly on the third stage of labour:

> If pains come on 20 minutes or half an hour after the delivery
> of the child, pull gently on the funis to extract the placenta; but
> in weak relaxed women with pendulous bellies, we should
> wait a long time before the uterus can recover its tone so as to
> be capable of contraction. If without attending to the state of
> the uterus . . . we should pull forcibly at the funis, the gaping
> sinuses may pour forth such a torrent of blood as to bring on a
> fatal syncope.

The key phrase here is 'without attending to the state of the uterus'. Far from putting forward a dogma or doctrine, Hunter was seeking to regulate practice by attentive observation: Sometimes, he held, manual removal of the placenta was appropriate, but at other times it was not. His famous anti-interventionism, then, consisted in a shift of emphasis and to some degree in self-presentation, rather than representing a total break with Smellie's teaching. Its rhetorical force was animated by Hunter's desire to demarcate himself from Smellie, to establish his own separate identity as a practitioner.

But if Smellie left a mark on Hunter, so too, in a different way, did James Douglas. The aristocratic practice in midwifery that Hunter initially owed to Douglas was largely made up of onset calls. This would have shifted the balance of Hunter's obstetric experiences sharply in the direction of normal birth and away from obstructed labours. Moreover, Hunter's consultancy work, too, would also have exposed him to normal births – and incidentally, through enhancing his reputation and status, probably helped him to develop his private onset practice as well. It is plausible to suppose that as Hunter gained more and more experience of normal birth, he became more and more conscious of those powers of nature that were to be a conspicuous theme of the argument of his lectures.

These experiences make it intelligible that Hunter's proclaimed approach to midwifery consisted in distancing himself from Smellie in the specific direction of arguing for less hasty intervention. But some-

thing more was to strengthen this attitude. Hunter's lectures reveal
an overwhelming concern with what he called the 'dress and address'
of the practitioner. In lecture after lecture he returned to such themes
as the reputation of the *accoucheur*, the devices needed to create and to
maintain the reputation, and the delicacy this enterprise required.
Hunter was, in fact, teaching his pupils man-midwifery, not merely
as a technical skill, but also as a social role. It was to this topic that the
last words of the lecture course were devoted: 'Advice to young accoucheurs' takes up several pages of the notes, and it ends with this
slogan: 'It is not the mere safe delivery of the woman will recommend
an accoucheur, but a sagacious well-conducted behaviour of tenderness, assiduity and delicacy.' Here we have the man-midwife who
wants to get into the delivery room, and to deliver normal births
amongst wealthy patients – a far cry indeed from the emergency
practice of a previous generation. And it seems likely that this
strengthened Hunter's reliance upon nature, his anti-interventionism: To touch a lady was a different matter from touching the wife
of a tradesman. At one point in the lectures this becomes explicit;
fittingly, this is one of Hunter's criticisms of Smellie. It concerns the
diagnosis of pregnancy:

> Smellie advises introducing a finger in ano which will more
> likely ascertain the pressure, but the indelicacy of this opera-
> tion has exploded its practice in private. Such practice is im-
> proper when you are called to satisfy a lady. Here you should
> for your own reputation's sake endeavour to use some ambig-
> uous answer, and by prescribing some inoffensive medicine
> . . . to amuse her a month longer.

Hunter's developing experience, his attitudes to technical obstetric
issues, and his approach to the social role of the man-midwife were
thus all of a piece. To some extent he inherited this particular niche
from James Douglas and (indirectly) from such predecessors as Hamilton and Manningham; but by his own lectures and by the force of
his own highly successful example, he must have enlarged it enormously. That he eventually delivered the queen herself was a fitting
symbol of his triumph.

The picture that has emerged here is consistent with the accepted
view that the 'revolution in obstetrics' was promoted both by the
forceps and by fashion, but it would seem that these two influences
worked within different spheres of practice. The role of the forceps
was primarily in emergency work; fashionable practice involved
onset and advance calls. What Smellie was for the obstetric surgeon,
the emergency practitioner, Hunter was for the physician-man-
midwife. With the distinction drawn between these different types of

practice, and with Hunter's own development understood in these terms, there is no longer a paradox about Hunter's attitude to the forceps.

Conclusion: man-midwifery and its historiography

It will be apparent that my approach to William Hunter, and to man-midwifery in general, differs in several respects from Professor Shorter's interpretation, elsewhere in this volume (Chap. 13). In the first place, we have different historiographical objectives: Shorter writes in evaluative terms, whereas I have limited myself to description. Second, we have different pictures of the long-term developments: Swayed as I am by Willughby's *Observations*, I do not find the anti-interventionism of the late eighteenth century a wholly novel development. I am inclined to believe that not all midwives were meddlesome, and I have claimed that midwives could influence male practitioners as well as learning from them.[10] Third, with regard to the eighteenth century, we have studied different things: Shorter has extracted from treatises specific doctrines about the management of the separate stages of labour, whereas I have focused upon the overall stance or approach of individual practitioners. Fourth, in contextualising our findings, we have again gone different ways: Shorter has related text to text, whereas I have sought the intelligibility of texts in obstetric practice. Finally, as to that practice, we have different underlying images of its nature: For Professor Shorter it is largely a technical, biological matter, whereas I have depicted it as a series of social acts. Our approaches, it seems, are not so much complementary as incommensurable – no doubt a tribute to the richness of the subject.

The burden of my argument has been that the word 'man-midwifery' conceals more than it reveals. It meant eight different things – different paths to childbirth, as I have called them – and these were themselves complex. Any individual practice comprised a specific mixture of these different elements, and there was great room for differences between different individuals. Not only were there changes over time (notably the publication of the forceps) and specificities of place (such as the different opportunities for practice in London and elsewhere), but also there were different attitudes on the

---

10 Jean L'Esperance suggests that it is the 'central message' of Professor Shorter's *A History of Women's Bodies* (New York, 1982) that 'women owe their current happy situation in society to the superior knowledge and kindness of the opposite sex'. See *Ontario History*, LXXV (1983), 98–103 (I quote from p. 100), and ibid. 298–9 for the author's reply.

part of the men-midwives themselves. Precepts and experiences were interwoven in complex ways: Given the wealth of treatises and case-records, together with the diversity of attitudes exhibited by male practitioners, there is ample scope here for further research.

If we are confused by the term man-midwifery, that is an artefact of our distance in time from the period. Contemporaries knew what they meant and would have experienced no sense of contradiction in using the same word in different ways. We do the same – witness how many different things are covered by such words as 'historian' or 'doctor' – but when studying the past, we stand outside the relevant speech-community and thus are misled by the appearances of words.

It is equally significant that a man could be, to all intents and purposes, a man-midwife – a man much engaged in delivering women – without ever being described as such. The most striking example of this is Percival Willughby, a specialist in deliveries in the 1660s. Willughby is more accessible to historical view than many other seventeenth-century practitioners (whether obstetric or not), yet the several ways he was described include no hint of his obstetric work. At different times and in different contexts he was called 'surgeon', 'physician', 'extra-licentiate', 'gentleman', and (on his tombstone, apparently erroneously) 'M.D'. Thus, just as we cannot read off the nature of man-midwifery from the word 'man-midwife', so too we cannot infer the absence of male obstetric practice from the absence of the word later used to describe it. This goes a long way to support the viewpoint, variously advanced by Roberts, Pelling and Webster, and Cunningham, that the content of practice is not to be naively inferred from any practitioner-label.[11] What such labels meant, at any point in the early-modern period, remains to be discovered – as does the full meaning of 'man-midwifery'.

Acknowledgements

I wish to acknowledge the help of Helen Brock, who has been very generous in supplying me with references and drew my attention in

---

11   R. S. Roberts, 'The Personnel and Practice of Medicine in Tudor and Stuart England', *Medical History*, VI (1962), 363–82, and VIII (1964), 217–34 (see particularly pp. 375–6 of the first of these two parts of the article); Margaret Pelling and Charles Webster, 'Medical Practitioners', in Webster, ed., *Health, Medicine and Mortality in the Sixteenth Century* (Cambridge, 1979), pp. 165–235 (see esp. p. 235); Andrew Cunningham, 'The Medical Professions and the Pattern of Medical Care: The Case of Edinburgh, c.1670–c.1700', in Wolfgang Eckart and Johanna Geyer-Kordesch, eds., *Heilberufe und Kranke im 17. und 18. Jahrhundert die Quellen- und Forschungssituation* (Münster, 1982), pp. 9–28. Cunningham writes (p. 17) that 'we just do not know which particular functions were undertaken by someone calling himself a "surgeon" or "apothecary": and we will not know them until such time as we try to discover them – from a position of confessed ignorance'.

particular to the Hunter lecture notes in the Royal College of Surgeons library; Andrew Cunningham, for his criticisms and advice; and the librarian and staff of the Royal College of Surgeons library, for facilitating my research. Where a reference is not supplied, supporting details will be found in A. F. Wilson, 'Childbirth in Seventeenth- and Eighteenth-Century England', (D. Phil. thesis, University of Sussex, 1982). This is to be published as *A Safe Deliverance* (Cambridge, in press).

Appendix: illustrative examples of different paths to childbirth

These cases are taken from the treatises of Willughby and Smellie (see footnote 4). References to Smellie's cases are to the case numbers supplied by McClintock to his edition.

One of the Willughby cases used here is described in both of the extant versions of his treatise, and I have reproduced both accounts since they give different though compatible details. These particular descriptions (example 3) are given in full. All the other examples are abridged to bring into greater prominence the theme with which I am concerned. I have modernised spelling and punctuation throughout.

Notice that in examples 2, 4 and 6 the absence of a midwife is not stated but can be inferred by contrast with examples 1, 3 and 5 respectively. In examples 5 and 6, the fact that the call was unbooked is inferred by contrast with examples 3 and 4. Again, in example 1 it is not stated explicitly who delivered the child (the midwife or Willughby), but it can be inferred that it was the midwife, both because there is no description of the birth itself and by contrast with his account of the third stage of labour. Finally, notice in examples 1, 7 and 8 the participation of two or more agents in bringing Willughby to the birth and getting him to act.

1.Advance call, with midwife (Willughby, Observations, *64–7)*

I was sent for by a Lady and kinswoman, who thought that she was within a fortnight of her account, but she continued above that time seven weeks . . .

Friday 29 November 1661 about four in the afternoon, she forced herself to have a stool in her closet. By this great striving . . . her waters did break . . . [but] she had no labour at all . . . I persuaded her, on Saturday night, to go to bed, and was called again to her [on Sunday] December 1 early in the morning . . . In the afternoon . . . she had a hard stool, but it must [have been] concealed from me.

Her labour being long and tedious, I entreated her to take the Earl of Chesterfield's powder to move the birth . . . The child was born . . . between four and five, that Sunday [afternoon].

The child was stillborn. The midwife made much ado to revive the child, but in vain. I caused her to separate it from the after-burden . . . The midwife was fearful to fetch the after-burden, so I was put upon the work by her husband, the which I quickly performed.

2. *Advance call, without midwife (Willughby,* Observations, *40–2)*

A young, good conditioned lady (the Lady Byron) . . . desired my company, and entreated me to be with her, and to assist her in the time of her travail, and in the mean space to direct her what was convenient to be done or observed by her . . . She had a thin and weak body, and was troubled with great fears, never having any child before.

August the thirteenth [1661] the moon changed; that night she had some grumbling disquiets, and the ensuing night they increased. Thursday, August the fifteenth, I came early in the morning to her, and finding some foregoing signs of labour, at her desire she was removed into another chamber, and laid into a truckle bed about seven in the morning.

. . . In the afternoon, about one o'clock, the womb began to open . . . About a quarter past four she was delivered of a daughter. It was troublesome to fetch the after-burden as she lay on her back. She was put to her knees, and then it was obtained easily, and so she was then removed to another bed.

. . . The child was baptized Aug. 22 1661 . . . Aug. 23, I left this lady, giving her thanks for her loving favours to me.

3. *Onset call, booked, with midwife (Willughby,* Observations, *37– 8; and British Library, Sloane MS 529, p. 3)*

Printed version. . . . being in Staffordshire with a worthy good man, I saw his wife great with child. [Lady Broughton, margin] She told me what terrible afflictions she had suffered in the birth of her first child, and wept much at the remembrance of them. She entreated me that I would come to her in the time of her labour, and for that purpose she would send good horses for me. I gave her instructions to lie quietly in or on her bed until I could come to her, and not suddenly put herself under her midwife's hands. She sent me horses. I went eight miles to her. In the mean time she kept her body warm, and lay quiet. So soon as I was come she sent for me into her chamber. Going with her midwife apart from the company, I asked how this gentlewoman was, and what she thought of the birth. She replied that she could not tell, and that in all her days she never was with so peevish a woman, and that she would not suffer her to touch her body. I sat by this gentlewoman a little space, and, perceiving that labour came upon her, I went forth of the room, putting her under the midwife's hands. The waters issued without enforcement, presently the child followed them, and she was easily and quickly delivered.

When I went away, she gave God thanks, and said that her pains were nothing in comparison to what she had formerly suffered.

Manuscript version. Anno 1648: There was a worthy good Lady, yet living, that had much suffered under the midwife's hands at the birth of her first child. As I walked with her, she made great moans, with tears in her eyes, thinking what afflictions she had suffered before she could be delivered, and feared what would become of her, being great with child. I comforted her and advised her not to let her midwife too suddenly meddle with her. Being not past 8 miles from her house, she sent 2 horses to bring me, and rejoiced at my coming. I asked the midwife how the labour proceeded; she said that she knew not, and that in all her days, she never came nigh so peevish a creature as this Lady was; and that she would not let her touch her. I was glad to hear it; I whispered the Lady in her ear, and went down into the parlour. I had not long been there, but the waters flowed, and the child followed, as she lay on her truckle-bed, and all sorrow was quickly past; for which when I came into the chamber to take my leave, with a smiling countenance she gave me thanks and rewarded my coming with gold.

4. Onset call, booked, without midwife (Smellie, case 100)

In the year 1748, I was bespoke to attend a woman in her first child; and received a call about the middle of the ninth month, when she complained of pains in her head and back . . . I found the os internum soft, but not open; from which circumstance I declared she was not in labour; then I ordered her to be blooded to a quantity of eight ounces; and a clyster being injected, she was relieved of her complaints. In a fortnight after this visit, I was again called, and found the labour begun . . .

For three or four days she had been subject to slight pains, which returned at long intervals; then they became more frequent, recurring every two hours; and by the time I was called, they had grown stronger, and came faster . . . I prescribed an emollient clyster . . . and then the labour proceeded in a slow and kindly manner . . . I did not confine her to any particular position, but allowed her to walk about, and undergo her pains whether sitting or lying in bed.

[Smellie then recounts the course of the labour in detail.]

I have given a particular detail of this case, in order to make young practitioners acquainted with the common method of acting in natural labours, these being the circumstances that usually occur to a healthy woman in bearing her first child.

5. Onset call, unbooked, with midwife (Smellie, case 186)

In the year 1742, I was called to a patient about the age of forty, in labour of her first child; though I was not permitted to examine, but was obliged to wait in another apartment, in case of accidents. By the midwife's information from time to time, I understood the child advanced very slowly . . . and that the pains, though seldom, were pretty strong.

In this manner labour proceeded for the space of twelve hours, at the expiration of which the midwife told me that . . . she was afraid [the child] was now dead . . . However, the child was delivered soon after she gave me this account, and appeared to have been but a very little time dead . . .

I afterwards learned that the shyness of the patient proceeded from the artful insinuations of the midwife, who terrified her with dreadful accounts of the use of instruments.

6. Onset call, unbooked, without midwife (Smellie, case 123)

I was called to a patient in labour of her first child. The membranes broke in the evening, and she had frequent pains all night; but would not allow me to examine till about eight o'clock next morning . . .

She enjoyed no rest all night, the pains grew excessively strong and frequent, and the child's head had not advanced in the least. Being apprehensive from her violent complaints of the abdomen that the uterus would burst by such strong efforts, I prescribed a paregoric draught to allay the violence of the pain and procure sleep . . .

About twelve that night, when the effect of the opiate was worn off, her violent pains recurring, I was allowed to examine again; and finding the head still in the same situation, the draught was repeated. This kept her tolerably easy till eight in the morning, when the pains returning, it was again administered; for the same reason it was repeated at six in the evening and four in the morning. About eight, I was permitted to examine the third time.

At length I was, in the evening, suddenly called from another apartment, and finding the head almost delivered, I had just time to prevent the laceration of the external parts . . . After delivery, her urine was obstructed for three days; and for eight weeks afterwards she lost the power of retention, which, however, returned with her strength. As for the child, it was probably lost by her timorous disposition, in consequence of which she refused all assistance at the latter end of labour.

7. Emergency call, booked (Willughby, Observations, 112–4)

January the 12 Anno 1669 I was entreated, and at that time engaged, by a worthy, good, loving gentleman, to be ready to attend his good wife [Mrs Alestry, margin], and to assist her and her midwife (if need required) in the time of her travail, with the best and utmost of my endeavours.

January the 30th, travail came upon her, about eleven o'clock at night, and so continued with throws and pains all that night and the next day, without any descent of the child. The pains continued all the time in her back only.

At night January the 31 I was sent for, and, upon discourse with her and the midwife, I conceived that the labour would be difficult, and full of danger . . . I entreated her to take a gentle clyster . . . and I stayed all that night in the house with her.

The next morning, Feb 1, I caused a Doctor of Physic to be sent for, and the Divines were entreated their prayers . . . [The Dr and I] concluded to appoint with external applications, to dilate the passages, and also internal medicines, to promote labour. But, through the ill position of her body, these ways nothing at all availing, I was earnestly entreated by the Doctor, from her husband, with several others of her relations, to use the operation of the hand, to try, if possible, the birth might be forced. Whereupon I did attempt it.

. . . I endeavoured to turn the birth, and would willingly have laid her by the infant's feet, but could not possibly effect it . . . [Subsequently,] by her husband, and friends, and the Doctor, with several women, I was much persuaded and entreated by them all to draw the child with instruments, and she was willing to submit, in hopes to be delivered.

But, through the narrow passage of her body, I could not get up my hand over any part of the head to fix the instrument, nor in any other part of it to make a breach . . . So I was necessitated to desist, without any hopes of delivery, not knowing which way to relieve her, and she died . . . And my not delivering her was occasioned by the straitness of the passages, and the unusual ill conformation of the bones . . . She had been afflicted, in her infancy, with the rickets. She had very great, swelled ankle-bones, she went waddling, and her left leg was shorter than the other, and the middle of her back was much inverted, from the hips to the shoulders. She was of a very low . . . stature.

8. *Emergency call, unbooked (Willughby,* Observations, *82–3)*

August 4 1668 Mrs Mary Harley of Walton in the Wolds, being in labour and having suffered much affliction; her husband, with her desire, caused me to be sent for. The child came right, with the head pitched towards the bones. She had, several times, strong forcing throws, but they nothing availed. To move more strongly the expulsive faculty, I gave her several doses of the midwife's powder, acuted with a large quantity of Borax.

Therefore I thought it good to put back the child's head, and to deliver her by the child's feet, the which I did about twelve o'clock that night . . . All of us thought the child had been dead. But . . . the child revived . . .

As for the good woman. She was very well for the space of an hour after her delivery, and for her preservation she gave God thanks and for my care of her she also thanked me.

After this time she fainted . . . But, through God's permission, with cordial spirits she was again restored . . . She was subject to a scouring, which I disliked. I gave her several medicines to prevent it . . . At her friends' desire I stayed with her ten days. I would willingly have stayed longer, for I feared her weakness. But, perceiving that they were willing to let me go, I took leave and departed, after I had left them some directions.

It was reported that she was afflicted with convulsions toward the end of the month, and so died.

13

The management of normal deliveries and the generation of William Hunter

EDWARD SHORTER

We have long known that eighteenth-century Britain saw a revolution in the management of obstetric complications. Terminating protracted labour, coping with placenta praevia, dealing with sudden post-partum haemorrhages – all found improved solutions amongst those 'man-midwives' who flourished in England and Scotland after the 1730s. What has been less clear to scholars, however, is that the medical management of *normal* deliveries similarly underwent a revolution in the eighteenth century. It changed from massive interventionism, in which the soft parts of the birth canal were fiddled with, manipulated, massaged and dilated, to a policy of non-intervention, in which the best wisdom insisted that normal labour be left strictly alone. Although obstetric complications offer a more dramatic story, relying on accounts of the rescue of dying mothers with forceps, version and other operations, the story of changes in normal delivery is of far greater import for the average woman, in the average, uncomplicated birth.

We shall discuss the normal delivery according to the various phases of the birth process. In each phase we shall see the generation of English and Scottish man-midwives that arose around the time of William Hunter implementing revolutionary advances, so that by the end of the eighteenth century the modern philosophy of non-interference in uncomplicated deliveries had been firmly established.

The first stage of labour: the labour pains dilate the cervix

As we pick up the narrative around 1700 we bear in mind the medical tradition, stretching from the ancient Greeks and Romans, of interference in normal labour. Dilating the introitus, vagina and cervix, massaging the perineum, lubricating the birth canal, manually detaching the placenta – all were traditions of centuries-old antiquity, not merely in academic medicine but in popular midwifery as well. Thus it will not surprise us to find officious intervention at every turn in the seventeenth century and before.[1] When does this tradition start to break? One historian of early-modern midwifery dates the reform – erroneously, I believe – with William Harvey's work in mid-seventeenth century.[2] While it is true that Harvey spoke admiringly of 'Nature' in his 1653 work on human reproduction, he gave no specific directions for supervising deliveries, and contented himself with rebuking 'the younger, more giddy and officious midwives'.[3] Moreover, the men who came directly after Harvey proved themselves to be quite meddlesome. The London MD John Maubray, who in 1724 began teaching midwifery in his home, instructed pupils to grease their hands, then manually to dilate the cervix,[4] a pernicious lesson on two counts: (1) the ointments used for this purpose could carry infection to the mother's uterus, as of course could the interfering hand; (2) manual dilatation of the soft parts of the birth canal risks lacerating them, thus further increasing the chance of infection and haemorrhage, to say nothing of the pain involved.

Nor was the London surgeon Edmund Chapman an improvement. He wrote in his 1733 text that cervical rigidity could, after 'many hours of strong pain', not better be overcome 'than with the finger to dilate and thrust back the ring or circle' that the cervix makes 'about the head of the child'.[5] Because he said nothing else about the management of normal labour, this vague counsel could only be taken as an invitation to interfere whenever the attendant, the mother herself, and the bystanders felt she had suffered enough.

The Dublin man-midwife Fielding Ould showed himself in 1742 to be even more interventionist. 'When labour is retarded by the thickness and hardness of [the cervix]', the forefinger must be introduced and 'the orifice must be gently dilated'. The attendant should then introduce several more fingers because 'this dilatation must be continued till the orifice gives passage to the head'. In addition, one

1   See on this Audrey Eccles, *Obstetrics and Gynaecology in Tudor and Stuart England* (London, 1982), pp. 86–100, and Edward Shorter, *A History of Women's Bodies* (New York, 1982), pp. 58–66.
2   Herbert R. Spencer, *The History of British Midwifery from 1650 to 1800* (London, 1927), p. 165.
3   William Harvey, *Anatomical Exercitations, Concerning the Generation of Living Creatures* (London, 1653), p. 488; on p. 509 he implies that Nature does best as he tells the story of the soldier's wife who gave birth alone.
4   John Maubray, *The Female Physician, Containing all the Diseases Incident to that Sex . . . Art of New Improv'd Midwifery* (London, 1724), p. 218.
5   Edmund Chapman, *A Treatise on the Improvement of Midwifery*, 3d ed. (London, 1753; 1st ed., 1733), p. 79.

might reach into the vagina to force the coccyx back out of the way. Ould also flattered himself for having invented a method of hastening labour: 'to introduce the thumb, being oiled, into the anus . . . whereby . . . the coccyx is pulled out . . . as far as is thought necessary'.[6] The possibilities for insinuating faecal contamination into the birth canal with this procedure are staggering.

Not until the early 1750s, almost a hundred years after Harvey wrote, did man-midwives finally begin advocating non-intervention in the first stage of labour. The York MD John Burton is technically entitled to priority here, for in his 1751 textbook he advised no vaginal examination before labour begins, for reasons of 'delicacy and tenderness', and went on to explain that 'the less the parts are handled, the better it is for both mother and child, because it always frets and stimulates them'.[7] But Burton was soon forgotten, and would live on only in Laurence Sterne's caricature of him in *Tristam Shandy* as 'Dr Slop'.

The most influential partisan of non-intervention in the first stage was to write a year later, William Smellie, who published the first volume of his *Treatise on the Theory and Practice of Midwifery* in 1752. Even if labour was slow, the attendant should not intervene, said Smellie, except perhaps for greasing the parts a bit with 'pomatum, hog's lard, butter, or Ung. althaea'. No matter how 'clamorous' the visitors or how 'anxious and impatient' the woman herself, Smellie advised against intervention and would only 'prescribe some innocent placemus, that she may take between whiles, to beguile the time and please her imagination'.[8] Thus the doctrine of non-intervention in the first stage was established.

Smellie's opinions were quickly taken up, even by such enemies as the midwife Elizabeth Nihell. Although she condemned every other aspect of Smellie's practice in her 1760 diatribe, Nihell praised non-intervention 'in the cases of natural and easy delivery [where] there is little or no actual occasion for the presence of the midwife, beyond that of receiving the fetus'.[9] (Nihell of course did not attribute this enlightened policy to Smellie, yet it must have come from some source in academic medicine since Nihell's female colleagues were at this time wildly interventionist.) The London surgeon George Counsell wrote in 1758 that 'in this natural and happy labour you will have

6 Fielding Ould, *A Treatise of Midwifery in Three Parts* (Dublin, 1742), pp. 40, 43.
7 John Burton, *An Essay Towards a Complete New System of Midwifery* (London, 1751), pp. 103–4.
8 William Smellie, *A Treatise on the Theory and Practice of Midwifery* (London, 1752), pp. 222, 224. 'Ung. althaea' from *Althaea officinalis*, or 'marsh mallow'.
9 Elizabeth Nihell, *A Treatise on the Art of Midwifery* (London, 1760), pp. 257–8.

little to do, besides receiving the child and taking proper care of the afterburden [placenta]'.[10] After the 1760s the historian will be hard put to find midwifery writers who advise doing anything more to the first stage of the uncomplicated delivery than 'lubricating the parts'.[11]

Second stage: the expulsion of the child

Progress in the management of the second stage of delivery came rather differently: The big break with meddlesomeness did not occur until the 1770s. The modern observer is, in fact, quite horrified to hear earlier advice on what to do normally as the infant's head passes through the cervix, into the vagina and out through the introitus. The older writers were quite brutal: As soon as they could reach the head, they would grab it with both hands and pull, moving it from side to side, as Maubray advised in 1724.[12] All this haste was thought necessary so that the uterus would not contract and make the delivery of the afterbirth impossible. John Burton wanted the birth attendant to slip the cervix over the child's head as it passed through.[13] Even Smellie offered the following bizarre strategy for a head that did not advance after 'several pains': 'one or two fingers' in the rectum 'ought to press upon the forehead of the child . . . great care being taken to avoid the eyes. This pressure detains the head till the return of another pain, which will squeeze it farther down, while the fingers pushing slowing and gradually, turn the forehead', all the while in the anus.[14]

William Hunter himself was unable to keep his hands out of the birth canal during the second stage of labour. As a student of Hunter's later explained, in Hunter's view, when the child's head was in the birth canal, 'a finger or two should be gently applied to dilate the passage'. One might also lift the cervix 'over the child's head'.[15]

Amongst Hunter's contemporaries the meddlesome practice arose of 'supporting the perineum', which meant at that time opposing with one's hand the progress of the child's head so that the mother's perineal body (the 'perineum') would be less rapidly stretched. Whether this kind of support actually reduces the incidence of per-

---

10 George Counsell, *The London New Art of Midwifery* (London, 1758), p. 18.
11 For the phrase, Thomas Cooper, *A Compendium of Midwifery* (London, 1766), p. 84.
12 Maubray, *Female Physician*, p. 219. Ould also advised pulling on the head, *Treatise*, p. 51.
13 Burton, *Essay*, p. 114.
14 Smellie, *Treatise*, p. 212.
15 Anon., *Lectures on the Gravid Uterus, and Midwifery; as Taught and Practised by the Late Dr. Hunter . . . By One Who Studied Him* (London, 1783), pp. 51–2.

ineal tearing is unclear.[16] But it risks bruising the muscles of the perineum, and moreover, in slowing the progress of delivery, exposes the infant to anoxia. 'Supporting the perineum' is therefore done hesitantly today. In the eighteenth century, however, even otherwise progressive figures such as London MD John Harvie were giving elaborate instructions for this support: Push against the perineum 'with a proper force' at every pain, said Harvie. Resist extension of the infant's neck as much as possible until, once the vertex is out, one may 'very cautiously with the palm of the left hand flip back the perineum over the child's face and chin'.[17]

So fiddling and meddling remained the order of the day until the advent of Charles White. The Manchester surgeon published his textbook in 1773, and only therewith did a British author propose almost complete non-interference with the second stage of labour. White opposed the 'greasy applications' so beloved of earlier writers. Although he did advocate support of the perineum, his minimal instructions lack Harvie's officious enthusiasm. White advised against the practice of grabbing the infant's head and pulling as soon as it appeared in the vagina or crowned, his motto being, 'Leave things to nature, and in general she performs her work best without assistance.' Finally, unlike many previous writers, he thought it unnecessary to pull on the child's armpits in order to deliver the shoulders.[18]

Thus, as Audrey Eccles has recently suggested, White's work stands as a major turning point in the history of obstetrics.[19] Most of the generation of textbook writers of the 1780s adopted these proposals. The Edinburgh surgeon John Aiken said in 1784, 'Officiousness is . . . not only odious, but injurious.' After a single vaginal examination the attendant should not interfere. 'The less handling the better.' Supporting the perineum was acceptable, but 'not strictly necessary'. Etcetera.[20] Another Edinburgh figure, the physician David Spence, called in 1784 for little more intervention than an en-

16 Some writers thought that it did reduce perineal tearing. The London MD William Osborn, who practised elaborate manoeuvres in the protection of the perineum, claimed that 'by strict attention to this management only, I have never once in my life, during thirty years practice, met with a laceration of the perineum to any extent'. *Essays on the Practice of Midwifery* (London, 1792), p. 37.
17 John Harvie, *Practical Directions, Shewing a Method of Preserving the Perineum in Birth, and Delivering the Placenta Without Violence* (London, 1767), pp. 3–8.
18 I have consulted the second edition of the work. Charles White, *A Treatise on the Management of Pregnant and Lying-In Women* (London, 1777; 1st ed., 1773), pp. 106, 108.
19 Eccles, *Obstetrics and Gynaecology*, pp. 86–7.
20 I consulted the second edition, John Aiken, *Principles of Midwifery* (Edinburgh, 1785; 1st ed., 1784), pp. 62–3.

ema at the beginning of labour and some support of the perineum at the end, believing that 'sliding [the perineum] gently over the face of the child' would help prevent tearing.[21] Whereas the Edinburgh midwifery professor Alexander Hamilton had, in the second edition of his textbook (1785),[22] called for lubricating the parts and slipping the perineum over the head, by the time the fourth edition was published in 1796 he had retreated to virtual non-intervention: 'Practitioners ought to be guarded against making too violent pressure on the perineum.'[23]

By the 1790s writers were already repeating the catechism that would guide birth attendants until the 1920s. The famous Thomas Denman wrote in 1794 that as the child descended through the pelvis, 'the practitioner should on no account interfere, provided the labour be natural'.[24] In that same year, the London MD Robert Bland catalogued the midwifery practices now considered useless:

1. Baths and herbs to soften the ligaments before delivery
2. Smearing the vagina and cervix with lard
3. Dilating the passages with the fingers ('still too generally used')
4. 'To this has been lately added, that of guarding the perineum' (by which he meant pushing the infant's head back with every contraction)[25]

Bland opposed this earlier meddlesomeness because it 'had the effect of intimidating and alarming the minds of women, and making them consider labour as an operation full of difficulty and danger'.[26] Thus the modern doctrine of not intervening if the mother was perfectly all right had been firmly established. (At this point no one thought of speeding up the birth for the sake of the foetus.)

Third stage: the delivery of the placenta

Medical officiousness in the first two stages of labour had undoubtedly been harmful, but it was probably not as risky to the mother as intervention in the third stage of labour: manual detachment and

21   David Spence, *A System of Midwifery* (Edinburgh, 1784), pp. 153–9.
22   Alexander Hamilton, *A Treatise of Midwifery*, 2nd ed. (Edinburgh, 1785), pp. 134–7.
23   Hamilton, *Outlines of the Theory and Practice of Midwifery*, 4th ed. (London, 1796), p. 195.
24   Thomas Denman, *An Introduction to the Practice of Midwifery*, 2 vols. (London, 1794–5), I, pp. 381–2; his italics.
25   Robert Bland, *Observations on Human and on Comparative Parturition* (London, 1794), pp. xii–xiii.
26   Ibid., p. xiv.

removal of the placenta. Only here did the attendant's hand actually enter the uterus, with the accompanying risk of infection.

The early eighteenth century man-midwives were fiercely interventionist. Maubray emphasised the urgency of getting out the placenta before the womb contracted, and thus insisted that the attendant go after it even *before* cutting the umbilical cord. Maubray recognised that the placenta often detaches immediately, but even in those cases the midwife should wrap the cord about the fingers of one hand, pass the other into the uterus and bring it out. If the placenta had not yet separated, the attendant should slip a hand under one edge and manually peel it off the wall of the uterus. An advantage of reaching into the uterus, Maubray thought, was being able to rectify malpositions, remove blood clots and generally tidy things up. Now the mother's 'womb is both duly purg'd and naturally shut again as it ought to be', he said after all the reaching in was done.[27]

The London surgeon and man-midwife William Giffard, progressive though he may have been in other areas, also went forcefully after the placenta. He tells us that after one delivery in 1728, he 'gave the child to the midwife to make a ligature upon and divide the navelstring, and at the same time I passed up my hand and separated the burden, which adhered closely to the lower side of the uterus. Afterwards I drew out some membranes and clods of blood that remained in the womb.'[28] Indeed Giffard criticises the female midwives for their timidity in only poking at the cervix with a finger or two, for 'if this opportunity is lost, the mouth of the womb soon contracts, after the protrusion of the fetus, by which the placenta, if it does not soon follow, is very often stopped in the passage'.[29]

The dramatic break comes with the Dublin man-midwife Fielding Ould in his 1742 *Treatise of Midwifery*. Thus, in all the innovations in the management of normal deliveries, Ould's is historically the first, for he writes ten years before Smellie and thirty before Charles White. The attendant should 'wait for her expulsion of it, [rather] than being too desirous to extract it'. He explicitly opposed manual detachment of the placenta, assailing the Dutch surgeon Hendrik van Deventer whose 1701 obstetrics textbook had encouraged doctors to renew an age-old aggressiveness towards the placenta. Said Ould, 'This fear of the womb closing makes many operators too hasty, which often pro-

---

27   *Female Physician*, pp. 220–3.
28   Edward Hody, ed., *Cases in Midwifery Written by the late Mr. William Giffard* (London, 1734), pp. 59–60.
29   Ibid., p. 67; see also p. 201.

duceth fatal accidents', a reference to the inversions of the uterus that occurred so frequently in those days.[30]

But sadly for the women being delivered, Ould's proposal was not immediately picked up. Explained John Burton in 1751, 'The next thing is to extract the placenta, which is certainly best done by introducing the hand into the womb immediately.' Indeed, said Burton, it was 'absolutely necessary to introduce the hand, and artificially to separate and extract the placenta', in order to forestall uterine prolapse.[31] Other men of Burton's generation felt likewise.[32] Even Smellie found himself advising tugging on the cord if the placenta had not yet detached by the time the birth attendant had finished busying himself with the newborn. After a wait of ten to twenty minutes Smellie assumed that it would not separate itself naturally and counselled going after it[33] – advice that is quite similar to our current views, but in those days far more dangerous to the mother because of the risk of infection.

Modern doctrines of the management of the placenta became firmly established only in the late 1760s with John Harvie (1767). Like Ould, he thundered against manual detachment, which he thought 'attended with great pain and danger', and associated with 'mortification' (meaning infection). Harvie as well opposed tidy-minded efforts to clean out clots of blood, which he called 'this horrid scooping work'. 'Of late' his students had been leaving the placenta entirely alone, and he felt this the best policy.[34] Whether William Hunter learned from Harvie, or vice versa, or whether both merely picked up on some suggestion abroad in the times, sown perhaps by Fielding Ould, is unclear, since Hunter left no big textbooks in his wake.[35] We know that Hunter could be fanatically non-interventionist, to the

30 Ould, *Treatise*, pp. 57–8; his critique of van Deventer, pp. 61ff. Van Deventer's *Dageraat der Vroedvrouwen* appeared in Leiden in 1696; his major obstetrics textbook *Operationes chirurgicae . . . obstetricantibus* was published in 1701, translated into English in 1716.
31 Burton, *Essay*, pp. 126–8.
32 See Cooper, *Compendium*, pp. 91–2; Counsell, *London New Art of Midwifery*, pp. 25–34; Chapman, *Treatise*, 3d ed., pp. 129–34.
33 Smellie, *Treatise*, pp. 232–8.
34 Harvie, *Practical Directions*, pp. 13, 18, 40. Note that Harvie was evidently the first to advise massage of the abdomen to assist in the expulsion of the placenta (pp. 45–6).
35 That non-interventionist ideas were in the air is clear from the manuscript notes of the lectures of the Edinburgh midwifery professor Thomas Young, who advised 'waiting for a quarter of an hour before delivering the placenta, and the hand is never to be introduced till *pulling on the cord* [my italics] is found to be ineffectual'. Spencer, *History of British Midwifery*, p. 92. Thus the *Zeitgeist* was not completely non-interventionist!

point of leaving genuinely accreted placentas behind for days, where they became foci of infection and may have caused several deaths.[36] In any event, after the late 1760s no major writer of whom I am aware advised routine manual detachment of the placenta or pulling on the cord to separate the placenta or reaching into the uterus to help pull the 'womb cake' out, unless it had stayed behind for quite a long time.

The 'generation of William Hunter'?

Thus our narrative has no single titanic figure towering over it, but consists rather of a number of men, somewhat scattered in space and time, making small contributions to what would, by the end of the eighteenth century, be a brilliant new synthesis. Ould in Dublin, Smellie, John Harvie and Hunter in London, White in Manchester – what ties them together? Why not, for example, 'the generation of William Smellie'?

It is not my purpose to downgrade Smellie's reputation, although his biographer Robert Johnstone's view that Smellie 'rendered to obstetrics something of the same order of service that Hippocrates had given to medicine some twenty centuries earlier'[37] seems a bit excessive in view of the meagreness of Smellie's contributions to the management of normal delivery. We might, however, recall that in London in the 1740s and 1750s many of these men probably influenced one another. Smellie, for instance, took William Hunter into his home as a boarder in 1740, just after Smellie had arrived in London, a nineteen-year medical practice in Lanark, Scotland, behind him. The following year Smellie began teaching midwifery in London. While in Scotland, Smellie had known the Scottish physician and chemist William Cullen. Hunter had also known Cullen, having apprenticed with him for three years before briefly studying medicine at Edinburgh. So here is a typical who-influenced-whom knot to be untied: Did Cullen preach to both men doctrines of 'naturalness'? Did Smellie come upon his views by pure inductive reasoning while in Lanark, as his biographer claims?[38] Did Hunter absorb his own 'hands-off' views as a young man living in Smellie's home and helping Smellie attend complicated labours, or as a later apprentice-surgeon with James Douglas, or in the London hospitals? These men all lived, worked

---

36 Hunter, *Lectures*, p. 53; Spencer, *History of British Midwifery*, pp. 125–6.
37 Robert W. Johnstone, *William Smellie: Master of British Midwifery* (Edinburgh, 1952), pp. 126–7.
38 Ibid., p. 127.

and attended coffee-houses so much in common that it is unrealistic to see any of them as the great teacher, the others as disciples.[39]

Both Hunter and Smellie were acknowledged as teachers of the next generation of man-midwives, those who wrote in the late 1760s and 1770s. (Smellie returned to Lanark in 1759.) Who was the more important of the two? Smellie had prominent pupils, amongst them Robert Johnson, author of a 1769 obstetrics textbook,[40] and John Harvie, whom we saw reinforcing Ould's views about not meddling with the placenta. Harvie in fact married the niece of Smellie's wife, and taught with Smellie for a while in Wardour Street,[41] so the two men must have been quite close.

Yet William Hunter also exercised an important influence upon a whole generation of British man-midwives. Even though Hunter published little of an obstetrical nature, Irving Cutter's judgement that he 'contributed little to obstetrics' strikes me as grossly inaccurate.[42] For one thing, one of the major writers in eighteenth-century midwifery, Charles White, fulsomely acknowledged Hunter as a mentor, dedicating his 1773 textbook 'to William Hunter . . . first among equals'.[43] It was as a young man in London in 1748 that White became friendly with John Hunter, and the two of them went together to William Hunter's lectures.[44] William Osborn, author of a 1792 textbook and a partner of Thomas Denman's, had also been Hunter's student.[45] We might also recall that Hunter circulated a lot in professional circles, in contrast to Smellie, and was rewarded for his visibility by becoming appointed 'Physician Extraordinary to Her Majesty' in 1762, after attending the queen in a delivery.[46] As a lion of the coffee-house medical community, it is inconceivable that Hunter's own extremely non-interventionist attitudes were without influence.

The proof of the pudding, however, is in the tasting. Smellie simply did not adhere closely enough to policies of non-intervention to

---

39   These facts are taken from Spencer, *History of British Midwifery*, pp. 67–70; Irving S. Cutter, "Historical," in Arthur H. Curtis, ed., *Obstetrics and Gynecology*, 3 vols. (Philadelphia, 1933), I, pp. 33–4; Johnstone, *Smellie*, pp. 18–24; George C. Peachey, *A Memoir of William and John Hunter* (Plymouth, 1924), pp. 55–71.
40   Robert Wallace Johnson, *A New System of Midwifery* (London, 1769).
41   Spencer, *History of British Midwifery*, pp. 61, 87; 'Harvey Graham' (pseudonym for Isaac Flack), *Eternal Eve: The Mystery of Birth and the Customs That Surround It*, rev. ed. (London, 1960), p. 160.
42   Cutter, 'Historical', p. 36. 'Certainly he did not influence clinical obstetrics to any great extent . . . He was far from being a master of clinical midwifery.' Cutter resents Hunter's reluctance to apply the forceps; p. 36.
43   I have seen only the second edition of 1777; 'first among equals', p. iv.
44   Charles J. Cullingworth, *Charles White* (London, 1904), p. 6.
45   Spencer, *History of British Midwifery*, p. 118.
46   Peachey, *Memoir*, p. 114; Hunter did not actually do the delivery.

be considered the guiding light of the movement. We have already witnessed his fiddling with the anus. Smellie also called for manual dilatation of the cervix in cases that later would be considered non-pathological. He wrote, for example, in 1752 that 'the mouth of the womb and *os externum* [introitus], for the most part, open with greater difficulty in the first than in the succeeding labours, more especially in women turned of thirty'. True enough. But then he went on to add, 'In these cases, the *os externum* must be gradually dilated in every pain, by introducing the fingers in form of a cone and turning them round.'[47] Smellie was, finally, a partisan of venesection *in labour*, if the labour was slow and 'if the patient is of a plethoric habit'.[48] Charles White, by contrast, largely rejected blood-letting in pregnancy and labour, unless the patient had an infection ('an inflammatory disorder').[49]

Consider the following. Smellie felt socially awkward whereas Hunter was the contrary.[50] Smellie left London in 1759 but Hunter was busy in the city until his death in 1783. Each man, finally, had large numbers of pupils. On balance, it seems just as apt to think of that crucial cohort of British obstetricians who in the 1750s and 1760s absorbed the doctrines of non-intervention as the generation of William Hunter, rather than as the generation of William Smellie.

The Enlightenment in action

We can find few better examples in the history of medicine of general cultural trends influencing specific medical practices than the impact of the Enlightenment upon obstetrics. The keyword to which these writers had time and again recourse in the eighteenth century was 'Nature'. And the essence of 'naturalness' in the birth process was leaving things alone, letting Nature take her course.

Whence does all this obstetrical talk about Nature originate? From the Continent and the *philosophes*, or from home-grown sources? Because men like Smellie had studied in Paris, and had both foreign and domestic authorities in their libraries, one is tempted to respond 'both'. Yet I have the impression that eighteenth-century man-midwives in Britain learned little about Nature from the Continent,

---

47 Smellie, *Treatise*, p. 223.
48 Ibid., p. 225.
49 White, *Treatise*, 2nd ed., pp. 67–73.
50 See, e.g., Smellie's letter to a Dr Clephane, apparently in 1759, explaining that he did not wish to see Hunter before his return to Scotland owing to 'Dr. Hrs glib tongue'. John Young, 'Dr. Smellie and Dr. W. Hunter: An Autobiographic Fragment', *British Medical Journal*, 29 August 1896, p. 514.

though they instructed themselves in all kinds of obstetric operations
from such authorities as François Mauriceau and Philippe Peu. It was,
as Roy Porter has pointed out, from home-grown sources that eighteenth-century British political philosophers drew, from Hobbes and
Locke.[51] And the seventeenth-century equivalent of Hobbes and
Locke in medicine was William Harvey. My argument would be that
Harvey, rather than the great authorities of the Continent, inserted
the discussion of Nature into eighteenth-century obstetrics.

In his 1653 book on reproduction Harvey had written, 'Let us blush
in this so ample and so wonderful field of nature to credit other men's
traditions . . . Nature herself must be our adviser.' Further, 'Nature's
book is so open and legible', that received authority, 'especially in the
secrets relating to natural philosophy', should be turned aside in
favour of 'following Nature's conduct with [one's] own eyes'.[52] Unfortunately, Harvey failed to link these general sentiments to precise
directions for the management of labour and delivery. But the eighteenth-century innovators we have reviewed here were quick to do
so.

It is interesting that the older generation of man-midwives saw
Nature as the enemy. John Maubray, discussing the placenta in 1724,
criticised 'they who leave all these things to mere nature'. 'For nature
itself most particularly requires our special assistance in this case.'[53]

But the newer men burbled with enthusiasm for all that was natural. Fielding Ould said of the management of the placenta that
'Nature designed its expulsion by the efforts of the mother . . . for
there are constant instances of women bringing forth both child and
burthen without any other assistance than that of Nature.'[54] Later
Smellie explained how he himself had been converted. After settling
in London he 'at first swam with the stream of general practice; till,
finding by repeated observation that violence ought not to be done to
nature . . . I resolved to change my method, and act with less pre-
cipitation, in extracting the placenta'.[55]

The young William Hunter wrote in 1745 to his friend William
Cullen, 'Since I begin to think for myself, Nature, where I am best
disposed to mark her, beams so strong upon me, that I am lost in
wonder.'[56] And indeed the mature Hunter evidently referred often to

51 Roy Porter, 'The Enlightenment in England', in Roy Porter and Mikuláš Teich,
eds., *The Enlightenment in National Context* (Cambridge, 1981), pp. 1–18.
52 Harvey, *Anatomical Exercitations*, pp. ii–v.
53 Maubray, *Female Physician*, p. 223.
54 Ould, *Treatise*, p. 61.
55 Quoted in Johnstone, *Smellie*, p. 52. From the context it appears that this
realisation dawned upon him in London, but the reference is ambiguous.
56 Quoted in Flack, *Eternal Eve*, p. 175.

Nature in demanding non-intervention. 'Labours should be treated naturally', he taught, 'left almost to nature.'[57]

It is curious that Elizabeth Nihell found so much to blame in the male midwives, for both were devoted to Nature. She wrote in 1760, 'Nothing can be more important to the well-doing of the patient than for no violence to be used to Nature, who loves to go her own full time, without disturbance or molestation.'[58] Thus do the paeans roll forth.

John Harvie stated in 1767, 'Nature, left to herself, will seldom fail to accomplish her own work; but when hurried' all kinds of disasters happened.[59]

Charles White's views, expressed in 1773, recalled those of William Harvey a century earlier. 'Reasoning from real facts and accurate observations has taken place of idle theory in almost every other science.' In midwifery too, hitherto governed by 'arbitrary custom and ignorant prejudice', he wanted Nature to prevail. Later in his book he said, 'Before we attempt to give aid to nature it is our duty to watch her operations, and to trace her through all her paths.'[60]

Enumerating all such encomia would be tiresome. But let me point out that on the threshold of the nineteenth century, we find Thomas Denman reminding his colleagues that parturition is like any other natural, physiological function, that in a normal delivery the birth attendant 'may with confidence rely upon the powers and resources of the constitution, which will produce their effect with less injury either to the mother or child and with more propriety than can be done by the most dextrous human skill'.[61] Recognising the naturalness of human birth constituted a revolution in obstetrics, and a direct line runs from Thomas Denman and his contemporaries to the American obstetricians of the 1920s.

This line, however, stops in the 1920s. At that time a second revolution, equally massive, began in the conduct of the normal labour, which from then on would be accompanied by a very substantial intervention indeed. The reason, however, was not the protection of the mother, but the protection of the foetus.[62]

57 Hunter, *Lectures on the Gravid Uterus*, p. 50.
58 Nihell, *Treatise*, p. 259.
59 Harvie, *Practical Directions*, p. v.
60 White, *Treatise*, 2nd ed., pp. viii, 95.
61 Denman, *Introduction*, I, p. 382; see also p. 407.
62 See Shorter, *Women's Bodies*, pp. 164–76.

14

Gender, generation and science: William Hunter's obstetrical atlas

L. J. JORDANOVA

An early nineteenth-century description of the Hunterian Museum in Glasgow lavished special praise on the exhibits illustrating the gravid uterus:

There are above five hundred Preparations under this division. They are prepared with the greatest taste and care, are exceedingly beautiful, making this department the most valuable perhaps of any in the world. Many splendid and valuable engravings were taken from these, and a volume of them published under Dr. Hunter's superintendence.[1]

This essay discusses the volume in question: William Hunter's *The Anatomy of the Human Gravid Uterus*, a folio volume published in 1774. Both the foregoing description, with its excess of superlatives, and the large, often dramatic plates of Hunter's obstetrical atlas suggest that the social and cultural meanings of images of pregnancy were complex, and that far from lying on the surface, they are deeply embedded in visual and verbal texts. What follows is an attempt to analyse Hunter's book, to place it in its cultural context, and to reveal the deeper meanings it contained.

Hunter made revealing scientific claims for his book. The assertion that seeing was knowing, which was integral to his project, raised the issue of how the mind acquires knowledge of nature. It also prompted the question, What sort of a phenomenon is nature? The explicit epistemology and the implicit notions of man and nature indicate that the illustrations to medical books such as Hunter's were not ornamental additions, nor were they convenient diagrams; they were their very *raison d'être*. The primacy of the visual was clear in Hunter's philosophy of education:

1 J. Laskey, *A General Account of the Hunterian Museum, Glasgow* (Glasgow, 1813), p. 51.

In explaining the structure of the parts, if a teacher would be
of real service, he must take care, not barely to describe but to
shew or demonstrate every part. What the student acquires in
this way, is solid knowledge, arising from the information of
his own senses. Hence his ideas are clear and make a lasting
impression upon his memory.[2]
Furthermore, Hunter was far from naïve where art was concerned.
Professor of anatomy at the newly founded Royal Academy between
1768 and 1783, he had decided views on art. For him 'the superiority
of Nature over Art seems to shine forth in almost every thing' – an
opinion many Academicians did not share. Hunter was also a collector and connoisseur who enthused over the rediscovered Leonardo
drawings at Windsor Castle and bought the work of such painters as
Rembrandt and Chardin.[3]

   The Anatomy of the Human Gravid Uterus has frequently been praised
in the highest terms as one of the great artistic achievements of medicine. It is indeed a remarkable book, not the least important aspect of
which is the large size of the plates, which Hunter took care to defend
in the preface. For him, the technical quality of the plates was of great
importance; they combine descriptive clarity with beauty. The work
contains thirty-four plates of different kinds; some depict several objects, others a life-size section of the human body – the female trunk
between the abdomen and the middle of the thighs (Fig. 14.1). Some
plates are packed with detail, others are more schematic, showing
large parts in outline only. Facing each plate are a short description
and a key to the letters placed on the engraving to mark specific
anatomical parts. The text, in both Latin and English, is arranged in
parallel columns. Hunter used words sparingly in the atlas, a feature
that serves to focus attention more completely on the images. The
plates show various stages of dissection from the open skin on the
pregnant abdomen to the empty womb and the placenta. The last two
engravings show 'abortions' and 'conceptions' from the early stages
of foetal development.

   There is no doubt that some of the plates have a peculiar force; they
arrest and may even shock the modern eye for reasons that may not
be immediately apparent. Their power derives in part from the way
the foetus is shown, with great attention to details like hair and fin-

2 W. Hunter, *Introductory Lectures Delivered by Dr. William Hunter to his Last Course
of Anatomical Lectures at his Theatre in Windmill Street* (London, 1784), p. 87.
3 M. Kemp, *Dr. William Hunter at the Royal Academy of Arts* (Glasgow, 1975), p. 38;
M. Kemp, 'Dr. Willim Hunter on the Windsor Leonardos and his Volume of
Drawings attributed to Pietro da Cortona', *Burlington Magazine*, CXVIII (1976), 144–8;
Laskey, *A General Account*, pp. 87–8.

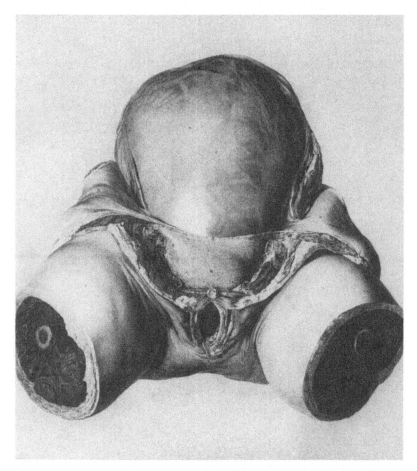

Fig. 14.1. William Hunter, *The Anatomy of the Human Gravid Uterus*, Plate IV
(Courtesy of the Wellcome Institute Library, London)

gers, and very tightly wedged into its mother's body (Fig. 14.2). This
differs strikingly from earlier representations of the foetus *in utero*,
which often showed it as a miniature adult floating in space.[4]

The impact of Hunter's images is further heightened by a technique
that was common in eighteenth-century anatomical pictures and
models. Parts of the body are shown realistically, often with great
attention given to facial features, hair and so on, while other parts are

4 Examples of early images of the foetus may be found in A. Eccles, *Obstetrics and
Gynaecology in Tudor and Stuart England* (London, 1982); J. L. Thornton and C.
Reeves, *Medical Book Illustration: A Short History* (Cambridge, 1983).

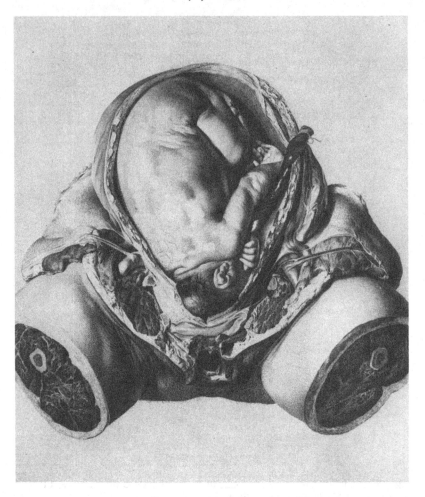

Fig. 14.2. William Hunter, *The Anatomy of the Human Gravid Uterus*, Plate VI (Courtesy of the Wellcome Institute Library, London)

cut off, such as the tops of thighs, giving a dislocated impression – the body is realistically whole, but also amputated to show human flesh resembling chunks of meat (Fig. 14.3). We can take the analogy with meat further, in that the human flesh of anatomical images is, like meat, between the full vitality of life and the total decay of death. The body was captured in visual form as it would have been at the moment of death: fresh, just as we desire the flesh we eat to be safely dead without being decomposed.

The startling effect of combining realism with butchery was commonly given by medical representations of the period. Anatomical

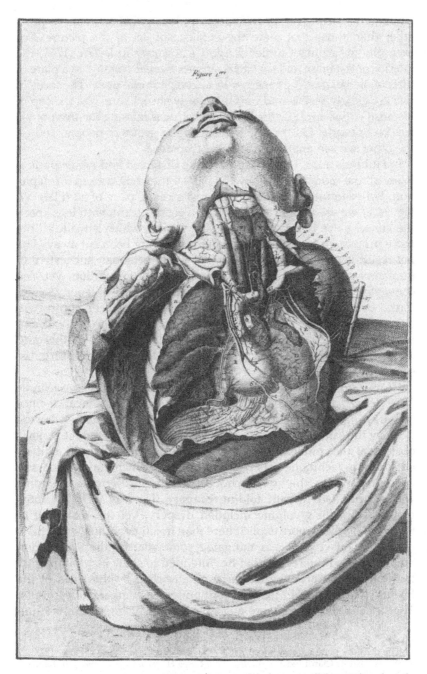

Fig. 14.3. Plate XVI from the volume of anatomy illustrations for the *Encyclopédie* (Courtesy of the Wellcome Institute Library, London)

illustrations frequently provided scrupulously lifelike detail in parts other than those that were the explicit subject of the picture. For example, in Jacques Gautier d'Agoty's *Anatomie de la Tête* (1748) the interior of the brain and the facial sinuses were illustrated in a plate of three male heads close together in a conspiratorial pose. The faces of two are clearly visible and naturalistically shown; one had the top of his head cut off to show the brain, the other is missing the front of his face on one side. On the one hand we see a group of people, and on the other we see anatomical objects displayed.[5]

In Hunter's atlas, this juxtaposition of dissected and whole parts is made all the more arresting by the part of the body chosen for depiction. For example, in perhaps the most striking plate of all (Plate VI; Fig. 14.2) we see a full frontal view of a female trunk with legs apart; the viewer's eye is drawn towards the vagina, which is made all the more prominent by the external genitals' having been cut away. The net result is an image that is intimate yet impersonal, suggestive of humanity yet butchered, celebrating the act of generation, yet also conveying violated female sexuality. This sense of violation is reinforced by Plate IV (Fig. 14.1) where the clitoris has been cut in two, although this has no relevance to the plate or, indeed, to the book as a whole. There is a notable contrast in the depictions of mother and child – the latter is treated tenderly while the former appears dissected and mutilated.

Hunter's plates can be compared with those in Jenty's *Demonstratio Uteri Praegnantis Mulieris* of 1761, a work of particular relevance since the drawings on which the plates of both books were based were done by the same artist, Jan van Rymsdyk, as were those for Smellie's obstetrical atlas published in 1754. In Jenty's work, however, a different printing technique was used, mezzotint, which emphasised soft contours, and the thighs were not sectioned. Furthermore, the torso was surrounded by soft folding drapery (Figs. 14.4, 14.5). Some plates in Smellie's volume included drapery, yet the treatment of female genitalia is more explicit here than in either Hunter's or Jenty's atlas. The effect of this is mitigated somewhat by the explanation Smellie offered the reader that he 'intended to shew in what manner the Perinaeum and external parts are stretched by the Head of the Foetus' (Fig. 14.6). Hunter and Jenty offer no comparable accounts. That a variety of ways were available for producing anatomical im-

5   The d'Agoty plate is reproduced in *La Decouverte du Corps Humain* (Paris, 1978), p. 18; see also R. Ciardi (ed.), *L'Anatomia e il Corpo Humano* (Milan, 1981); B. Lanza et al., *Le Cere Anatomische della Specola* (Florence, 1979).

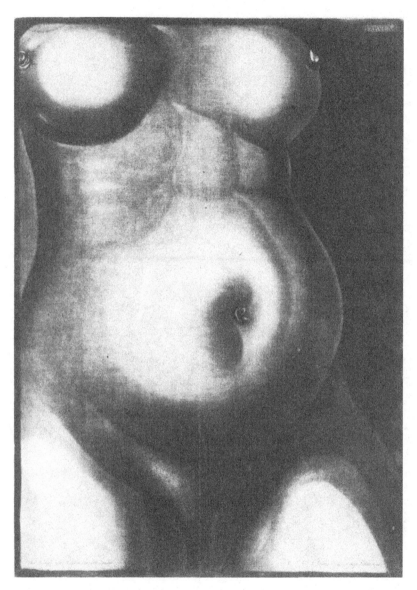

Fig. 14.4. J. N. Jenty, *Demonstratio Uteri Praegnantis Mulieris*, Plate I (Courtesy of the Wellcome Institute Library, London)

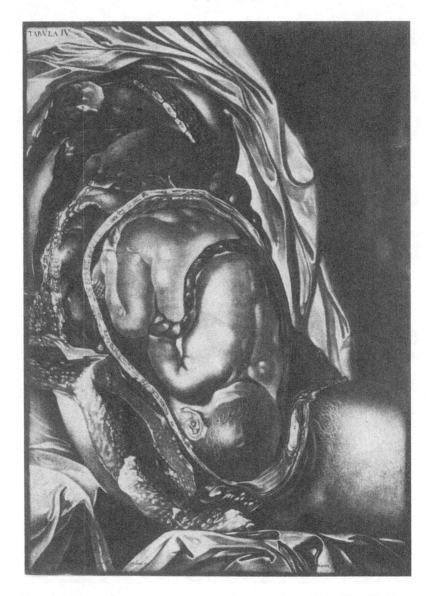

Fig. 14.5. J. N. Jenty, *Demonstratio Uteri Praegnantis Mulieris*, Plate IV (Courtesy of the Wellcome Institute Library, London)

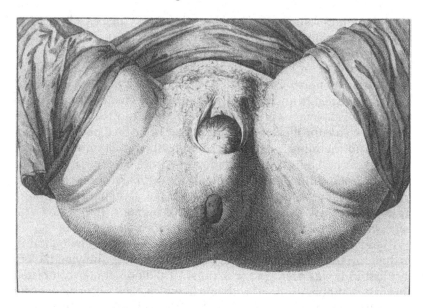

Fig. 14.6. William Smellie, *A Sett of Anatomical Tables*, Plate XV (Courtesy of the Wellcome Institute Library, London)

ages heightens the significance of those chosen by Hunter, his artists and engravers.[6]

The preface to *The Anatomy of the Human Gravid Uterus* shows that Hunter was quite deliberately putting certain views across in the book:

> The art of engraving supplies us, upon many occasions, with what has been the great desideratum of the lovers of science, an universal language. Nay, it conveys clearer ideas of most natural objects, than words can express; makes stronger impressions upon the mind; and to every person conversant with the subject, gives an immediate comprehension of what it represents.[7]

Hunter, of course, begs the most important question: What *is* being represented? He wished to suggest that this was self-evident; we must refuse his suggestion. Images, he is asserting, are vital means

6 J. N. Jenty, *Demonstratio Uteri Praegnantis Mulieris* (Nuremberg, 1761); W. Smellie, *A Sett of Anatomical Tables, with Explanations, and an Abridgement of the Practice of Midwifery, With a View to Illustrate a Treatise on that Subject, and Collection of Cases* (London, 1754), the quotation is from the commentary facing plate XV; J. L. Thornton, *Jan van Rymsdyk: Medical Artist of the Eighteenth Century* (Cambridge, 1982).
7 W. Hunter, *Anatomia Uteri Humani Gravidi* (Birmingham, 1774), Preface.

for the communication of natural knowledge. Seeing is itself an act of understanding and knowing. It is the immediate perception of un-acted-upon nature, which Hunter holds up as an epistemological ideal. As he said of Plate VI, 'Every part is represented just as it was found, not so much as one joint of a finger having been moved.' Hunter appealed to an apparently unambiguous nature through simple naturalistic images of physical reality. We can see this as an attempt to create the illusion that there need be no mediations between nature and the human mind – for him truth was all on the surface. There were no limits to the imitation of nature, so that 'a painter or sculptor in executing a single figure in the ordinary situation of quiet life cannot copy Nature too exactly, or make deception too strong'. Thus scrupulously exact bodily details, including surface blood vessels, were essential for giving a 'natural appearance'.[8]

There were, according to Hunter, two traditions of anatomical illustration. The first made simple portraits of nature showing the object just as it was seen, in the manner of Bidloo. Hunter contrasted this first tradition, his own, with one in which nature is imaginatively reconstructed in the minds of anatomists and artists. Although he could see disadvantages with the first tradition and advantages with the second, in the last analysis pictures 'which represent what was actually seen' are the ones carrying 'the mark of truth', and are 'almost as infallible as the object itself'.[9] Despite such assertions, Hunter's work did not reflect nature but fabricated it. For example, the bodies from which the pictures were drawn were dead, and had often been so for a long time. The plates strive to give an impression of vitality, as in the way the umbilical cord seems to gleam as if it were still wet.

A lifelike effect was partly achieved by injecting blood vessels with wax to keep their shape.

> Filling the vascular system with a bright coloured wax, enables us to trace the large vessels with great ease, renders the smaller much more conspicuous, and makes thousands of the very minute ones visible, which from their delicacy, and the transparency of their natural contents, are otherwise imperceptible.[10]

In general, Hunter found anatomical preparations to be of great value for revealing both structures requiring 'considerable labour to anatomize' and those not commonly seen. Although he preferred wet

---

8 Kemp, *Dr. William Hunter at the Royal Academy*, pp. 39, 35.
9 Hunter, *Anatomia Uteri*, Preface.
10 Hunter, *Introductory Lectures*, p. 56.

preparations to dry ones, he was enthusiastic about making wax models from dead bodies. Wax enjoyed a considerable vogue in this period for modelling and sculpting purposes as well as for anatomical ones. The Italians specialised in producing wax figures designed to be beautiful ornaments as well as anatomically informative, although Hunter was sceptical about waxworks not cast from real subjects.[11] But however they were made, these models suggest an urgent search for verisimilitude, and wax, with its potential for resembling human flesh, was a particularly attractive medium.

For Hunter anatomical pictures ought to reveal 'true nature, that is, the peculiar habit and composition of parts, as well as the outward form, situation and connection of them'.[12] The plates in the *Gravid Uterus* show the extent to which Hunter was concerned with the topography of the body, the spatial relationships between parts, their surface features and particularly their texture. Anatomy, for Hunter, was a study of three dimensions, like sculpture, wax modelling or landscape painting. He had little of the architect's concern with inner structure – the skeleton – as the German anatomist Soemmerring had. Rather, Hunter's enterprise was closely akin to that of a cartographer, lovingly recording all the details of the terrain – flesh and tissues. There was no smoothing out here but, rather, corrugations depicted in loving detail. When the mapping had been completed, the human body would, in some significant sense, be known and understood.

Hunter himself employed a topographical analogy, and considerably developed it by likening the physician to a general and the sick body to a country under civil war or invasion:

> To do his duty with full advantage, a general, besides other acquirements, useful in his profession, must make himself master of the Anatomy and Physiology, as we may call it, of the country. He may be said to be master of the *Anatomy* of the country, when he knows the figure, dimension, situation, and connection, of all the principal constituent parts; such as, the lakes, rivers, marshes, mountains, precipices, plains, woods, roads, passes, fords, towns, fortifications, etc. By the *Physiology* of the country, which he ought likewise to understand, is meant, all the variety of active influence, which is produced by the inhabitants.[13]

The notion of topographical exactitude was of considerable impor-

11 Ibid., pp. 89–91, 56. See also Lanza et al., *Le Cere.*
12 Hunter, *Anatomia Uteri*, Preface.
13 Hunter, *Introductory Lectures*, p. 70.

tance in British art during the eighteenth century, especially among landscape painters and portraitists.[14]

Hunter's epistemology was fundamentally a visual one. There is no space here for refined, abstract analysis. Instead, all was known by means of sight. It may be worth considering the significance of the sense of sight and of ideas of light for conceptions of human knowledge in this period. Not only were these three elements (vision, light, knowledge) commonly associated, but light was the dominant metaphor of the progress of the human intellect. The connection between light and science was, of course, commonly made, for example, in references to Isaac Newton.

The themes of vision, light and knowledge, and the relationships between them, were taken up in the visual arts by Joseph Wright of Derby, who consistently called into question diverse kinds of human knowledge by depicting the scientist, philosopher, alchemist, anatomist and artist contemplating their objects of study. Light itself and its various sources were clearly of considerable interest to Wright. But looking, and more generally vision, is also explored in his paintings. Seekers after knowledge, and those who expound knowledge, are frequently depicted in the company of others whose view of their activities is radically different. Many of his pictures allude to the problem of comprehending death, a problem most sharply brought into focus by the horror that awaits those who plunder graves in *Miravan Opening the Tomb of his Ancestors* (Fig. 14.7). It shows a young nobleman who has broken into an ancestral tomb in search of treasures. What he finds is a skeleton – death – and, with new awareness, turns away, covering his eyes.[15]

Wright's distinctive manner of treating light pictorially was closely connected with his exploration of the ways in which human beings understand nature, their attitudes to knowledge and the gender differences involved. In *An Experiment on a Bird in the Air Pump* (c. 1767–9), he hinted at a tension between the search for scientific knowledge and femininity. While the natural philosopher demonstrates the air pump, one girl turns away from the apparatus, fearing that the bird will die in the experiment, and a smaller girl looks on in puzzlement. Wright would seem to be drawing on the idea, frequently articulated by thinkers of the Enlightenment, that there was an inherent incom-

14 *Polite Society by Arthur Devis 1712–1787: Portraits of the English Country Gentleman and his Family* (Preston, 1983), p. 12; R. Paulson, *Literary Landscape: Turner and Constable* (New Haven, Conn., and London, 1982), pp. 40–1.
15 B. Nicolson, *Joseph Wright of Derby: Painter of Light*, 2 vols. (London, 1968); Paulson, *Literary Landscape*, pp. 49, 58, chap. 8, p. 113; M. H. Nicolson, *Newton Demands the Muse* (Princeton, N.J., 1946).

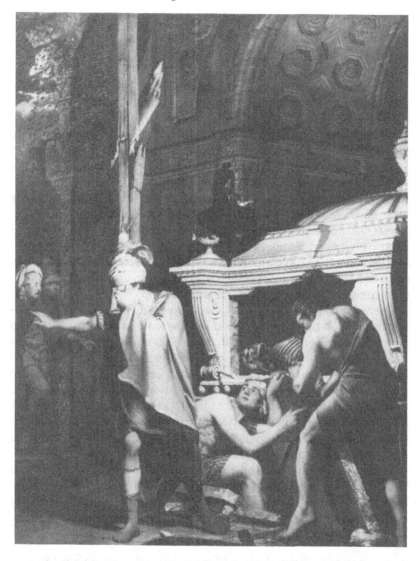

Fig. 14.7. Joseph Wright of Derby, *Miravan Opening the Tomb of His Ancestors* (1772) (By kind permission of the Derby Art Gallery)

patibility between women and scientific knowledge. Often this was done by associating the feminine with nature and the male with reason; the former became thereby objectified and passive, the latter active and enquiring.[16]

Hunter's epistemology was soon challenged, even by those who saw themselves as extending his work. Samuel Thomas von Soemmerring, for example, prepared his *Icones Embryonum Humanorum* (1799) as a supplement to Hunter's *Gravid Uterus*. It showed mainly embryos in the early stages of pregnancy. Soemmerring's approach to anatomy was governed by a notion of the *ideal*, in contrast to Hunter's emphasis on the *natural*. Thus, Soemmerring was allied with the tradition of anatomical illustration that Hunter associated particularly with Bartholommeo Eustachi. According to Soemmerring, the anatomist should select from his material the most beautiful, perfect and undamaged specimens in order to 'find the true norm of the organs'. Furthermore, 'we have to let our intelligence detect and remedy such deviations as occur in specimens taken from cadavers, in consequence of death, preparation, or preservation'.[17]

The espousal of the ideal as a goal in science and art was widespread. It took the form of the 'classicisation of anatomical study' to which Kemp refers. In *The Nude Male*, Walters suggests that the neoclassic nude was accepted only at its farthest remove from the naked human body – signs of organic life such as veins and sinews were smoothed away. Her statement 'The nude is idealised almost to death' is particularly applicable to the Italian wax anatomical models mentioned earlier.[18] By contrast, Hunter wished all such details to be faithfully depicted. Another form of the 'ideal' was the assertion of the priority of imagination over reason, which was such a fundamental aspect of critiques of the Enlightenment in the 1790s. Such critiques were a vital part of debates within the British artistic community of the period, and they found powerful expression in the works of William Blake and his friend John Flaxman, whose admiration for Hippocrates and Galen was part and parcel of his classicism.[19]

16 L. J. Jordanova, 'Natural Facts: A Historical Perspective on Science and Sexuality', in C. MacCormack and M. Strathern (eds.), *Nature, Culture and Gender* (Cambridge, 1980), pp. 42–69.
17 Soemmerring is quoted by L. Choulant, *History and Bibliography of Anatomic Illustration* (New York and London, 1945), pp. 302–3; Hunter, *Anatomia Uteri*, Preface.
18 M. Walters, *The Nude Male: A New Perspective* (Harmondsworth, 1979), p. 206; Kemp, *Dr. William Hunter at the Royal Academy*, pp. 26–7; see also H. Honour, *Neo-Classicism* (Harmondsworth, 1968).
19 J. Flaxman, *Lectures on Sculpture* (London, 1829); J. Hagstrum, 'William Blake Rejects the Enlightenment', in N. Frye (ed.), *Blake: A Collection of Critical Essays* (Englewood Cliffs, N.J., 1966), pp. 142–55.

Hunter saw nature's truths as being on the surface, ready to be received by the trained, observant mind, whereas Soemmerring saw them as being below the surface, requiring the active intellect of the medical scientist to bring them out in their pure form, a form in which they might never actually exist. There can be no doubt of the general cultural significance of the positions held by Hunter and Soemmerring respectively, going back as they do to Aristotelian and Platonic traditions. Soemmerring's view, indicative of the growing antirationalism of the time, was informed by an intense dislike of what he took to be the materialism of much contemporary physiology – a point that came out clearly in the hostile stance he took towards the guillotine during the French Revolution.[20] Soemmerring's attack on materialism and the French Revolution was linked to his anatomical and aesthetic views that led him to an epistemology in marked contrast to that of Hunter with its stress on the visible, material world. This does not mean that Hunter was a radical materialist. On the contrary, he was an ardent defender of the king and held orthodox religious views, extolling the works of the Supreme Being who was the creator and director of the universe. Yet it was the real world of nature in all its infinite variety that captured Hunter's interest, and especially the 'machinery' of the human body. Real detail, not ideal form, was his object of study.

The relationships between words and images are varied and intricate. In the case of Hunter's volume, it is by no means obvious how the book was to be used, which groups it was intended for, or, indeed, what kind of work Hunter intended to produce. At one level, the images are clearly medical in that they show anatomical preparations carefully designed to display internal organs, and we have seen the emphasis Hunter placed on such demonstrations when teaching. However, unlike Smellie, Hunter does not structure the book around the needs of a young *accoucheur*. The anatomical tables in Smellie's volume were designed to accompany his midwifery textbook. Both were aimed at the young male practitioner, as is clear from the plates explaining the use of forceps.[21] To the extent that Hunter's atlas can be labelled 'medical', commentators tend to disregard the other elements it contains.

Medicine is a form of culture in that, like all social phenomena, it contains meanings that must be interpreted in relation to myths,

20   L. J. Jordanova, 'Medical Mediations: Mind and Body in the Guillotine Debates during the French Revolution', *Kos* X (1984).
21   Smellie, *A Sett of Anatomical Tables*, esp. plates XVI–XIX, XXI, XXIV, XXVI, XXXV; W. Smellie, *A Treatise on the Theory and Practice of Midwifery*, 2 vols. (London, 1752–4.

symbols and beliefs. Furthermore, medicine in general, and *The Human Gravid Uterus* in particular, raises such issues as death, birth, production and creativity – all these combine elements of human experience with the mythical and symbolic, which are deeper than the conscious level. The historical relationship between art and anatomy bears out this point. It is misleading to construe this as a continuous, progressive joint quest for technical perfection. Male and female figures were commonly depicted as Adam and Eve, female figures with children as madonnas, while reminders of death abound in anatomical images. These were part of iconographical traditions, and are best understood in the same terms as art historians or historians of culture have developed. By implication, 'realism' can no longer be seen as the unproblematic commitment of art and anatomy, nor must it be allowed to develop into a spurious criterion of value. Realism is, in fact, itself a historical contruct, not an unproblematic and self-evidently valuable analytical term.[22]

To acknowledge the presence of mythic and symbolic elements in anatomical images is also to say that they are mediations in that they present social and cultural relations in an experiential form. For example, anatomical depictions may assist in papering over, accommodating and exploring tensions and contradictions not fully explicit in the image itself. Such latent levels may be about sexual modesty or desire, fear of death, disease and mutilation, the bonds between parents and children, or the sexual act itself.

Anatomical images of pregnancy mediate gender and family relations in particular. Family and gender are ideological contructs as well as powerful human experiences, and medicine has played a central role in constructing familial relationships, especially that between mother and child. Hunter produced *The Gravid Uterus* at a time of intense medical concern with domestic medicine – the health practices of families, of which the wife and mother was the main architect.[23]

The clusters of ideas around male and female, nature and science, also underlay anatomical treatments of women's bodies. Early anatomical images were rather discreet generally when it came to sexuality. The genitals, particularly of women, were mostly veiled or cov-

22 N. Bryson, *Word and Image: French Painting of the Ancien Régime* (Cambridge, 1981), and *Vision and Painting: The Logic of the Gaze* (London, 1983).
23 W. Buchan, *Domestic Medicine* (Edinburgh, 1769); C. Lawrence, 'William Buchan: Medicine Laid Open', *Medical History*, XIX (1975), 20–33. W. Hunter's other work in the area of reproduction is outlined in C. H. Brock (ed.), *William Hunter 1718–1783: A Memoir by Samuel Foart Simmons and John Hunter* (Glasgow, 1983), pp. 12, 17, 20–2, 23, 47, 59, 63.

ered in some way. Female sexual characters were often removed, as in the omission of pubic hair, which was shown in a sketchy way and without relentless naturalism if present at all. Similarly breasts were not emphasised, and on occasion the whole body was masculinised, leaving only the head hair as unambiguously feminine. But Hunter and some of his contemporaries showed female genitals in unrelenting detail. This revealed to open view what was normally concealed, and revealed it furthermore in a context of dissection, mutilation and death – a situation commonly construed at the time as one of violation, as Hogarth's *Stages of Cruelty* made clear. Anatomical illustrations linked medical knowledge to sight, and, in the case of eighteenth-century depictions of women, to seeing parts of nature previously deemed private, thereby forging additional links with sexual-cum-intellectual penetration and with the violence of the dissecting-room.[24]

Hunter made aesthetic claims for his atlas just as Laskey did when he described the Hunterian Museum in Glasgow. Yet the content of the images and the manner in which they had been composed diverged most markedly from the normal canons of taste in the period, unlike many other anatomical illustrations. Those by Albinus, for example, were set against elaborate backgrounds of plants, trees, hills, animals, lakes and buildings. Joseph Wright made an exact copy of one figure for his *The Old Man and Death* (1774).[25] Hunter's plates are not at all comparable to contemporaneous 'polite art', nor do they seek to be decorous. By making a public proclamation about the legitimacy of all natural objects being known and seen, Hunter was countering the mystification and concealment of certain anatomical parts, which was justified by reference to religious convention and modesty, and he was also basing his aesthetic firmly in nature. Whatever the eye could see was true, and it was beautiful because it was natural: 'What imitates Nature most is most striking; and . . . it will be likewise *more pleasing* if the subject be properly adapted to our passions.'[26] Artificial convention should give way to the reality of nature. There was a precedent for this approach in the anatomical drawings of Leonardo, and Hunter saw himself in this tradition. Furthermore,

---

24 Examples of women in anatomical illustrations can be found in Thornton and Reeves, *Medical Book Illustration*, and in A. Hahn et al., *Histoire de la Médecine et du Livre Medical* (Paris, 1962). On the broader significance of such images see Jordanova, in MacCormack and Strathern, *Nature, Culture and Gender*, and 'Body Image and Sex Roles in the Eighteenth Century: Anatomical Models and Pictures', *Kos*, no. 2 (1984), in Italian; the Hogarth prints are in S. Shesgreen, *Engravings by Hogarth: 101 Prints* (New York, 1973), plates 77–80.
25 Nicholson, *Wright of Derby*, p. 56.
26 Kemp, *Dr. William Hunter at the Royal Academy*, p. 39.

such affinities with Renaissance art served as a powerful legitimation for later practices.[27]

Our understanding of the implications of anatomical models and illustrations so far as gender is concerned can be furthered by comparing them with 'polite art'. For example, the Italian wax models that functioned as collectors' items, with their glass coffinlike cases, pearl necklaces, luxuriant hair and ecstatic facial expressions, are reminiscent of Bernini's statue of Saint Theresa (Fig. 14.8). There the saint's face suggests both religious ecstasy and sexual transports. The use of such recognisable patterns in anatomical models and illustrations shows that gender differences and the perception of sexuality were important elements in the medical realm also. Thus, in the case of women we can demonstrate the close relationships between medical images and those in the culture more generally, and conclude that there was a mixture of eroticism, violence and idealisation in the drive to know and see more of feminine nature.[28]

The case of the foetus is altogether more complex and elusive than is that of women. Few depictions of children prior to the eighteenth century satisfy our canons of naturalism, and perceptions and theories of childhood underwent some dramatic changes between the seventeenth and nineteenth centuries. Many early pictures of foetuses treat their bodily shape as being essentially similar to that of an adult. An alternative way of expressing these ideas would be to say that earlier it had not seemed so pressing to present an accurate, naturalistic depiction of a foetus as it did to Hunter, for example.

Placing changes in medical illustrations of embryos, babies and children in the context of changes in portraiture can be revealing. The two seem to follow a similar pattern. Hunter's full-term foetus strives to be realistic – it has long elegant fingers and magnificent hair. It is almost too perfect, and it was the perfection, completeness and beauty of the new-born child that contemporary medical opinion stressed. The plates in the *Gravid Uterus* showing the full-term child nearly bursting out of the womb are very different from the tiny adult body floating in an enormous cavity in a variety of postures, found in early illustrations, and persisting in some popular eighteenth-century prints (Fig. 14.9).

Children, of course, were also important in images of the family in the eighteenth century. Whereas for Blake, for example, there was no natural identity of interest between parents and children, for the vast

27   M. Iversen, 'The New Art History', in F. Barker et al. (eds.), *The Politics of Theory* (Colchester, 1983), pp. 212–19, esp. pp. 213, 215–6; Kemp, 'Dr. William Hunter on the Windsor Leonardos'; Hunter, *Introductory Lectures*, pp. 37–9.
28   Jordanova, in MacCormack and Strathern, *Nature, Culture and Gender*.

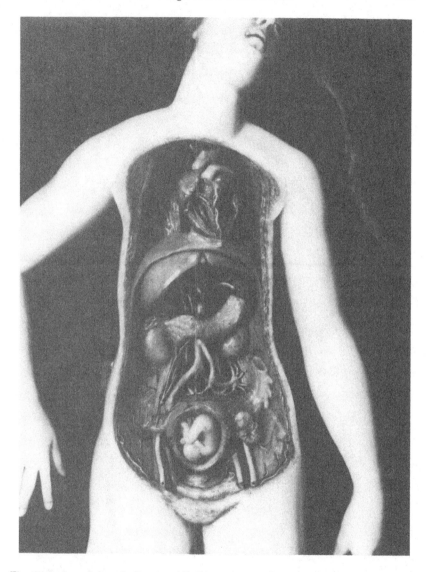

Fig. 14.8. A wax female figure with the covering of the trunk removed (Courtesy of the Wellcome Institute Library, London)

majority of writers and artists there was a natural fusion, an organic link between the different family members, particularly between mother and child. This fusion was represented visually by showing an intertwining intimacy between women and their offspring. Sometimes this was achieved by actually blending figures together, as

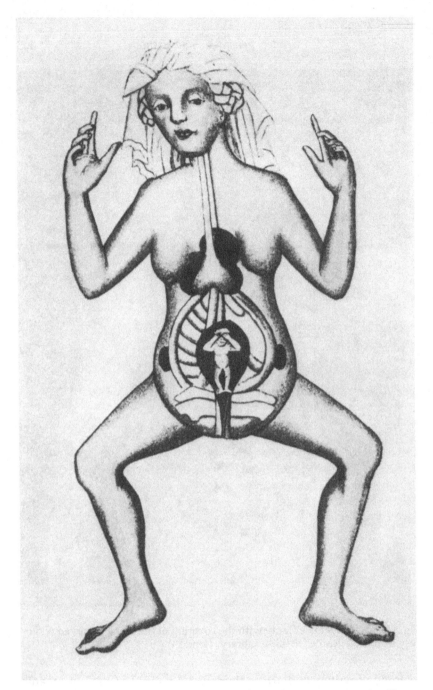

Fig. 14.9. From a miniature painted about 1400 in a Leipzig manuscript (Courtesy of the Wellcome Institute Library, London)

Gainsborough did in *The Baillie Family* (c. 1784), where the clothes of the mother and those of the baby she is holding on her knee appear continuous. Reynolds produced a similar effect in *Lady Cockburn and Her Three Eldest Sons* (1774) by encircling the mother with her children and showing them scantily dressed, which serves to emphasise their 'naturalness'. This fusion is all the more effective when women's sexuality and their reproductive powers were treated as inseparable. This is particularly marked in the work of the French painter Greuze, as in his *La Mère Bien Aimée* (*The Much Loved Mother*) (c. 1765–9), where the wife rapturously greets her husband while children throng around embracing her.[29]

To return to the foetus, it is worth recognising both the difficulties of imagining life before birth and how highly charged such ideas are. Two issues are present here: the nature of the birth process and the way in which the foetus develops before its passage to the outside world. Birth is an event that marks, in an apparently natural manner, a fundamental transition. All societies see birth as a dramatic moment infused with magical significance, as the heroic myths associated with those born through Caesarean section bear witness. Images of the foetus evoke beliefs about the act of birth. They also represent ideas about growth and development.

Hunter's atlas must therefore also be placed in the context of ideas about embryology. In order to understand the changes in the ways foetuses were shown, a brief discussion of theories of preformation and *emboîtement*, which enjoyed a wide following during the eighteenth century, may be helpful. These theories presumed 'that the gradual appearance and apparent creation of the parts observed, as the ovum turned into the embryo and then into the adult, were simply due to an increase, in size and in hardness, of parts that were already present'.[30] All living things were created at the beginning, later generations being enclosed within earlier ones. The formation of an individual was simply the growth of an already existing being. Although not new in the seventeenth century, these theories came to prominence with the work of Swammerdam in the 1660s, and remained influential throughout the eighteenth century.

Preformationism, where the baby is essentially like an adult, therefore removes the need to think about foetal growth and the human

29 S. F. Damon, *A Blake Dictionary: The Ideas and Symbols of William Blake* (Providence, R.I., 1965); W. Blake, *Songs of Innocence and Experience* (London, 1970); Bryson, *Word and Image*, chap. 5, esp. pp. 136–7; C. Duncan, 'Happy Mothers and Other Ideas in 18th Century Art', *Art Bulletin*, LX (1973), 570–83; L. Hautecoeur, *Les Peintres de la Vie Familiale: Évolution d'un Thème* (Paris, 1945).
30 E. Gasking, *Investigations into Generation 1651–1828* (Baltimore and London, 1966), p. 41.

status of the child. Within this framework, the child was always human and complete; it merely had to grow bigger. For those committed to the alternative hypothesis, epigenesis, the full-term foetus had emerged gradually from a beginning that was radically distinct from its final form. It is worth remembering how preposterous this latter view seemed to many, so that Claude Perrault could say in 1680, 'If the egg consists of homogeneous matter as is presumed on this hypothesis (epigenesis), it can only develop into a foetus by a miracle, which would surpass every other phenomenon in the world.'[31]

The uterine space around the 'preformationist' embryo, as we may call the little men of early images, possibly suggests the further growth yet to come. But it might also suggest a separation between the would-be adult and its immediate environment (its mother, that is), whereas Hunter's plates, in contrast, convey an almost oppressive intimacy between mother and child, an intimacy ceaselessly expressed in medical writings of the period. Although birth scenes – that is, the room and its occupants during or soon after a birth – were common, particularly in the sixteenth and seventeenth centuries, the actual process of birth was rarely depicted. Smellie, however, did show the head just appearing in his *Sett of Anatomical Tables*. This absence of depictions of the moment of separation gives Blake's portrayal of birth as an act of releasing untameable human energy a peculiar power. In *The Marriage of Heaven and Hell* (1790, Plate 3; Fig. 14.10), he showed a child half out of its mother, already actively embracing life with its outstretched arms. Blake's picture is notable because it expresses so forcefully a particular conception of childhood. In its moment of birth, the new being affirms its vitality and energy, those elements of the human spirit that Blake's works celebrate in so many different forms. In this sense the child was an emblem or symbol for Blake, playing an important role in his metaphysical and mythological systems.[32] Children and foetuses in medical illustrations represent equally complex ideas.

The vitality of generation appears in Hunter's *Gravid Uterus* not as force or energy but in the fullness and texture of the internal organs.

31 Gasking, *Investigations*, p. 37. I am most grateful to Dr Helen Brock for her advice on what Hunter's own views about the preformation *versus* epigenesis debate may have been, for he never stated them unequivocally. Dr Brock suggests that Hunter inclined towards epigenesis, and this has been my assumption in this essay. She says, 'All Hunter's drawings of early stages of human embryology give no suggestion of a complete individual – nor did John Hunter's drawings' (personal communication).
32 W. Blake, *The Marriage of Heaven and Hell* (London, 1975), plate 3; Damon, *A Blake Dictionary*, esp. pp. 81–2; P. Coveney, *The Image of Childhood: The Individual and Society. A Study of the Theme in English Literature* (Harmondsworth, 1967).

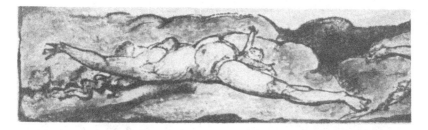

Fig. 14.10. William Blake, *The Marriage of Heaven and Hell*, detail redrawn from Plate 3 (Copyright of the Fitzwilliam Museum, University of Cambridge)

He used the bodies of a number of women who had died at different stages of pregnancy. The outer layers of tissues were carefully peeled off to reveal the foetus beneath, just as the wax modellers made removable flaps and organs for their female figures, which invariably contained a pregnant uterus at their deepest layer.

Clearly, Hunter was fascinated by different tissues and their textures. The importance he attached to stripping off layers can be seen in Plate XXI, taken from a drawing by Alexander Cozens. Hunter described it as 'from a seventh subject, at seven months. The womb opened by a crucial incision, and the four corners carefully separated, . . . so as to shew the child, and waters, through the enclosing membranes.' The result is an indistinct and blurred effect whose very lack of clarity conveys the sense of looking *through* tissues, of the foetus being contained by them, even pressing against them. Simultaneously, the viewer sees the anatomical closeness of foetus and womb, and acquires a sense of the deep recesses of the body marked by layers of tissues. Smellie's atlas contained a similar plate.[33]

In the anatomical plates, the mother's body framed and moulded the foetus, the two lives being portrayed as a single interconnected system.[34] Both Hunter's and Jenty's plates displayed these features, which were absent, however, in those made by Stubbs at the very beginning of his career for John Burton's *An Essay Towards a Complete New System of Midwifery* (1751). Stubbs made the uterus into an abstract capsule connected with other physical objects only through a disembodied hand reaching up into the womb in one of the etchings (Fig. 14.11, left). However, Stubbs's later work on human and animal

33 A. S. Marks, 'An Anatomical Drawing by Alexander Cozens', *Journal of the Warburg and Courtauld Institutes*, XXX (1967), 434–8; Smellie, *A Sett of Anatomical Tables*, plate XI.
34 Hunter's interest in the relationship between the circulatory systems of mother and child and in the nature of the placenta is discussed in Brock (ed.), *William Hunter*, pp. 47–8.

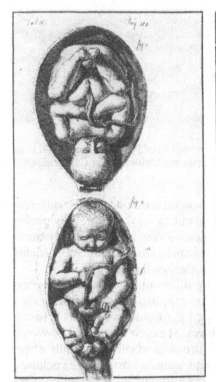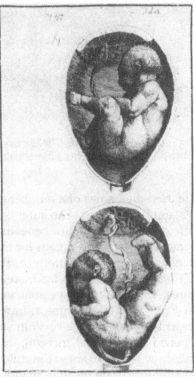

Fig. 14.11. John Burton, *An Essay Towards a Complete New System of Midwifery*, Plates 10 (left) and 13, etchings by George Stubbs (Courtesy of the Wellcome Institute Library, London)

anatomy, some of it for William Hunter himself, suggests the same relentless search for a form of realism as we find in the *Gravid Uterus*.[35]

The sense of the woman and child being as one was particularly strongly asserted when it appeared in danger of violation, as for example in the case of illegitimate children. Significantly, ambiguities about property and inheritance were the most threatening aspects of illegitimacy. These were children who were more likely to be killed, abandoned or otherwise deprived than those born to legally married parents, although marriage itself was far from being unambiguous, both in theory and in practice. To be more precise, the special mater-

35 Two of Stubbs's plates are reproduced in B. Taylor, *Stubbs* (London, 1971), plates 1 and 2; see also W. Gilbey, *Life of George Stubbs* (London, 1898), pp. 6–8; R. Paulson, *Emblem and Expression: Meaning in English Art of the Eighteenth Century* (London, 1975), chap. 10, esp. p. 173.

nal relationship was to be expressed only within the confines of civil law. For example, for Rousseau, children conceived in a wife's adulterous relationship violated natural rights, making them robbers. Legitimate children, by logical extension, were lawful possessors of their parental heritage; the common family interest consisted of shared and natural rights to property.[36]

Hunter's foetuses possess and confidently inhabit their mothers' bodies. In contrast, earlier, protoadult 'preformationist' foetuses lived in a different world, where they seemed lost in the waters of the womb. They appeared as temporary tenants, with no 'natural' rights of possession. From the point of view of imagery, they were born into a looser family structure, one that easily permitted children to leave home for work or training without shattering a bond with the mother, which was construed in the late eighteenth century as at once natural, legal and social. Also connected are the general acceptance of child labour, which was beginning to be seriously questioned for the first time at the end of the eighteenth century on the grounds that children required parental protection by virtue of their very nature, and the common practice of informal adoption in earlier periods. Both child labour and informal adoption made sense in a culture where the death of parents before children reached adulthood was common, making parents temporary custodians of their progeny. The medical literature of the second half of the eighteenth century, in contrast, emphasised the intertwining of maternal and child welfare, and furthermore, sought to woo fathers into greater responsibility for the upbringing of children.[37]

The 'preformationist' image of the foetus appears to us to be manifestly 'artificial', whereas the Hunterian portrayal seems more 'natural'. This difference prompts us to see the latter as an unmediated representation of nature. Yet this would be a mistake. Both are cultural products, and as such they carry within them levels of meaning: the ideas, assumptions, tensions and contradictions of their times. There is no unmediated nature, only different mediations, some of which conform more closely to our current conceptions than others. If we compare Hunter's obstetrical atlas with that of Jenty, both dif-

36 J.-J. Rousseau, *Emile* (London, 1911), esp. book 1; C. Brinton, *French Revolutionary Legislation on Illegitimacy* (Cambridge, Mass., 1936); S. M. Okin, *Women in Western Political Thought* (London, 1980).
37 P. Ariès, *Centuries of Childhood* (Harmondsworth, 1973); J.-L. Flandrin, *Families in Former Times, Kinship, Household, and Sexuality* (Cambridge, 1979); the role of fathers is emphasised in W. Cadogan, *An Essay upon the Nursing and the Management of Children* (London, 1748); and in S. Tissot, *An Essay on Onanism* (Dublin, 1772). J. Hanway, *A Sentimental History of Chimney Sweepers* (London, 1785), outlines some of the arguments against child labour.

ferences and similarities emerge, and both are equally important. They share a precise naturalism and an emphasis on the identity of mother and child. They differ in that Hunter's is more impersonal and reifying where Jenty's, partly by virtue of its different printing technique, is both softer and more holistic. This contrast is clear in the comparison between the cross-sectioned thighs shown in Hunter's book and the more complete ones depicted in Jenty's.

These works share many features that clearly separate them from anatomical pictures in different and earlier traditions. It is the search for satisfying portrayals of the human body, a quest that unites art and anatomy, that lies behind the work of men like Hunter and Jenty: 'In Painting and Sculpture the power of representing the human body in all the variety of its circumstances as near as possible to the original reality must be an acquisition of the greatest consequence, because it is so essential to the effect of the work.'[38] The history of portrayals of the human body can be understood only by reaching for a more fundamental level of human experience – that of myth and symbol. The religious reasons for attempts to capture human form are of special importance. John Flaxman made this clear when he lectured on sculpture at the Royal Academy in the early nineteenth century. His fourth lecture, 'On Science', stressed 'the circle of knowledge', an expression he used to imply the need for a synthesis of art and science if the human figure were to be properly represented. He approvingly quoted Socrates as saying, 'The human form is the most perfect of all forms, and contains in it the principles and powers of all inferior forms.' He reinforced the point by referring to the view of the ancients that man was a microcosm, to 'Revelation', and to the general assent given, even in pagan countries, to the idea that the most beautiful human form was divine.[39]

Once it can be agreed that naturalism and realism must be analysed and not taken for granted, as the vast majority of works dealing with medical images do, then more detailed themes can be examined. Some possibilities relating to Hunter's atlas have been suggested in this essay. They include the gamut of factors from epistemology and metaphysics, on the one hand, to law and political theory, on the other, and include such topics as style, tradition and patronage. The most important point is that societies have profound, if concealed, stakes in their boundaries and in those cultural artefacts that sustain them and give them meaning. The *Gravid Uterus* touched on a number of such boundaries, most easily expressed through their related

38 Kemp, *Dr. William Hunter at the Royal Academy*, pp. 40–1.
39 Flaxman, *Lectures on Sculpture*, pp. 102–3.

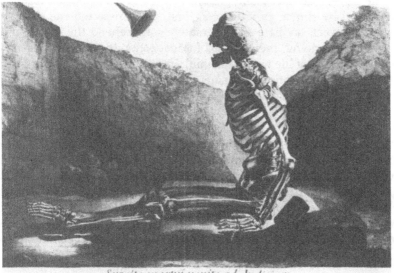

Surgite mortui venite ad Judicium

Fig. 14.12. Plate from J. Gamelin, *Nouveau Recueil d'Ostéologie et de Myologie* (Courtesy of the British Museum)

dichotomies: male/female, life/death, foetus/child, child/adult, science/nature. Of these dichotomies, the divide between life and death was of exceptional importance in a society where the finality of death was being called into question, especially by the medical community in their investigations into the possibilities for reviving the drowned or hanged. It is surely important that so many anatomical pictures served as *memento mori*, as is most obvious in those that contain skulls and skeletons, particularly where the latter are sitting up in response to the trumpet blast that heralds the Last Judgement (Fig. 14.12). Lessons about death are often contained in the gesture and position of the figure, and the background and accompanying objects. These are far from extraneous to the image: On the contrary, it is they that render it meaningful. They frame the image, give it a location, and guide the viewer as to what he should attend to.[40]

40 J. McManners, *Death and the Enlightenment* (Oxford, 1981); *La Decouverte du Corps Humain*, esp. p. 20; J. Hall, *Dictionary of Subjects and Symbols in Art*, rev. ed. (London, 1969); *memento mori* are discussed under 'Skull', p. 284 and 'Still Life', pp. 291–2; on attempts to revive the drowned see L. J. Jordanova, 'Policing Public Health in France 1780–1815', in T. Ogawa (ed.), *Public Health* (Tokyo, 1981), pp. 12–31, esp. pp. 23–5.

The life–death dichotomy was raised in two forms by Hunter's work and by similar productions. First, they dissected the dead in order to reveal, lay bare and ultimately comprehend the living, and second, in so doing, they opened for inspection the process of gestation, the giving of life and the coming into life. In producing his book Hunter did not capture an image of nature with an 'innocent eye'; instead he unveiled cultural constructs and social relationships.

Acknowledgements

I am deeply endebted to the following people for their generous help and encouragement: Catherine Crawford, Karl Figlio, Margaret Iversen, Elaine Jordan, Thomas Puttfarken and William Schupbach. I greatly benefited from the comments of the members of the Social History Seminar, King's College, Cambridge, on an earlier version of this essay. Don Smith prepared the drawing from Blake with admirable care. The editors of this volume also offered useful comments.

INDEX

413

Index

Printed in the United States
By Bookmasters